Monitoring Training and Performance in Athletes

Monitoring Training and Performance in Athletes

Mike McGuigan, PhD

Auckland University
of Technology

Auckland, New Zealand

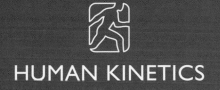

HUMAN KINETICS

Library of Congress Cataloging-in-Publication Data

Names: McGuigan, Mike, 1971- author.
Title: Monitoring training and performance in athletes / Mike McGuigan.
Description: Champaign, IL: Human Kinetics, [2017] | Includes
  bibliographical references and index.
Identifiers: LCCN 2016021011| ISBN 9781492535201 (print) | ISBN 9781492535393
  (e-book)
Subjects: | MESH: Athletic Performance--physiology | Physical
  Fitness--physiology | Stress, Physiological
Classification: LCC RA781 | NLM QT 260 | DDC 613.7--dc23 LC record available at
  https://lccn.loc.gov/2016021011

ISBN: 978-1-4925-3520-1 (print)

The web addresses cited in this text were current as of September 2016, unless otherwise noted.

Acquisitions Editor: Roger W. Earle
Developmental Editor: Melissa J. Zavala
Managing Editor: Karla Walsh
Copyeditor: Patsy Fortney
Indexer: Tips Technical Publishing, Inc.
Permissions Manager: Dalene Reeder
Senior Graphic Designer: Keri Evans
Cover Designer: Keith Blomberg
Photographs (interior): © Human Kinetics, unless otherwise noted
Photo Asset Manager: Laura Fitch
Photo Production Manager: Jason Allen
Art Manager: Kelly Hendren
Illustrations: © Human Kinetics, unless otherwise noted
Printer: Walsworth

Printed in the United States of America   10   9   8   7   6   5   4   3   2   1

The paper in this book was manufactured using responsible forestry methods.

Human Kinetics
Website: www.HumanKinetics.com

United States: Human Kinetics
P.O. Box 5076
Champaign, IL 61825-5076
800-747-4457
e-mail: info@hkusa.com

Canada: Human Kinetics
475 Devonshire Road Unit 100
Windsor, ON N8Y 2L5
800-465-7301 (in Canada only)
e-mail: info@hkcanada.com

Europe: Human Kinetics
107 Bradford Road
Stanningley
Leeds LS28 6AT, United Kingdom
+44 (0) 113 255 5665
e-mail: hk@hkeurope.com

E6859

CONTENTS

PREFACE

Monitoring systems for athlete training and performance are becoming commonplace, particularly in high-performance sport programs. This has corresponded with an explosion in research in this area as well as in information on blogs and other social media platforms. Practitioners are increasingly asked to collect, analyze, and interpret information on their athletes. Despite all of these developments, practitioners are without a resource that provides an evidence-based summary of current best practices for athlete monitoring. *Monitoring Training and Performance in Athletes* links the research- and science-based concepts of athlete monitoring with practical strategies to use with athletes and clients.

This book will appeal to sport coaches, strength and conditioning coaches, sport scientists, physical therapists, and athletic trainers working across a range of sports and athletes from secondary school to professional levels. It provides a thorough overview of the contemporary evidence in athlete monitoring as well as examples of best practice from high-performance sport. A unique feature is the blending of rigorous scientific evidence with the art of coaching to provide a one-stop shop for anyone overseeing an athlete monitoring program. Practitioners will learn the science underlying athlete monitoring approaches, general principles of application, and how best to implement these methods in practice. All of this has been done without losing sight of the realities of working in sport

environments. This book will help practitioners ask better questions about the rationale and uses for athlete monitoring while challenging them to consider how to use monitoring data to inform the programming and coaching of their athletes.

Chapter 1 sets the scene by answering the question "Why monitor athletes?" Chapter 2 presents a variety of simple analysis techniques for investigating individual monitoring data in detail. In chapter 3 the physiological effects of training stress are explained, as are the concepts of overreaching and overtraining. Methods for monitoring training stress and measures of fitness and fatigue are presented in chapters 4 and 5. Chapter 6 reviews practices currently used in athlete monitoring, along with technology. Blending the art and science of coaching has particular importance for monitoring, and these principles are addressed in chapter 7. Finally, chapters 8 and 9 provide guidelines, approaches, challenges, and solutions for monitoring athletes in individual and team sports, respectively. Case studies and examples throughout the book show how the information can be used in practice.

The information currently available on athlete monitoring can be overwhelming. This text provides relevant and practical information that practitioners can use to make an impact on their athletes' preparation and performance.

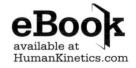

ACKNOWLEDGMENTS

First, I would like to thank the many athletes and coaches I have had the opportunity to work with over the years. I don't think it would be possible to write a book on athlete monitoring without significant interactions with athletes, coaches, and practitioners from a range of sports. In particular, I had the opportunity to work with three world-class coaches. Waimarama Taumaunu, Ruth Aitken, and Jean-Pierre Egger, thank you for the insights and conversations.

I would also like to thank Roger Earle, Melissa Zavala, Karla Walsh, and all the team at Human Kinetics behind the scenes for their help throughout the process of developing and writing this book.

I have been involved with many research projects on athlete monitoring over the years. Thank you to the many athletes who have been participants in these studies. Also, thanks to all the wonderful colleagues and postgraduate students I have worked with—in particular, Mike Newton, Stuart Cormack, David Tod, Matthew Sharman, Sophia Nimphius, and Nic Gill.

I have also been fortunate to have had several excellent mentors. I was lucky enough to work with and learn from three of the best researchers in the world in the areas of athlete training and monitoring. Carl Foster, Robert Newton, and William Kraemer have been extremely generous with their time over the years, and I will always be thankful for their support.

Finally, and most important, thanks to my family. My wife, Kathryn, and daughters Rachel, Emma, and Nicola inspire me every day.

1

Why Monitor Athletes?

Athlete monitoring has become an integral component of total athlete preparation. Elite sporting programs that do not do some type of monitoring are rare; most invest substantial resources in monitoring systems. Also, many new technologies and companies target the athlete monitoring market. As a result of these developments, sport coaches, sport scientists, and strength and conditioning practitioners need to be familiar with the principles of athlete monitoring, starting with a good understanding of the reasons for doing so.

Over the last several decades, sport scientists have been collecting a great deal of information about athletes. For example, monitoring athletes using technologies such as global positioning systems (GPS) and accelerometry is now widespread in elite sport. As a result,

practitioners need at least a basic understanding of these technologies. Added to this is the increasing body of research on athlete monitoring. Practitioners' challenge is to avoid collecting data for no reason but to instead use all of this information to help their athletes better their performances.

Historically, there has been a great deal of interest in quantifying the training of athletes (32). For many years, coaches have been systematically recording the training of their athletes using training diaries. Track and field coach Clyde Littlefield (1892-1981) and swimming coach James "Doc" Counsilman (1920-2004) were known to keep detailed records of the training and competitions of their athletes and to adjust their training programs based on this information (4). In fact, research from the 19th century documents strength and fatigue responses (although not in high-level athletes) (36). Systematically monitoring the physiological and psychological variables related to performance helps practitioners measure the effectiveness of their training programs and decide how to revise or update those programs. Recent times have seen frequent discussions in the media and a steady stream of research on the topic.

As noted, practitioners need to understand the reasons for monitoring athletes and how to use the information to improve their performances. Buy-in on the part of both athlete and practitioner will also increase the effectiveness of any monitoring program.

Figure 1.1 depicts monitoring issues and how monitoring helps athletes. When examining the figures in this book, keep in mind an important quote from British statistician George Box: "All models are wrong, but some are useful" (5). The models in this book provide a starting point for discussions of key concepts. As shown in figure 1.1, the ultimate outcome in sport is performance. To have any effect on an athlete, a monitoring program needs to have performance as its underlying consideration. Traditionally, physical and psychological factors were monitored. However, technical and tactical components are extremely important to overall athletic performance. The monitoring program attempts to quantify factors such as training dosage (also known as load), variables of training, and lifestyle factors (e.g., sleep, nutrition, life stress). Subsequent chapters address these factors and methods for monitoring them. A solid understanding of these factors

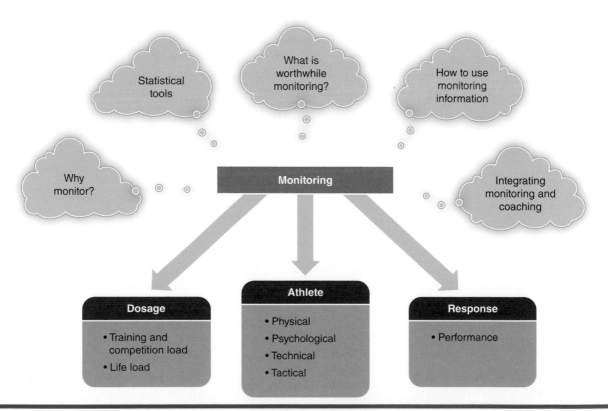

Figure 1.1   Monitoring issues and how monitoring helps athletes.

and how they are related is the basis of a good athlete monitoring program.

Stress Response to a Training Session

How an athlete ultimately performs is the result of the accumulation of individual training sessions. Thus, a key purpose of monitoring is to evaluate the stress response to individual training sessions, which are the building blocks of the overall training program. Practitioners need to know how hard their athletes are working in both training sessions and competition.

One of the challenges facing practitioners is the plethora of methods and technologies available for monitoring athletes. A method can be as simple and cheap as measuring the duration of the session and keeping a record of the elements of the session in a training diary (32). More complicated and expensive methods include analyzing biochemical markers such as cortisol (a stress hormone) and measuring athlete movements using GPS and inertial sensors. However, expensive does not necessarily mean better; simple tools often provide as much, if not more, information than more sophisticated methods (50).

Practitioners also need to know the effect of physiological loading on athletes during and following training sessions. The relationship between the training dose and the athlete's response largely determines the adaptations to the training program as those sessions accumulate (14). An athlete's return to a state of homeostasis is affected by the training dosage. The greater the training stress is, the longer the recovery period must be (51).

Two important factors to assess when determining the stress response to training sessions are training readiness and nontraining parameters.

Assessing Training Readiness

Monitoring helps determine the impact of individual training sessions on athletes' physical performance states and **training readiness**. Many practitioners assess the training readiness of their athletes at the beginning of training sessions to determine whether they need to make adjustments to the session. For example, an athlete experiencing excessive fatigue might benefit from a reduction in intensity. However, evidence supporting the use of a specific test to assess training readiness is lacking. Rather than relying on a sophisticated test, practitioners may do something as simple as asking the athlete "How do you feel?" This type of subjective information has been shown to be very effective for monitoring the well-being and fatigue levels of athletes (50). Subjective monitoring methods and wellness scales are discussed in more detail in chapter 4. A combination of subjective and objective measures often provides an overall picture of the athlete's readiness for the training session.

Training readiness can be assessed using high-velocity movements such as vertical countermovement jumps or drop jumps. The practitioner establishes a baseline result from when the athlete is in peak condition and uses it as a benchmark for subsequent assessments. If, for example, an athlete falls 10% or more below the peak performance value, the practitioner may adjust the session. Some practitioners use high-force movements such as isometric mid-thigh pulls or isometric squats as monitoring tools. Decrements in force production (e.g., greater than 5%) could indicate the need to change a training session. Movement screening and observing athletes during the warm-up provide key information about their readiness for training sessions. Practitioners also use manual therapies such as massage or joint manipulation to determine athlete readiness; however, research evidence for the efficacy of this type of approach is lacking.

Another monitoring tool that is becoming more widely used for assessing training readiness is **heart rate variability (HRV)** (46). HRV provides information about the neural influence on the heart—in particular, the regulation of the sympathetic nervous system. HRV is discussed in more detail in chapter 5. One benefit of methods such as HRV is that they are noninvasive and data can be collected at rest using smartphone applications (19). An increasing body of research is emerging in this area, providing guidelines for the use of HRV in training monitoring (47).

Assessing Nontraining Parameters

In addition to measuring the acute response to the training session, monitoring systems allow practitioners to measure what is happening outside of training and competition (e.g., nutrition, hydration, sleep, and wellness). This gives practitioners the full picture of what is affecting athletes' performance. The total stress on the athlete—not just the stress of training and competition—

needs to be considered. Research has shown that factors such as stress can play a role in the risk of developing injury (30, 37). One study in the United States found that university American football players were at greater risk of developing injury during periods of academic stress (37). This was in addition to high levels of physical stress from increased training and playing loads. Practitioners need to be aware of not only the physical demands on their athletes but also other stressors.

An interesting question to consider at this point is what practitioners should do when a monitoring tool reveals significant levels of fatigue. Should the session continue as planned, or should it be modified? The answer depends on several factors. It might be appropriate to continue with the training session as planned during a heavy training block. However, if the session is close to a major competition, it might be more appropriate to use a reduced **training load** (the measure of total training stress experienced by the athlete) or even to drop the session altogether. These concepts are explored in more detail in chapter 7.

Adaptation to a Training Program

One of the fundamental reasons for monitoring athletes is to gauge their progress in response to a training program. A practitioner may decide to test athletes at the beginning of a training cycle and then again at the end. This can provide valuable information about the response of the athletes to that particular block of training. However, if the window of time between these testing periods is too long (greater than 6 weeks), the practitioner might miss crucial information about the athlete's responses. Pretesting and posttesting is the standard way of gauging an athlete's progress because it does the following:

- Provides objective data on the effects of the training program
- Assesses the impact of a specific type of intervention
- Helps the practitioner make informed decisions about changes to the training program
- Identifies the physical strengths and weaknesses of the athlete
- Maximizes the practitioner's and athlete's understanding of the needs of the sport
- Adds to the body of knowledge on high-performance athletes

However, physical capacities such as strength and power can change rapidly, particularly in developing athletes and those with a low training age. Research has shown a great deal of variability in how much untrained people can increase muscular strength following a resistance training program (18, 33). A classic study by Hubal and colleagues (33) showed that 1-repetition maximum (1RM) strength gains could change up to 250% (range = 0-250%) following 12 weeks of progressive resistance training. Another study by Bamman and colleagues (3) showed a large variation (0-60%) in muscular hypertrophy after 16 weeks of resistance training. Even in elite athletes, levels of strength and power can increase across a training cycle (1, 2). A practitioner who is

prescribing training based on measures of strength such as 1RM, then, will need to regularly monitor the athletes' strength levels. A relatively simple way to do this is to use training loads to estimate the athletes' maximal strength. Other capacities such as power might be more challenging to measure. In terms of exercise prescription, regular monitoring should allow the practitioner to make informed decisions based on how the athlete is responding to the training program. With other physical capacities such as aerobic endurance, fast adaptations can occur, particularly in less-trained athletes with a low training age (8). Gathering regular feedback about how the athlete is adapting can help the practitioner adjust the training program to optimize that adaptation.

Regular monitoring gives practitioners detailed information for reporting purposes. Sport is a results-driven business, and although an effective monitoring system does not guarantee success, it can certainly contribute. Monitoring data also assists practitioners working in elite sport with reporting and accountability. Objective information helps to build a case for the effectiveness of a program. For example, a strength and conditioning practitioner may be able to demonstrate that the program changed athletes' physical characteristics, reduced injury rates, and contributed to competitive performance. This could be especially important during an end-of-season review of the strength and conditioning program. Although monitoring information may not guarantee staff retention, at least the practitioner will know that he or she did everything possible to prove the worth of the program and will have information that can be used to secure future opportunities.

Risk of Overreaching, Overtraining, Sickness, and Injury

One of the major reasons sport invests so much time in athlete monitoring systems is to keep athletes playing and reduce the time lost to injury and illness. Particularly in professional sport, in which so much money is invested in players, those players need to be available to compete in the most important events. The goal of athlete monitoring is to reduce the risk of overreaching, overtraining, sickness, and injury. Research has shown that high training volumes are not necessarily the cause of maladaptation to training; rather, the issue is how the athletes get to that point and how they have accumulated the volume (21). The destination is critical, but practitioners need to consider the journey the athlete has undertaken to get there.

It is important to consider the relationship between the acute stimulus of a single training session and the cumulative effect of training (14, 31). Fatigue is a normal and expected response to training. Under normal circumstances the athlete experiences acute fatigue in response to the training session and recovers within a period of hours to days. This acute fatigue, when followed by adequate recovery, should result in adaptation and improved performance (14). Problems can arise, however, when a mismatch exists between the stress of training and recovery. Some practitioners induce a state of overreaching in athletes by using intensified training. This can result in high levels of adaptation following the supercompensation period. With the overreaching state a decrement in performance can last from several days to several weeks (14).

However, if the mismatch between the cumulative training load resulting in fatigue and the level of recovery continues for an extended period, the athlete may enter into an overtrained state. **Overtraining** is a state characterized by decrements in performance accompanied by psychological disturbances that remain for an extended time despite significant reductions in training load (40). The restoration of the capacity to perform may take from several weeks to several months. This has crucial implications for the availability of athletes for major competitions. These important concepts are discussed in more detail in chapter 3.

As well as resulting in significant reductions in performance, excessive training loads that result in prolonged fatigue can place athletes at a higher risk of injury and illness (30). This has very serious implications for athlete monitoring. A great deal of interest exists in how to predict injury or illness in athletes. A monitoring system that can help reduce the risk of injury or illness would provide significant performance benefits.

Figure 1.2 shows factors that can affect training load as well as contribute to overreaching, overtraining, illness, and injury. A monitoring system needs to take these factors into account and, where possible, quantify them. Factors outside of training and competition, referred to as life load, also need consideration: work demands, study demands, relationships, and the general stress of life. Training and competition load are affected by factors such as volume, intensity, duration, frequency, and type of exercise. The combination of training load and life load determines the acute response to the training session. As these sessions accumulate, athletes will experience a chronic response to training. If a period of intensified training without sufficient recovery occurs, a state of

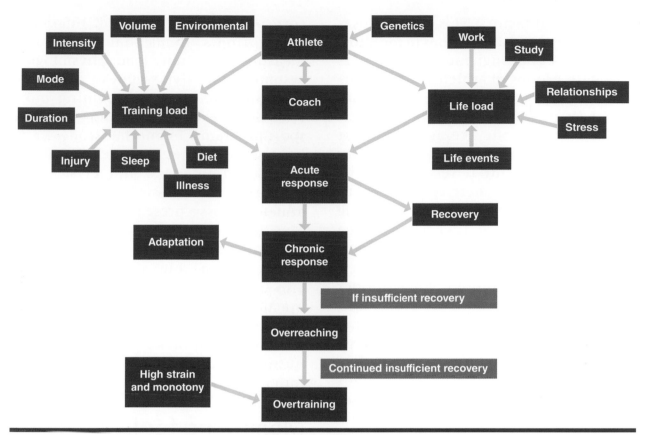

Figure 1.2 Factors that affect training load and their relationship to overreaching, overtraining, illness, and injury.

overreaching can occur. If this continues, athletes could enter an overtrained state (14).

When an athlete is suffering from performance fatigue, it is important to determine whether that fatigue is the result of overreaching or overtraining. Criteria for diagnosing overtraining syndrome, as well as exclusion criteria for the condition, have been developed to guide practitioners (40). It is important to note that no single diagnostic tool exists to identify overtraining syndrome. This diagnosis can be made only by excluding all other possible influences on the changes in performance and mood state (40). Signs to look for include unexplained underperformance, persistent fatigue, increased perceived exertion in

training and competitions, and disturbed sleep. Many tools for athlete monitoring are discussed in more detail in later chapters.

Importance of Individualized Monitoring

An individualized approach to athlete monitoring is critical to get the best results from a training system. The relationship between training dosage and performance varies between athletes, most likely as a result of factors such as genetics, training history, and psychological factors. This book focuses on individualized approaches to monitoring athletes. Although most practitioners deal with groups of athletes, it is important to focus on each athlete's responses rather than just on the group's results. Looking only at the average results for a group of athletes can result in missing important individual responses. The approach proposed here is no different from the approach used when designing a training program. Rather than taking a one-size-fits-all approach and creating a generic program for a squad of athletes, a strength and conditioning practitioner should take into account individual athletes' strengths and weaknesses (38, 45).

When implementing a monitoring system, it is equally important to allow for individual athlete variation. For example, some athletes tolerate increases in training load better than others do (23, 30). Monitoring individual athletes allows practitioners to identify those who are not responding to the training program. Solid evidence now demonstrates that people have individual responses to training (10, 33). This is true not only for physical capacities such as muscular strength (33) and aerobic endurance (10) but also across a range of physical capacities and markers. Practitioners need to be aware of these differences to ensure a full understanding of total athlete preparation.

An increasing body of research now includes regular monitoring data from elite athletes (6, 9, 29, 41). For example, Buchheit and colleagues (9) monitored the fitness, fatigue markers, and running performance of Australian rules football players during a preseason camp. Over 14 days the athletes were monitored using ratings of perceived exertion (RPE) and GPS during all training sessions. Daily measures of fatigue, sleep quality, muscle soreness, stress and mood, and salivary cortisol were also obtained. Integrated monitoring systems that incorporate measures of training load, physiological systems, subjective wellness, and physical performance are becoming more commonplace in high-performance sport programs. In another study, Bradley and colleagues (6) tracked training load, nutrition intake, and physical performance in professional rugby union athletes across a preseason. Tracking this type of information throughout a period of training permits researchers to observe trends across a group of athletes. This can also be useful for answering questions practitioners might have. For example, Bradley and colleagues (6) were able to observe and make suggestions about nutrition intake and training demands for professional rugby union athletes.

Monitoring for Injury Risk

Monitoring training also has an important role to play in the area of injury prevention (34). In particular, monitoring has huge potential for uncovering information about injury risk and its relationship to training load. For example, several studies from contact sports such as rugby league (23-25, 35), rugby union (15), and Australian rules football (12, 49) show a relationship between changes in cumulative training load and risk of injury. A study by Cross and colleagues (15) showed that rugby players were at a higher risk of injury if they had high 1-week cumulative training loads or a large week-to-week change in training load. These are similar to observations made in other contact sports (35, 49, 56). Not only do excessive loads need to be monitored, but also inadequate exposure to training load can be an issue (56). Being undertrained is often a bigger concern for many athletes than being overtrained. In elite sport, the issue is not necessarily the high volumes of work themselves but rather how the athletes get to that point. The implication is that by monitoring training loads weekly, practitioners will be much better informed about the changes in training. As a result, they can manipulate the program design to ensure that players are not exceeding thresholds that put them at increased risk of injury (22).

Monitoring for Illness

In addition to injury, athletes are at increased risk of developing illnesses such as upper respiratory tract infections during heavy periods of training (16, 44, 53). Not a great deal of research exists on the relationship between training load and illness in team sport athletes (56). However, a number of researchers who investigated this relationship in mainly aerobic endurance–based sport discovered increased susceptibility to upper respiratory illnesses after prolonged strenuous exercise (28). Monitoring immune markers such as salivary immunoglobulin A (IgA) and cytokines may hold some promise for identifying athletes at risk of developing these illnesses (26-28). Prolonged and strenuous bouts of exercise during training and competition have been shown to impair immune function (27). This can put athletes at greater risk of developing upper respiratory tract infections as a result of decreased levels of salivary IgA and cytokines (27). Thus, monitoring these types of markers is logical.

Monitoring Recovery

Recovery strategies are an increasingly important part of high-performance programs. Many studies have shown an individualized rate of recovery in response to contact sport (57). For example, West

and colleagues (57) investigated the neuromuscular, hormonal, and mood responses in 14 professional rugby players following match play. At 60 hr postmatch, seven players had not fully recovered to baseline levels for peak power on a vertical countermovement jump. However, the average results for the squad of players revealed full recovery of the squad to baseline levels. Examining the individual ratios of salivary testosterone to cortisol demonstrated that at 60 hr postmatch, five players showed recovery or a slight increase over recovery levels, whereas nine players showed a decrease, ranging from −6% to −65%. Only by monitoring each athlete's response to training and recovery will a full picture emerge. Postexercise recovery strategies could be individualized; for example, athletes who recover more slowly might use more aggressive and intensive recovery strategies. Practitioners need to be mindful about balancing recovery and adaptation and any negative effects associated with excessive recovery in their athletes (43, 48).

Monitoring Training Load

Individualized monitoring determines the degree of agreement between the training load prescribed by the practitioner and the load experienced by the athlete. Research suggests that a lack of agreement often exists between practitioners and athletes in terms of perception of the workload intensity (7, 20, 42). Problems can occur when intended easy sessions become hard sessions, and vice versa, which can lead to adverse effects such as overreaching or a lack of adaptation. Using a systematic monitoring system with objective measures such as heart rate and GPS makes these adverse effects less likely to occur. However, the true value of this information emerges only from observing individual responses.

Monitoring Effects of Training and Competition Schedules

Monitoring athletes may also provide information about the impact of competition schedules on individual player availability (11, 39). This can be a particular issue in sports with heavy competitive schedules such as football (11, 17) and baseball (52). Carling and colleagues (11) investigated the effects of match congestion on a professional football team competing in domestic and European competitions over a 4-year period. They documented the impact of players being rested at key periods, which highlighted how the coaching staff rotated and rested key players. The authors noted that the systematic monitoring of the players during match recovery periods using measures such as RPE, wellness, and recovery of muscle strength enabled practitioners to make evidence-based decisions on whether to rest players from subsequent matches (11). McLean and colleagues (39) investigated the neuromuscular, endocrine, and perceptual responses to varying durations of recovery in elite rugby league players. The results showed that as a playing group the athletes tended to recover fully within 4 days of match play, but the results were highly individual. This highlighted the need for practitioners to use individual monitoring to make decisions about appropriate approaches to training and potential adjustments to training load, particularly in elite athletes. Monitoring can assist with reducing

training errors when a mismatch occurs between the prescribed training load and the athlete's ability to tolerate it safely. Avoiding such mismatches is possible only when monitoring occurs on an individual basis. These concepts are explored more in chapters 8 and 9.

It is exciting to see more data being published about elite athletes (41, 54, 55). Sport science researchers have traditionally published research on recreationally trained athletes, which may have more limited application to athletes in high-performance sport. One of the challenges in this era is the increased use of data analytics or analyzing large amounts of data to make conclusions and find patterns (13). Looking at this at the level of the individual athlete makes interpretation of data even more challenging. Practitioners now need skills to process, interpret, and implement the tsunami of available information into their programs (13). One important skill is being able to filter out information that is not important. Individual monitoring can add value to a high-performance program by giving practitioners a more complete understanding of how the athletes are tracking. Monitoring data can then be used to aid decision making in areas such as load management, training program design and manipulations, and competition peaking. If done well, this should increase athlete availability by reducing incidences of injury and illness.

Monitoring appears to be extremely important for athlete and practitioner education by providing data to support decisions and identify best practice approaches to athlete preparation. Athlete and practitioner buy-in to the monitoring program is a fundamental contributor to the system's success. A key aspect of any monitoring system is that it must ultimately inform decision making. Data that are not used are simply data collected for the sake of it. Athletes in particular are less likely to take monitoring seriously if they do not understand why the information is being collected.

Practitioners must always question the reasons for gathering information in their monitoring programs. They must weigh the cost of the monitoring program and consider the value of the information (cost-benefit analysis). Chapter 7 describes a systematic process to help with making these decisions.

INDIVIDUAL RESPONSES IN A SQUAD OF ATHLETES

In this example, a range of monitoring measures is presented for an elite international squad of netball athletes. During a 10-day training camp, the coaching staff implements a monitoring system to assess how the athletes are responding to each training session (two or three per day). The coaches want to adapt the training program across the 10 days and detect early signs of overreaching, excessive fatigue, or both. The monitoring program for the training camp includes measuring RPE (training load) and heart rate during all training sessions as well as using daily wellness questionnaires (for muscle soreness, sleep quality, fatigue, and mood), salivary cortisol (stress marker), a drop jump test (neuromuscular fatigue), nutritional intake, and body weight measures.

One of the tests (drop jump) reveals little average change in neuromuscular fatigue in the group of 20 athletes across the training camp (mean = –1.5%). However, a look at the day-to-day variation of individual athletes for each test reveals a different picture. Taking just one day of the training camp as an example, changes in drop jump results from baseline range from –27% to +8%.

Meetings are held each evening with all of the coaches and support staff to discuss the individual players' data from the previous 24 hr. These meetings also include discussions about the coaches' perceptions of how the players performed in training and match play. Any injuries or limiting factors are also presented and discussed. Closely examining each player's response allows the coaching staff to see which players are experiencing excessive fatigue and to make necessary adjustments to their training loads. For example, the training load of an athlete who has exhibited excessive levels of fatigue over the previous 1 to 2 days might be reduced for the next day.

Alternative methods or increased recovery could also be considered. It would also be important for the coaches and support staff to delve deeper into any reasons for excessive fatigue. Issues as simple as poor sleep patterns over the preceding days or outside stresses in the athlete's life could be contributing factors. All factors need to be considered at an individual level.

Finally, this type of monitoring information can also be used in team selections. For example, coaches can see which players cope well with the demands of back-to-back matches played in similar formats to major competitions such as world championships.

Conclusion

High-performance sport programs are now investing a significant amount of resources in athlete monitoring systems. Therefore, it is critical that those working in sport understand why athlete monitoring is important. Practitioners should monitor their athletes for compelling reasons. Athlete monitoring can provide information about areas such as acute response to a training session and adaptations to a training program. Monitoring can also help determine whether overreaching and overtraining are occurring. If done effectively, it may also be used to predict illness and injury in athletes, thus minimizing the time that athletes miss training and, most important, competition. An effective monitoring system can reduce the risk of training errors resulting from a mismatch between the prescribed training load and athletes' ability to tolerate that load. This can only be done using individualized athlete monitoring. Clearly, understanding the reasons for monitoring athletes will assist practitioners in implementing effective systems that can effect change in their sporting performance programs.

2

Research Tools for Athlete Monitoring

Because athlete monitoring generates a great deal of data, practitioners need research tools to help them analyze the data effectively. **Statistics** is the science of collecting, classifying, analyzing, and interpreting numerical data (8, 39). Practitioners are typically not familiar with or overly enthusiastic about statistical analysis, but it can help them make use of monitoring information. A basic understanding of statistical concepts is important, particularly for those who use statistics on a regular basis. Practitioners must be aware that applying research tools incorrectly can result in misinterpreting data and making incorrect conclusions.

Traditional statistical methods are often not the most appropriate for analyzing data in sport environments because they focus on the group rather than the athlete. Traditional methods address statistical significance, whereas practitioners are more interested in practical or clinical significance. Fortunately, contemporary techniques, which provide helpful insights into how athletes respond to training and competition, are becoming more widely used. These methods enable practitioners to take into account many of the issues they face in sporting environments. This chapter provides simple explanations of these methods and examples of how these contemporary methods can be used in practice. Although a basic understanding of these statistical methods is sufficient for most practitioners, a more in-depth understanding can be useful. Practitioners who invest time in learning about these techniques in greater detail can be richly rewarded. More technical explanations are available (21).

Basic Statistical Tools for Practitioners

What are the basic statistical tools practitioners can use to enhance their athlete monitoring (8)? Figure 2.1 depicts the basic tools that all practitioners should have in their monitoring toolboxes, even though they may not always need all of them. These tools are discussed in more detail throughout this chapter.

Two branches of statistics are descriptive and inferential (39). **Descriptive statistics** provide a summary of data and are a good starting point for analyzing monitoring data. They are simply a way to describe the data. **Inferential statistics** allow one to use a random sample taken from a population to make inferences about that population. Recently, scientists and practitioners in sport science have made increasing use of **magnitude-based approaches**, which can be more practical because they address the meaningfulness of change to athletes (2). Practitioners may be more interested in understanding whether a change in a monitoring variable is prac-

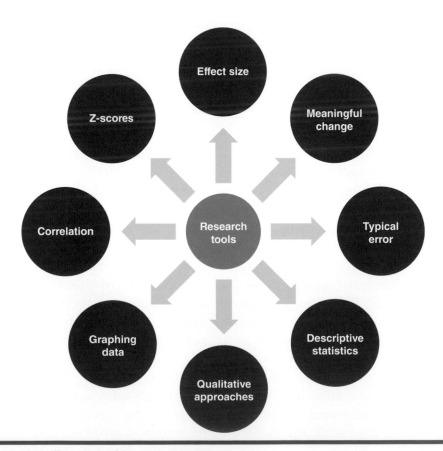

Figure 2.1   Statistical toolbox for athlete monitoring.

tically meaningful rather than statistically significant. That is, can the change be applied practically in the sporting environment? Statistical measures of central tendency, variability, percentile rank, smallest meaningful change, effect size, and standard scores all can be useful for monitoring a group of athletes, but more important is monitoring the athletes in the group.

Descriptive Statistics

Descriptive statistics summarizes or describes a large group of data and is used when all the information about a population is known. For example, if all the members of a squad of athletes are being monitored, statements can be made about the entire team with the use of descriptive statistics. The categories of numerical measurement in descriptive statistics include central tendency, variability, and percentile rank. In the sections that follow, these terms are defined and examples of how to calculate the values and scores are presented. At the most basic level, descriptive statistics such as mean and standard deviation can be used to report monitoring data. However, at times these may not be the most appropriate statistics or convey enough meaningful information. Practitioners often also use simple statistics such as **minimum** (lowest data value), **maximum** (highest data value), and range (the difference between the maximum and minimum, which represents the overall spread of the results) when reporting monitoring data. However, the first step is to have a solid understanding of how to classify types of monitoring data.

Classification of Data

Administering performance monitoring tests and recording the results are relatively straightforward aspects of any athlete monitoring program. However, an understanding of the types of data is necessary to ensure that the results are evaluated correctly. Rating scales used in athlete monitoring include rating of perceived exertion (RPE), Profile of Mood States (POMS), Recovery-Stress Questionnaire for Athletes (RESTQ-Sport), and Daily Analysis of Life Demands for Athletes (DALDA). Some of these scales use numerical data, some use verbal descriptors, and others use simple checklists (39). Data generated from athlete monitoring can be generally grouped into four categories: nominal, interval, ratio, and ordinal.

Nominal Scale

A **nominal scale** is used to group athletes into categories (3). Examples are classifying athletes as men or women or by position, such as quarterback or wide receiver in American football.

Interval Scale

An **interval scale** has equal intervals or units (6). There is no absolute zero, so negative scores are possible. An example of an interval scale is temperature measured in degrees.

Ratio Scale

A common type of scoring used in athlete monitoring is the **ratio scale** (6). It possesses an absolute zero, is based on order, and has equal distances between points. Measurements such as distance, time, and force are based on ratio scales.

Ordinal Scale

Sometimes referred to as a **rank order scale**, an **ordinal scale** ranks scores rather than providing any indication of the magnitude of difference (3). For example, an ordinal scale might rank scores from top to bottom or highest to lowest.

Measures of Central Tendency

Measures of **central tendency** are values about which the data tend to cluster. The three most common measures of central tendency are mean, median, and mode.

Mean

The **mean** refers to the average of the scores (i.e., the sum of the scores divided by the number of scores) (8). This is the most commonly used measure of central tendency. Because it uses all the data values of the sample, it provides information on the entire sample. However, the mean, or average, is greatly affected by the presence of extreme values (also called outliers).

Median

The **median** is the middle score when a set of scores is arranged in increasing order of magnitude (8). When there is an even number of scores, the median is the average of the two middle scores. Half of the scores fall above the median, and half fall below the median. In some cases, the median is a better measure of central tendency than the mean because of the distribution of the scores (e.g., a few athletes in the group have very high or very low scores). Extreme scores can raise or lower the squad mean to the extent that it does not adequately describe the status of most of the athletes.

Mode

The **mode** is the score that occurs with the greatest frequency (8). If each numerical score appears only once, there is no mode. If two or more scores have the greatest frequency, then all of these scores are modes. The mode is most useful for informing the practitioner of a score that occurs most regularly. The mode is generally regarded as the least useful measure of central tendency for athlete monitoring.

Variability

Practitioners often want to know the spread of data around the center of the distribution. The degree of dispersion of these data points within the group is called **variability** (3). Two common measures of variability are range and standard deviation.

Range

The **range** is the difference between the smallest (minimum) and the largest (maximum) data values or scores. This represents the overall spread of the scores. The advantage of the range for practitioners is that it is easy to understand. The major disadvantage is that it may not be an accurate measure of variability because it uses only the two extreme scores and therefore is greatly affected by outliers. For this reason, the range has limited application in practical settings. For example, the range could be the same for a group with widely dispersed results as for a group with narrowly dispersed results and a single extreme result (i.e., one athlete achieves a particularly high or low score). However, the range can be useful for showing the spread of scores for a particular measure in the group of athletes.

Standard Deviation

The **standard deviation** is a measure of the variability of a set of results around the mean (3). A small standard deviation indicates that a set of data values is closely clustered around the mean. A large standard deviation indicates a wider dispersion of the data values around the mean. Generally, the mean and standard deviation are reported alongside each other as mean ± standard deviation (e.g., 77.5 ± 6.7 kg could be the descriptive statistic reported for the body weight of a group of athletes). Reporting a summary of a squad of athletes in this way is a good way to show the group average while also providing some indication of the spread of the data. The standard deviation is most useful when the data values are normally distributed, forming a bell-shaped curve as shown in figure 2.2.

The normal bell-shaped curve is the foundation and starting point of many statistical techniques (3). As figure 2.2 indicates, when data are normally distributed, about 68% of the scores are within 1 standard deviation of the mean.

About 95% are within 2 standard deviations, and 99.7% are within 3 standard deviations of the mean. Although many statistical calculations are based on this normal distribution, practitioners are often dealing with nonnormal distributions in athlete monitoring. In fact, this curve almost never occurs in real-life data. What this means is that a certain amount of error is built into all statistical techniques; practitioners should be mindful of this when using these methods.

The normal curve is a frequency **histogram** (a graph that plots data according to the frequency of occurrences) that demonstrates that the greatest number of scores occurs in the middle of the curve and fewer and fewer scores occur out to the sides (figure 2.2). A normal curve with a long, low tail on the left is called a **negatively skewed** curve. When the tail of the curve is on the right, it is referred to as **positively skewed**. Outliers can change the shape of this curve. This is a common occurrence in many athlete monitoring situations, particularly because practitioners often deal with

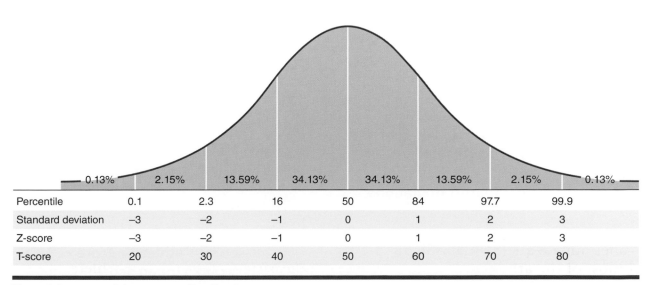

	0.13%	2.15%	13.59%	34.13%	34.13%	13.59%	2.15%	0.13%
Percentile	0.1	2.3	16	50	84	97.7	99.9	
Standard deviation	−3	−2	−1	0	1	2	3	
Z-score	−3	−2	−1	0	1	2	3	
T-score	20	30	40	50	60	70	80	

Figure 2.2 Normal frequency distribution curve.

small sample sizes. For example, coaches often deliberately modify training so that programs include heavy and light weeks or days. These periods of loading and unloading are examples of extreme but important outliers that need to be taken into account.

Standard deviations (and the degree of skewness) are often calculated using a spreadsheet. However, a basic understanding of how they are calculated is useful for understanding these measures. Following are steps for calculating the standard deviation of a group of data:

1. Calculate the deviation of each score from the mean by subtracting the mean from each **raw score** (actual score obtained by the athlete).
2. Square each deviation score.
3. Sum all of the squared deviations.
4. Divide the sum by $N - 1$ to get the variance.
5. Take the square root of the variance to find the standard deviation.

For example:

Resting heart rates for an athlete over 8 days = 55, 62, 57, 51, 62, 65, 71, 58 beats/min

Mean = 60.1 beats per min, so the deviation score for each day = −5.1, 1.9, −3.1, −9.1, 1.9, 4.9, 10.9, −2.1

Squared deviation scores = 26.01, 3.61, 9.61, 82.81, 3.61, 24.01, 118.81, 4.41

Sum of all the squared deviations = 272.88

$272.88 \div (8 - 1) = 38.98$

Square root of 38.98 = 6.24 beats/min

More advanced techniques for analyzing data can provide some interesting information about the patterns of athlete monitoring data. Using data mining can give a more in-depth mathematical description of patterns. **Data mining** refers to the process of deeper exploration using analysis techniques of large data sets that practitioners typically encounter in athlete monitoring. Looking at the clustering of group data according to similarities in the data is one approach. At the simplest level, the clustering can consist of classifying athletes by position, playing standard, or level of experience.

Z-Scores

The extent of unusualness of a data point is determined by calculating the **z-score**—the number of standard deviations away from the mean. The z-score is an example of a standardized score and is useful in athlete monitoring because it provides much more information than just the raw score (42). Practitioners can use the z-score to express the distance of any athlete's result in standard deviation units from the mean. When scores are transformed into z-scores, normally distributed z-scores have a mean of 0 and a standard deviation of 1 (see figure 2.2). The z-scores will range between −3 and +3. The z-score indicates how many standard deviations below or above the mean the athlete's score is. For example, a z-score of +1.5 would indicate that the athlete's score is 1.5 standard deviations above the mean for the group of athletes.

The z-score can be calculated as follows:

Z-score = athlete's score − group's mean score ÷ group's standard deviation

For example, if an athlete has a result of 55 watts/kg for peak power during a vertical countermovement jump, and the mean and standard deviation for the group are 60 watts/kg and 5 watts/kg, respectively, the preceding equation can be used to determine the z-score for that athlete as follows:

$$Z\text{-score} = 55 - 60 \div 5 = -1.0$$

In other words, the athlete's score is 1 standard deviation from the group mean. Because the z-score is negative, the athlete's score is 1 standard deviation below the group mean.

T-Scores

T-scores, which are derived from z-scores, are essentially modified z-scores. Calculating the t-score requires multiplying the z-score by 10 and then adding 50. Practitioners and athletes often find t-scores easier to understand than z-scores because they are always positive values. T-scores generally range from 20 to 80; 50 represents the mean score (see figure 2.2). If an athlete has a z-score of −1.5, the t-score would be calculated as follows:

$$T\text{-score} = -1.5 \times 10 + 50 = 35$$

T-scores are not used as widely in athlete monitoring as **z-scores** are. Practitioners could use them if they believe the coach and athlete would understand them better.

Standard Difference Score

Standard difference scores are z-scores derived from a change in the variable. These scores help identify athletes who have had large changes in a particular measure. The standard difference scores can help practitioners track changes in

response to a training intervention (i.e., pretraining versus posttraining), but they can also be used for regular athlete monitoring. An advantage of this approach is that it takes into account large differences in the rank order of the scores.

Standard difference scores can be calculated by finding the difference between the premeasure and postmeasure for each athlete and then dividing it by the standard deviation of the difference score or using a baseline standard deviation (32). The standard difference scores can then be sorted by rank and plotted on a graph. A more in-depth discussion of standard difference scores and methods of calculation is available (32). Here is how the standard difference score could be calculated for an athlete who scored 23 out of 40 on a wellness questionnaire and who, the week before, scored 28 out of 40 with an established baseline standard deviation of 3:

$$\text{Standard difference score} = \text{posttesting value} - \text{pretesting value} \div \text{baseline standard deviation}$$

$$= 23 - 28 \div 3$$

$$= -1.67$$

Percentile Rank

An athlete's **percentile rank** refers to the percentage of athletes being monitored who scored below that athlete. As with calculating the median, percentile ranking requires arranging monitoring results in order from lowest to highest (also known as arranging the data **ordinally**). For example, if an athlete is ranked in the 50th percentile, 50% of the group produced scores below that athlete's score. Norms based on large samples are sometimes expressed in evenly spaced percentiles. This approach is more useful for testing capacities such as muscular strength and endurance and tends to be less widely used for athlete monitoring.

Effect Size

Effect size is one of the most useful statistics for practitioners (11). It allows the data to be reported as a standardized metric that can be understood regardless of the measurement scale used. It is a very insightful method for reporting changes in monitoring variables and highlights the practical significance of any changes; more complicated methods rely on statistical significance, which is much more difficult to understand. A variety of methods can be used for interpreting effect sizes (see the section Using Effect Size).

Confidence Limits

Confidence limits (or confidence intervals) are the range within which the actual score from the monitoring tool will fall. They provide meaningful information about how large the change or difference is and whether it is increasing or decreasing (19). A common approach is to use 90% or 95% confidence limits, which means that the value will most likely fall within this range 90% or 95% of the time. In other words, they represent the practitioner's level of confidence that the true value in the group of athletes is contained within the specified interval. When using 95% confidence limits, if a practitioner did the monitoring 100 times, the athlete's score would fall within that interval 95 times.

Reliability

Three vital considerations for practitioners when developing protocols for monitoring athletes are the reliability, validity, and sensitivity of the tools. Monitoring is useful only if the tools are repeatable (**reliability**), measure what they are supposed to (**validity**), and can detect change in the athlete (**sensitivity**). These components often are discussed interchangeably, but they are factors that need to be considered individually when selecting monitoring tools for athletes. The reliability of the monitoring tools is often considered the most important factor because it affects the precision of the monitoring of athletes (1). For example, in elite athletes the degree of change in many of the measures can be very small; practitioners working with this population need a reliable monitoring tool. When measuring the wellness of athletes using a **questionnaire** on a daily basis, the practitioner needs to know what change on the measurement scale would indicate a meaningful change.

When performing any type of monitoring, establishing the reliability of the method is crucial. One approach is to look at current research to see whether researchers and practitioners have found the measure to be reliable using statistics. However, practitioners must also try to establish the reliability of monitoring tools with their own groups of athletes. For example, there may be differences in reliability between developmental and elite athletes. Research across a range of sports and athlete populations seems to suggest that this is the case (28, 29). In one study, high school athletes in the United States were shown to have higher variability on jump monitoring variables compared to university-level and elite athletes (28).

A variety of methods for measuring reliability are available to the practitioner. The most common are correlations, typical error of measurement, coefficient of variation, and change in the mean. Practitioners do not need to use all of these methods; calculating the typical error of measurement and subsequently determining the coefficient of variation (expressed as a percentage) is a good starting point.

Correlations

Measures used in athlete monitoring need to be repeatable. **Retest reliability** refers to how reproducible a measurement is. All things being equal, the measurement of an athlete on day 1 should be the same as the measurement on day 2. A test–retest correlation is a common method for measuring reliability. **Correlation** is a statistical method used to determine the magnitude of the relationship between two variables. A correlation of 1.0 means that a perfect relationship exists between two variables; 0.0 represents no relationship whatsoever. **Pearson correlation coefficients** and **intraclass correlation coefficients (ICC)** are used for quantifying retest reliability. Of the two, ICC is the more suitable measure, especially when tests are repeated more than twice (a desirable approach when establishing retest reliability and when monitoring athletes). Online spreadsheets can be used to calculate measures of reliability (16).

Typical Error of Measurement

Typical error of measurement is a very useful method for assessing changes in monitoring variables with athletes (15). This provides a direct measure of the amount of error associated with the test. Measurement error refers to variation in the monitoring tool from any source. Therefore, it includes factors such as equipment error and the biological variation of the athlete.

Coefficient of Variation

The **coefficient of variation (CV)** is an important type of typical error of measurement. The CV refers to the typical error expressed as a percentage of the athlete's mean score for the monitoring tool. This can be useful for calculating the reliability of monitoring tests, and it is recommended that practitioners use this for all their monitoring tools. The CV can be used to look at the consistency of differences between athletes. The more common approach is to calculate the CV using the team average.

The typical error can be calculated as follows:

Standard deviation of difference scores ÷ square root of 2

To calculate the CV, the following equation can be used:

CV = 100 (standard deviation ÷ mean)

Practitioners can use this approach to calculate typical error for all the measures used in their monitoring batteries. From this they can determine whether the changes seen as a result of training are meaningful. Online spreadsheets can be used to calculate typical error and CV (16). The typical error and CV can be expressed relative to the meaningful change calculation to give insight into the sensitivity of the test (discussed in the sidebar Testing for Reliability on page 23).

Change in the Mean

The **change in the mean** is another measure of reliability that has two components: random change and systematic change. The random change in the mean is due to sampling error. The systematic change is the nonrandom change in the value between trials that can be the result of factors such as athlete motivation. One way to calculate this is to perform a **paired t-test** between the pairs of trials. A t-test is a statistical test that allows a comparison between two means. A paired t-test can also be used when comparing groups of athletes who have been monitored more than once with repeat testing. This test can be performed using Excel or a variety of statistics programs.

Maximizing Reliability

Practitioners should use monitoring tools with small **learning effects** (i.e., the degree to which athletes are familiar with them). Athletes should have at least four familiarization trials to reduce any learning effects. The differences between two sets of monitoring results can be a result of several factors including interrater and intrarater reliability.

Interrater Reliability

Interrater reliability refers to the degree to which different people conducting the monitoring agree in their test results over time or on repeated occasions. Using a clearly defined scoring system and assessors who are trained and experienced with the test are essential to enhance interrater reliability. For example, if the quality of movement in an overhead squat is being used as a monitoring tool at the start of a training session, it is important to have clear and accurate monitoring criteria. In an ideal world, the same practitioner should perform the monitoring of the group of athletes.

Practitioners should be aware of other sources of interrater differences as well, such as variations in calibrating technologies, how the athletes are prepared for the monitoring, and how the monitoring test is performed. For example, in a vertical countermovement jump test, differences could occur based on the type of warm-up the athletes perform prior to the test. Personality differences may result in different testers motivating athletes to different degrees. For example, larger interrater variability may occur if an intern performs some of the monitoring tests and the head strength and conditioning coach performs others.

Intrarater Reliability

Intrarater reliability refers to the consistency of scores in repeated tests conducted by a single tester. Poor intrarater reliability can be a result of inadequate training in the monitoring methods, a lack of concentration, or an inability to follow standardized procedures for calibration, athlete preparation, and test administration. One easy way to reduce this variability is to ensure that those performing the monitoring are well trained in all aspects of the assessment.

Reducing Measurement Error

Measurement error can be reduced by paying attention to the likely sources of error and using appropriate methods and analysis techniques to reduce error. When developing a monitoring system, investing time early on to identify sources of potential error and coming up with strategies to minimize these can go a long way in enhancing the quality of the system. In addition, practitioners can improve reliability and validity to reduce error in monitoring by making monitoring conditions as consistent as possible. Following are guidelines to use with monitoring that involves some type of physical test:

- Ensure a consistent and adequate warm-up before the test.
- Provide consistent instructions and verbal encouragement.
- Perform the monitoring test at the same time of day to reduce the effects of diurnal variation (38).

- Perform the monitoring under the same environmental conditions as much as possible. Because environmental conditions can be controlled best indoors, attempt to perform monitoring indoors if possible. Recording the environmental conditions (e.g., temperature, humidity) can be useful.

TESTING FOR RELIABILITY

An important first step when implementing a monitoring program is to establish the reliability of the measures. Let's say, for example, that a vertical countermovement jump test is one of the monitoring tools. The practitioner would like to use the test to track jump height in the group of athletes at the start of the week as an indicator of training readiness. The tests are repeated on 4 days at the same time of day. Practitioners should always aim for more than one repeat test to determine the reliability of their measures.

The following mean results are obtained from the group of 12 athletes:

Day 1 = 60 cm

Individual results for day 1 were 61, 55, 58, 67, 49, 65, 60, 54, 57, 63, 68, and 58 cm. The mean is calculated by taking the sum of the results (715) and dividing by the number of athletes ($N = 12$) to give a mean of 59.6 cm. The standard deviation of these scores is 5.6 cm.

Day 2 = 62 cm

Day 3 = 64 cm

Day 4 = 64 cm

The difference scores are 2 cm (62 cm from day 2 minus 60 cm from day 1), 2 cm (64 cm from day 3, minus 62 cm from day 2), and 0 cm (64 cm from day 4 minus 64 cm from day 3), and the standard deviation of these difference scores is 1.2 cm.

The typical error is then calculated as the standard deviation of the difference scores divided by the square root of 2, or 1.2 ÷ square root of 2 = 0.85 cm.

The CV can be calculated as 100 times the standard deviation of the results (days 1 to 4) divided by the mean of the results (days 1-4). In this example the CV is $100 \times 1.9 \div 62.5 = 3.0\%$.

In an ideal situation the reliability would be calculated based on results from multiple athletes and using several time points. The time of day the testing occurs would be consistent. Also, the practitioner would try to replicate the conditions under which the monitoring test is used in practice and aim to have at least 10 athletes complete the reliability testing (more is even better!). The practitioner would also try to establish the reliability of the tests across various cohorts of athletes if working in different sports and with different levels of development (e.g., youth athletes versus more experienced athletes). Using this approach, it should be possible to build up an in-house database of reliability measures, including typical errors and CVs for the monitoring tests used.

- Provide plenty of familiarization trials to reduce learning effects. As previously suggested, provide at least four trials.
- Standardize the premonitoring conditions (e.g., sleep, nutrition, training) as much as possible in the period leading up to the monitoring.

What Is Acceptable Reliability?

A commonly asked question in athlete monitoring is "What is an acceptable level of reliability for a measure?" In short, the answer is that practitioners should use measures that are as reliable as possible. Although no preset standards for acceptable reliability measures in athlete monitoring are widely adopted, it is often suggested that ICC values above 0.75 may be considered reliable; this index should be at least 0.90 for most monitoring applications. Practitioners can use a category system to determine the level of reliability, in which >0.90 is considered extremely high; 0.70 to 0.90, very high; 0.50 to 0.70, high; 0.30 to 0.50, moderate; and <0.30, low. Practitioners and scientists often use arbitrarily chosen targets for the CV of less than 10%. It is not clear how appropriate this target is for athlete monitoring, and it would seem to be a fairly liberal interpretation (1, 38). Where possible, practitioners should use monitoring tests with extremely high reliability. Aiming to have the CV below 5% has also been suggested (42). Again, the reliability of the test should be as high as possible.

High reliability is a prerequisite for monitoring minor yet significant changes in an athlete and for measuring the effect of a training program on a team. If the reliability of a monitoring tool is poor, the practitioner may never know the true status of the athlete or the effect of training sessions. Monitoring methods need to be good enough to detect any changes in the status of the athletes.

Validity

Validity deals with determining whether the monitoring tool assesses what it is supposed to assess (i.e., is it accurate?). For example, does a method chosen to track fatigue provide a valid measure of fatigue? Validity also deals with the issue of how well the monitoring tool relates to the athlete's competition performance.

As with reliability, several types of validity exist, including ecological validity, construct validity, face validity, content validity, and criterion validity. The types of validity most critical for athlete monitoring are construct and ecological validity. These have to do with whether the variable being monitored has any application to the setting in which it is collected. Another important consideration is whether the variable is theoretically linked to a factor such as athlete fatigue and training load (see chapter 4).

Ecological Validity

Ecological validity refers to how well the monitoring tool relates to actual athlete performance and how well the findings can be applied in real-life settings. Ecological validity is particularly important when looking at research studies of athlete monitoring. Consider the recommendation that practitioners wait 30 min following a training session before taking the session RPE measure to get a global rating of an athlete's perceived exertion (see chapter 4). Thirty minutes is a long time to ask athletes to wait around after a training session to provide more monitoring information. However, research by Singh and colleagues (35) has shown that 10 min is sufficient, which increases the practicality of this monitoring tool.

Construct Validity

Construct validity refers to overall validity, or the extent to which the test actually measures what it was designed to measure (3). Construct validity also refers to the test's ability to represent the underlying construct (the theory developed to organize and explain some aspects of existing knowledge and observations). It is also a measure of the test's ability to discriminate between groups of athletes. For example, the POMS questionnaire is used to measure the overall construct of mood. The construct validity of the POMS questionnaire refers to how well it measures what it purports to measure (i.e., the athlete's mood). Another example is using session RPE to represent the global perceived exertion by matching the average of RPE measures taken during the session (see chapter 4). Other forms of validity (e.g., face validity, content validity, criterion-referenced validity) are secondary and provide evidence for construct validity. Given a choice between two valid athlete monitoring tests, practitioners should consider the simplicity and economy of test administration.

Face Validity

Face validity is the appearance to the athlete, coach, and other practitioners that the test measures what it is purported to measure (6). For example, a wellness questionnaire that contains questions about fatigue and sleep quality would likely have high face validity for coaches and athletes for monitoring fatigue.

However, a vertical countermovement jump test to monitor swimmer fatigue might not have high face validity because coaches and athletes may question the relevance of this movement for their sport (this does not mean it is not a useful test of neuromuscular fatigue, though). If the monitoring tool has face validity, the athlete is more likely to respond to it positively. The assessment of face validity is generally informal and qualitative. However, it is important because it creates athlete buy-in. For monitoring tests, face validity is particularly desirable based on the assumption that the athlete performing the monitoring test wants to do well and will theoretically be more motivated by a test that serves a valid purpose and appears to measure something that is relevant.

Content Validity

Content validity refers to expert assessment that the monitoring tool measures what it claims to measure (6). A test for athlete assessment that has high content validity includes all the abilities needed for a particular sport or sport position. For a practitioner creating an athlete monitoring system, content validity helps to determine the components that need to be included to ensure validity. The practitioner should list the components to be assessed and make sure they are all represented in the monitoring battery. Although the terms *face validity* and *content validity* are sometimes used interchangeably, the former relates to the appearance of validity to nonexperts, whereas the latter refers to actual validity.

Criterion Validity

Criterion validity refers to the relationship between the scores on a test and scores on a criterion measure (3). A **criterion measure** is a test that is widely accepted as a gold standard and valid test. For example, the gold standard test for body composition is dual X-ray absorptiometry. Criterion validity can be divided into two parts: concurrent validity and predictive validity. **Concurrent validity** refers to the validity of a test for measuring a construct at a particular time. In most cases, the test is correlated with another, more accurate measure of the construct that is not feasible in most sport situations. An example is comparing a performance test and competition performance. It would be difficult to conduct a performance test such as a 3-km time trial on the day of competition. **Predictive validity** refers to the ability of a test to predict some construct or outcome in the future (6). This type of validity is important for athlete monitoring because it deals with future performance, which is fundamental in sport. Obvious areas in which this would have application are injury prediction and fatigue monitoring. Practitioners and coaches are always interested in valid tools that will

enable them to predict how athletes will respond to a given training stimulus. Even more important is optimizing conditions to achieve peak performance in competition.

A crucial aspect for criterion validity is choosing a suitable criterion measure. Obviously for sport, performance in the event would be a well-accepted criterion measure. In sport science, well-established criteria such as laboratory-based measures of body composition and 1RM can be used. However, in athlete monitoring less consensus is available on what constitutes gold standard measures for things such as training load and fatigue. For example, researchers have studied the validity of methods such as session RPE relative to other measures of training load such as heart rate–based methods (12, 43).

Figure 2.3 shows a validity correlation between peak force produced during an isometric mid-thigh pull (IMTP) test and 1RM squat. The high correlation ($r = .90$) and the linear correlation in the scatter plot suggest that these two tests measure a similar construct. This indicates that

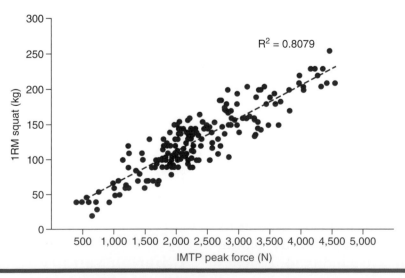

Figure 2.3   Validity correlation of IMTP versus 1RM squat.

both proved similar information and thus either could be used. It should be noted that for a test to have high validity, it needs to have high reliability. However, a test can be highly reliable but not valid.

Different factors can affect the validity of athlete monitoring. A key consideration is to reduce the effect of potential confounding variables (13). Areas that practitioners often overlook include instructions on how to perform the monitoring test, the consistency of verbal encouragement, the number and gender of observers, and even music played during the monitoring (13). A good strategy is to keep the conditions as consistent as possible whenever monitoring is performed. A spreadsheet available online can be used to calculate validity (21).

Meaningful Change

The sensitivity of a monitoring tool refers to its ability to detect small but important changes in performance or an aspect such as fatigue. This relates to both reliability and validity. Practitioners need to determine the worthiness, or the meaning, of a change in the monitoring tool results. Meaningful change is defined as the smallest practical change that is important (18). In other words, is the change in the measure provided by the monitoring tool meaningful? A reliable monitoring tool may provide consistent results, but if it is not sensitive to changes in the athlete's performance, its value is questionable.

Practitioners must know how much change constitutes practical data about both the athlete and the group of athletes. This requires evaluating the size of the change in the context of unrelated factors that may have affected the outcome of the test. This process depends on the nature of the athlete population and the test selected (27, 38). Practitioners need to determine the typical error of measurement and CVs for the monitoring tests they use.

A meaningful change is an important consideration when monitoring an athlete's level of preparation. By determining the smallest meaningful change, the practitioner can calculate the amount of change that will indicate that the athlete is not responding positively to the training stimulus or is becoming excessively fatigued.

Determining the Smallest Meaningful Change

The smallest meaningful change can provide helpful insight, especially when used to compare athletes at similar performance levels. In this context, **smallest meaningful change** refers to the degree of change required to determine differences between competitors in a specific event. For example, in the 100-m final at the Olympics, what is the difference between fourth place and getting a medal? This comparison approach has been investigated using several athlete populations (25) and involves calculating the value of the CV for elite athletes in the particular event. Similar concepts can be applied to athlete monitoring. Research has shown that practitioners want to be confident about measuring approximately half the value of the smallest meaningful change when testing elite athletes (19). Practitioners can calculate the smallest meaningful change for the monitoring tools that are specific to the type of athletes they are working with. Table 2.1 shows examples of CVs from studies of a variety of sports (25). Practitioners can use these results as a guide, but they will get a great deal more

TABLE 2.1   Typical Coefficients of Variation for Some Sport Events

Sport	Event	Gender	Variability
Athletics	Track	Combined	1.1
	Field	Combined	1.4
Rowing		Combined	0.9
Track cycling	Sprint/pursuit	Combined	1.2
	Time trials	Combined	0.8
Swimming		Combined	0.8
Weightlifting	Snatch	Men	1.9
	Clean and jerk	Men	2.0
	Total	Men	1.7
	Snatch	Women	3.6
	Clean and jerk	Women	3.7
	Total	Women	3.3

Data from Malcata and Hopkins (25).

value from their monitoring programs if they take the time to establish their own criteria.

It is also important to put the smallest meaningful change in the context of the reliability of the monitoring tool. Prior to doing this, the smallest meaningful change can be calculated using the following formula (19):

Smallest meaningful change = 0.2 × between-athletes standard deviation

The 0.2 refers to the smallest meaningful, or important, effect statistic (see the section Using Effect Size) (19). Between-athletes standard deviation refers to the standard deviation that has been calculated for a group of athletes. It is also possible to use the standard deviation for a single athlete using a series of monitoring test results.

Ideally, the smallest meaningful change should be greater than the typical error or CV of the monitoring test. That way the practitioner can be confident that any change is not simply due to the error or noise associated with the test. Another approach is to simply apply the CV of the test as the benchmark for a meaningful change. Multiplying the CV by a factor of 1.5 or 2 can be a way to be certain of a real change in the monitoring measure (42). It is important to work out these scores of smallest meaningful changes using the same (or a similar) population of athletes, in addition to using as many athletes as possible. This ensures that outlying, or extreme, scores do not have too great of an effect on the overall score.

Practitioners can also apply a set of criteria when looking at these values. For many years the Australian Institute of Sport rated tests as "good" if the technical error was less than the smallest meaningful change. If the typical error was approximately the same as the smallest meaningful change, the test was rated as "OK." Finally, if the typical error was much higher than the smallest meaningful change, the test was rated as "marginal." These ratings can give the practitioner some indication of the usefulness of the test. Practitioners should be aware that just because a test has poor reliability does not mean that it has no value. The sensitivity of the test may be of more concern when the measures of interest undergo large changes. For example, recent work has suggested that some variables during jump monitoring (e.g., eccentric rate of force development) may be sensitive to fatigue despite having large typical errors that exceed the smallest meaningful change (28).

Using Effect Size

As alluded to earlier, using standardized change or difference can reveal the degree of change observed with monitoring tools. Effect size can be useful for calculating performance changes following a training program or for comparing groups of athletes (11). It can also be used in day-to-day or week-to-week athlete monitoring. For example, a practitioner could use effect size to compare jump velocities in a group of athletes from week 1 to week 2. This measure, also known as **Cohen's effect size**, is useful in meta-analyses to assess the magnitude of differences or changes in the mean in different studies (9). Effect size is similar to a z-score. With this method, the practitioner expresses the difference, or change in the mean, divided by the between-subjects standard deviation using the following formula:

$$\text{Effect size} = \text{mean 2} - \text{mean 1} \div \text{standard deviation 1}$$

where 1 and 2 = day, week, or time point 1 or 2.

For example, mean vertical squat jump velocity for week 1 is 2.94 m/s and the standard deviation is 0.19 m/s. For week 2 the mean is 3.04 m/s and the standard deviation is 0.23 m/s. The equation would be as follows:

$$\text{Effect size} = 3.04 - 2.94 \div 0.19 = 0.53$$

It is also possible to use the pooled standard deviation in the calculation (9). In the preceding example the pooled standard deviation is 0.21 m/s, so the calculation would look like this:

$$\text{Effect size} = 3.04 - 2.94 \div 0.21 = 0.48$$

Practitioners can use either approach as long as they are consistent in the application and do not switch between methods, which will give slightly different results.

No clear guidelines exist about what constitutes a smallest meaningful difference or change with this measure, but 0.2 has been suggested (19). Several scales have been provided to compare the magnitude of the effect (9, 19). The original classification system proposed by Cohen suggested <0.2 as a trivial effect, 0.2 to 0.5 as a small effect, 0.5 to 0.7 as a moderate effect, and >0.7 as a large effect (9). However, these are somewhat arbitrary and don't need to be rigidly followed. The scale suggested by Hopkins and colleagues (19) has become more widely accepted, and the reference values for small (0.2), moderate (0.6), large (1.2), and very large (2.0) can be a useful starting point for practitioners.

Consider a group of athletes that has a week 1 mean broad jump result of 205 cm (standard deviation of 9.7 cm); a week later the mean broad jump

TABLE 2.2 Classification Scale for Effect Sizes

Magnitude	Effect size
Trivial	<0.2
Small	0.2-0.6
Moderate	0.6-1.2
Large	1.2-2.0
Very large	2.0-4.0
Extremely large	>4.0

Data from Hopkins et al. (19).

result is 208 cm. The effect size would be calculated as follows: (208 − 205) ÷ 9.7 = 0.31. The practitioner would interpret the effect size of 0.31 as a small effect, or change, from week 1 to week 2. Table 2.2 shows a suggested scale for classifying the effect sizes (calculated as difference in the means) that could be used for athletes with varying degrees of experience. Another key point is that small effects can have large consequences in athlete monitoring. More in-depth discussions of effect sizes and their application are available (9, 11, 23).

Comparing to Baseline

Determining whether a monitoring variable has changed depends largely on the baseline value it is being compared with. Practitioners must have multiple baseline values with which to compare athletes' results. Having multiple baseline measures also improves the reliability of the measure. However, comparisons must be meaningful, particularly when monitoring for athlete fatigue. For example, during an intensive period of the com-petition season, a practitioner should compare test results against a value that represents a relatively fatigue-free state in the athlete.

Understanding Meaningful Change in Athlete-Reported Questionnaires

In addition to physical performance tests, questionnaires and subjective responses of athletes are commonly used for monitoring. However, determining what constitutes a meaningful change in these athlete-reported questionnaires is challenging (see chapter 4). Wellness questionnaires often require subjective ratings on a scale that broadly represents categories from poor to excellent. A potential problem with interpreting scores on these scales is that athletes can give automated responses, particularly if they are answering these questions on a regular basis. Problems can sometimes occur with athletes who regularly report high or low values despite having had the scales explained in detail and following correct anchoring procedures. Anchoring procedures involve providing a series of verbal cues prior to beginning the questionnaires so the athletes understand the ratings (see chapter 4).

Solutions to these problems with questionnaires have been suggested (10). One is to determine the degree to which each athlete's response is above or below normal. Another solution is to compare the athlete's result on that day to a value that represents what the athlete regularly reports. This had been done by using a modification of the z-score or standard difference score, calculated as follows (10):

TESTING FOR MEANINGFUL CHANGE

Let's say you are interested in calculating the smallest meaningful change in relative peak power on a vertical squat jump test. Ten athletes complete the testing and get scores of 66, 49, 56, 65, 61, 54, 53, 69, 62, and 55 watts/kg. The between-athletes standard deviation is 6.5 watts/kg. The smallest meaningful change for this test is 6.5 × 0.2 = 1.3 watts/kg. For the purposes of monitoring, you round this down to 1 watt/kg. On a repeat test the following week, you would consider a change in the test results of greater than 1 watt/kg to be meaningful. In the follow-up testing of the group 1 week later, the athletes get scores of 68, 50, 56, 62, 58, 54, 51, 66, 62, and 53 watts/kg. Immediately, you can identify which athletes have experienced a meaningful change based on the calculations. For example, athlete 1 went from 66 to 68, indicating a positive change, whereas athlete 4 went from 65 to 62, indicating a negative change (remember that any athlete with a change greater than ± 1 watt/kg would be considered to have had a smallest meaningful change). You can also perform an effect size calculation on the two time points to give an indication of the magnitude of change in the group.

Week 1: Mean = 59; standard deviation = 6.5

Week 2: Mean = 58; standard deviation = 6.3

So the effect size would be calculated as 58 − 59 ÷ 6.5 = −0.15, indicating a trivial effect (see table 2.2). This is a good way to look at how the group of athletes as a whole has responded to the week of training.

You could also simply compare the typical error of the test against the change in the test measure. For example, if the observed change is greater than the typical error, this can be rated as a real change (this could be an improvement or a decline depending on the measure). Where the observed change is less than the typical error, the measure can be considered stable. You don't just have to concern yourself with smallest meaningful change. It is possible to apply these principles to an evaluation of the magnitude of moderate and large meaningful change. Here you would use moderate effect size (0.6) or large effect size (1.2) to perform the calculation.

(Current score − baseline score) ÷ standard deviation of individual baseline scores

where the standard deviation of baseline scores could be made using scores collected during the preseason phase. For example, a practitioner working in the National Football League in the United States could use the results collected during the 4 weeks in which preseason games are played.

What this score does is convert the athlete's score to a standard deviation from the baseline. Practitioners can set their own thresholds to determine how many standard deviations are practically important. It has been suggested that a threshold z-score of >1.5 is effective for identifying scores considered to be at risk (10). This is based on the fact that it represents 1.5 standard deviations away from the baseline score. A survey of monitoring practices in high-performance sport found that some practitioners used 1 standard deviation as a threshold for monitoring (37). However, more research is needed to confirm the validity of this approach. Practitioners also have the option of maintaining a fixed baseline throughout the monitoring year or of having a rolling baseline against which to compare results.

Assessing Chronic Change

Practitioners are often faced with the challenge of determining the importance of between- and within-athlete change. Although the response of the athlete is of primary concern, looking at a lack of change or change of a different magnitude in comparison to the group can also provide insights (10). For example, as part of the periodized program, the group mean of a monitoring variable may suggest an overreached state in response to a heavy loading phase. However, one athlete's results from one point to the next may have remained stable. If the group members are showing fatigue, the lack of response in an individual may suggest that the athletes are responding differently to the loading phase. Thus, appropriate adjustments may need to be made.

A more advanced technique for investigating change in a monitoring variable is **time series analysis** (5). It is used extensively across many disciplines but has received relatively little attention in athlete monitoring. It involves calculating a moving average to analyze time series data, thus allowing practitioners to determine when performance is increasing or decreasing (7). Athlete monitoring is suitable for time series analysis because it consists of time series data with a systematic pattern and random noise (5).

The analysis can be quite sophisticated, but it essentially involves calculating a moving average of the data and looking for patterns. Because a great deal of noise and variability is often associated with monitoring data, methods such as time series analysis can help to control for this and allow for a systematic analysis of patterns.

In one study Chiu and Salem (7) tracked power produced in repetitions of clean pulls to determine systematic patterns and reduce variability. Let's say a practitioner is interested in monitoring peak power (in watts) during a bench throw on a weekly basis and obtains the following values over the course of 12 weeks: 850, 903, 901, 876, 834, 904, 977, 1,011, 800, 911, 876, and 923. To calculate a moving average, the practitioner would calculate the mean values as appropriate. To do a 3-point moving average, the practitioner would do the following:

Week 1 = 850

Week 2 = 877 (mean of weeks 1 and 2)

Week 3 = 885 (mean of weeks 1-3)

Week 4 = 893 (mean of weeks 2-4)

Raw values could be plotted on a graph along with the moving average values.

Another technique for identifying trends in monitoring data is **split middle analysis** (36). This can be useful for looking at trends in athletes. It involves splitting the data into halves based on days or weeks and then determining the median for each half. The practitioner takes the first 50% and then the second 50% and determines the median for each period. These two medians can then be plotted on a graph that includes all the data points to visualize any trend in the results. For example, results from a wellness questionnaire over the course of 4 weeks could be plotted on a graph. However, doing this every day will result in a great deal of data, and the graph may appear very noisy. Median values for weeks 1 and 2 and weeks 3 and 4 could be calculated to reveal any general trend in those two data points.

Identifying sudden changes in athlete monitoring measures can also be useful. Stone and colleagues (36) proposed that using **statistical process control** can provide valuable information for identifying spikes in monitoring variables. Statistical process control is used extensively in other fields such as business and manufacturing as a method of quality control (26). By calculating means and standard deviations and graphing this information, including thresholds for standard deviations (e.g., ±2), the practitioner can visualize extreme scores.

Acute Versus Chronic Monitoring

Another athlete monitoring approach that is becoming more widespread involves looking at the ratio of acute to chronic monitoring variables. For example, investigators have compared absolute training load performed in 1 week to average chronic training load over 2 to 4 weeks (4, 22). This acute-to-chronic workload ratio can be calculated simply by dividing the acute workload for 1 week by the average for any given number of weeks (22). Z-score calculations are also useful here for identifying thresholds such as low and high athlete workloads (22).

Correlation and Relationships

Practitioners are often interested in relationships between monitoring variables. As discussed briefly in the section on reliability, correlation is a statistical method used to establish the degree of relationship between two variables. For example, a strength and conditioning practitioner might want to know whether a relationship exists between peak force produced during an isometric squat and some measure of fatigue during a training session. Measuring the magnitude of the relationship can be relatively simple to do. However, correlation is often a misunderstood concept and should be used with some caution with monitoring systems. Although practitioners often associate correlation with causation, the two are fundamentally very different. It is possible to find a relationship where none exists. Table 2.3 shows how the strength of correlations between two variables can be interpreted and used as a guide. The strength of the relationship is represented by an *r*-value, which

TABLE 2.3   Classification Scale for Correlation Coefficients

Magnitude	Correlation coefficient
Small	0.1
Moderate	0.3
Large	0.5
Very large	0.7
Extremely large	0.9

Data from Hopkins et al. (19).

can range from −1.0 (a perfect negative relationship) to 1.0 (a perfect positive relationship); 0 indicates no relationship.

It is also possible to square the *r*-value to calculate **R-squared**, also known as the **coefficient of determination**. This is a measure of the amount of variability in one variable that is explained by another. It is usually expressed as a percentage by multiplying by 100. If we take the example from figure 2.3, the correlation between 1RM squat and peak force on the IMTP was $r = .90$. Therefore, R-squared = 81% (.90 × .90 × 100). This means that 81% of the variability in the 1RM squat is explained by the variability in the IMTP. Because most of the variability in each test is explained by the other, only one is needed because they essentially measure the same thing. However, the calculation also shows that 19% of the variability is accounted for by other variables. There may be aspects such as differences in the type of contraction (i.e., dynamic versus static) that could account for this.

Sample size is also a potential issue when calculating correlations; sometimes misleadingly high relationships can be seen with small sample sizes. However, this can also be an issue with very large data sets, or "big data," in which false relationships can be found. Practitioners should be careful when interpreting these relationships and be aware that correlation does not necessarily indicate causation. Exploring relationships in these large data sets with more advanced techniques may be more appropriate.

Exploring relationships between only two variables is rather simplistic given that sport performance is affected by multiple factors. When exploring relationships between data, practitioners can use more advanced techniques such as regression and modeling. **Regression** is a statistical technique or model that is used to explain variability in one variable based on one or more other variables (3). By using this technique, it is possible to predict or estimate an athlete's score on one measure based on his score on one or more other measures. Taking the example in figure 2.3, it is possible to predict the athlete's 1RM based on the results of the IMTP test. However, the accuracy of this estimate depends on how good the relationship and model are because of the variability. Regression calculations can be made using Excel or statistical software. **Modeling,** in relation to monitoring training load using methods such as training impulse (TRIMP), is discussed in chapters 3 and 4.

Presentation of Results

An important first step when dealing with monitoring data is to take the time to organize and summarize it. The process of attempting to discover the meaning within the data is critical. Once this front-end work is done, a monitoring system can be implemented that will provide the most valuable information about the athletes.

Exploratory data analysis using the methods described previously can be useful for identifying patterns, trends, and relationships in the data. This initial step should also involve visualizing the monitoring data in some form. Displaying the data in a graph provides a visual summary of the information that may be easier to interpret than numbers. The practitioner can see whether any patterns exist. For example, are the results in the group of athletes tending to increase, decrease, or stay the same?

It is also valuable to look for any outliers or clear exceptions to the pattern of the data. This can indicate the presence of interesting cases in the results or simply an error in the data. A good knowledge of what typical numbers look like and a usual range for the variable are critical here. Some practitioners just accept the numbers produced by a piece of technology, which can be problematic. Once graphical representations of the data are created, numerical summaries and concise descriptions can be produced.

Graphing Monitoring Data

A good first step when analyzing monitoring data is to graph the results in some way. For example, z-scores lend themselves well to being presented in graphs. This can help practitioners compare physical capacities and decide which areas to modify in a training session, an overall training program, or both. The approaches discussed in this chapter need to be combined with a strategic approach to the presentation of the results to coaches. It is not enough to have developed a reliable and valid monitoring battery, collected data, and determined whether the changes are meaningful. To assist with the interpretation of the results, the practitioner also needs to assess the magnitude of the change, taking into account the reliability and sensitivity of the test. Then it is important to present the results in a way that coaches and athletes can understand. Otherwise, the information is unlikely to make a difference in the performance of the athlete.

Reporting can be done in several ways and using a combination of methods. Typically, numbers alone are not very helpful or well understood by coaches and athletes. Graphing data may reveal trends in the results or large changes in the monitoring variables that make sense to these key stakeholders.

The main types of graphs practitioners use are line graphs, bar graphs, scatter plots, stem and leaf plots, radar plots, and pie graphs (33). Many research papers report results using traditional

GUIDELINES FOR CLEAR REPORTS ON MONITORING DATA

A key part of the reporting process is giving the results to coaches and athletes in a timely manner. Just as poor presentation of testing data can limit the potential for improving athlete performance, taking excessive time to deliver the information to the key stakeholders can have a negative impact. Monitoring data need to be reported as quickly as possible so that practitioners have time to implement changes in the training and correct any identified issues. Ideally, reporting would involve some type of real-time feedback. To have any chance of informing practitioner decision making, monitoring should occur immediately following the training session. In some instances the reporting and analysis of monitoring data can occur within the session itself. For example, velocity-based training can add greatly to the value of power training in the gym. Practitioners should aim to provide monitoring reports that are meaningful and timely and that provide specific recommendations for coaches and athletes.

line graphs or bar graphs. However, these are not always ideal for looking at monitoring data. Scatter plots, line graphs, histograms, and stem and leaf plots are very useful for looking at the overall distribution of data (44). Histograms are generally used for large amounts of data (see figure 2.4 later in this chapter). **Line graphs** can show trends or abrupt changes in monitoring data (see figures 4.4 and 4.8 in chapter 4). With small numbers of athletes (<50), the best option is to show the full data set. **Scatter plots** are a great way to visualize the relationship between two variables (see figure 2.3).

Creating Figures and Tables

The following general guidelines can help practitioners design effective figures and tables:

- Ensure that visuals are suitable for users; think about the target audience (in most cases, coaches and athletes).
- Make the message clear.
- Include important information.
- Make data values visually clear.
- Make visuals easy to read and understand.
- Avoid "chartjunk," or clutter in the graph. Chartjunk refers to anything in a figure that does not add anything to the key information being conveyed (41).
- Value importance over beauty. The key message and readability should be primary considerations.

Many resources are available to help practitioners improve data presentation (41, 44, 45).

Following are guidelines to follow when putting together a graph:

- Put all of the data into some type of table format or spreadsheet.
- Choose the most appropriate format for presenting the data (using the previous guidelines).
- Create a concise title that describes what the graph is showing.
- Decide which variables are plotted on the respective axes, and select an appropriate scale for each axis.
- Write appropriate descriptions for the axes.
- Include the units of measurement used for each axis.
- Plot the data points using graphing software (or even go old school and draw by hand).

Several methods for analyzing athlete monitoring information have been presented. The following sections address additional key considerations.

Percentage Change

A simple percentage change calculation is a popular way to present monitoring results. Following is the formula:

Percentage change = [(postmeasure − premeasure) ÷ premeasure] × 100

For example, the power output for a track cyclist is 1,911 watts in week 1 and 1,866 watts in week 2. The percentage change calculation is as follows:

$$\text{Percentage change} = [(1{,}866 - 1{,}911) \div 1{,}911] \times 100 = -2.4\%$$

This could also be reported along with the noise of the test (expressed as typical error or CV) and the smallest meaningful change. When extreme precision is required for interpretation, spreadsheets available online can be used to discover the exact chances that the observed change in the monitoring variable is greater than the smallest meaningful change (20).

Likely Limits

Another useful approach is to use likely limits or confidence limits for the true value of the monitoring variable. The simplest way to report likely limits is to use the observed change plus or minus the typical error (15). For example, an athlete has changed by +3%, and the typical error of the test is ±1%. If the smallest meaningful change was 1.5%, then a positive change likely occurred since the last test. This is because the change seen in the athlete's result is greater than both the typical error and the smallest meaningful change. Importantly, the smallest meaningful change is greater than the typical error.

It is possible to perform simple calculations of confidence limits. For example, these can be calculated for technical error of measurement by multiplying the value by 1.96 (rounding up to 2 makes the calculation even simpler). This represents ±2 standard deviations based on the normal distribution curve. The results can then be interpreted using qualitative terms such as *possibly harmful, very likely, substantially positive,* and *unclear but likely to be beneficial* (19). This type of magnitude-based inferences approach is becoming more widely used in athlete monitoring. Spreadsheets are available that can precisely calculate confidence limits and the associated clinical chances (17).

Z-Score Plots

Using z-scores by calculating the athlete's score minus the average score divided by the standard deviation to show the relative change is discussed in an earlier section. These numbers have little impact unless put into context. **Radar plots** or histograms are often a good way to present z-scores visually to coaches and athletes. The advantage of presenting these statistics as graphs is they can demonstrate where the athlete falls within the group. When monitoring a range of measures, graphing the z-scores using radar plots or histograms provides a pictorial representation of the athlete's strengths and weaknesses relative to the group. This can be a useful tool for identifying areas that need to be addressed. Determining whether the athlete is excessively fatigued or not responding to the training stimulus as expected enables the practitioner to make appropriate adjustments to the program.

Figure 2.4 shows a weekly athlete monitoring profile that includes measures of IMTP, reactive strength (from a drop jump), sleep quality, soreness, fatigue, overhead squat movement rating, global positioning system load, and saliva cortisol. The profile provides a snapshot of the athlete from that week, from which the practitioner may conclude that the excessive muscle soreness and some indications of fatigue and stress may require attention.

Practitioners often use z-score radar plots to show the results of one-off monitoring and testing. However, an important part of the athlete monitoring process is retesting and comparing the results to previous results. Problems can arise when testing groups if particular athletes are not available for monitoring as a result of injuries or other commitments. With small sample sizes (common in high-performance sport settings), a particularly strong (or weak) athlete in a particular monitoring test can result

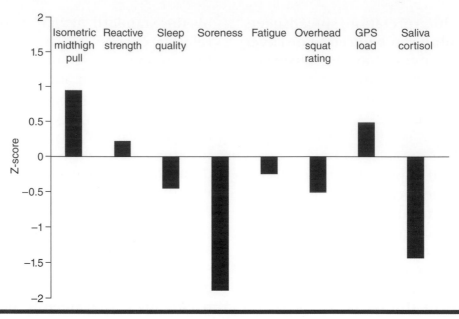

Figure 2.4   Athlete monitoring profile.

in significant changes in means, standard deviations, or both. This can make the results more susceptible to extreme values, or outliers.

An alternative approach can be to use modified z-scores by determining benchmark means and standard deviations for the monitoring tests. Practitioners can determine these benchmarks, or targets, based on sources such as published literature on a similar population, previous testing data with that group or similar athletes, discussions with other support staff, and feedback from the coaches. Over time the practitioner should be able to build a database of historical data on the athletes. This allows for more sophisticated analysis using categories such as playing position and training age. Once these benchmarks are determined, the modified z-scores can be calculated as previously described but with the slight modification of using a benchmark score rather than the squad or team average, as follows:

Modified z-score = (athlete's score − benchmark score) ÷ standard deviation

Figure 2.5 shows the z-scores for an athlete monitored using this approach. The monitoring program includes measures of neuromuscular fatigue (vertical countermovement jump mean power), wellness (a questionnaire), training load (RPE × session duration), injury risk (movement screen tests), and immune status (salivary IgA). The team average is the average of all the z-scores, so this will always equal zero using the traditional calculation. The practitioner can set benchmarks depending on the relative importance on particular aspects of the monitoring program.

Athletes can also be monitored over time for monitoring variables, as shown in figure 2.6. In this plot, the athlete's results are graphed over 3 weeks of a particularly heavy training block to observe the changes in the monitoring areas. The practitioner may observe that the pro-

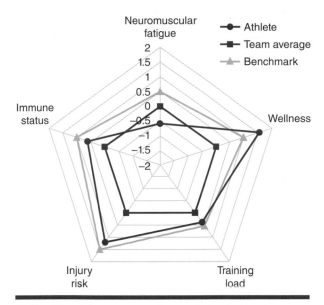

Figure 2.5 Comparison of an athlete's monitoring profile to the team average and benchmarks using a radar plot.

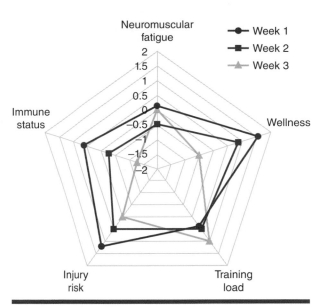

Figure 2.6 Monitoring an athlete over time using a radar plot for physical capacities.

gressive increase in loading is resulting in negative outcomes and make necessary adjustments (e.g., introduce a deloading week).

These graphs allow the practitioner and coach to visualize the changes in variables over time. It is important to note that for some measures a negative z-score would be produced by athletes who performed better on a monitoring test. A good example of this is measures of speed over 20 m, in which a faster (shorter) time would be better. To standardize the radar plots when using measures such as speed and body composition, the practitioner can multiply the z-score by −1. More in-depth discussions of the use of z-scores are available (31).

Standard Ten Scores

Numerous other methods can be used to present monitoring data. Those who find z-scores confusing, for example, could use an alternative such as a standard ten (STEN) score, which reports results from 1 to 10. These can be calculated from z-scores or the original monitoring data. To calculate STEN scores, practitioners can use either this formula:

$$STEN\ score = (z\text{-}score \times 2) + 5.5$$

or this one:

$$STEN\ score = [(\text{monitoring result} - \text{mean monitoring result}) \div \text{standard deviation}) \times 2] + 5.5$$

Consider an athlete who scores 23 out of 40 on a wellness scale (1-10 scale for four items: stress, muscle soreness, sleep quality, and fatigue). The mean for the group is 32 out of 40, and the standard deviation is 4.5, so:

$$STEN\ score = [(23 - 32) \div 4.5) \times 2] + 5.5 = 1.5$$

Creating Spreadsheets

The problem with many statistical programs (e.g., Statistical Package for the Social Sciences [SPSS], Statistical Analysis System [SAS]) is that learning to use them to their full potential requires a significant investment of time. Because practitioners tend to be short on time, mastering statistical software packages may not be feasible. However, for most, spreadsheets are sufficient. Spreadsheets can provide very powerful analyses, and a program such as Excel should be able to do everything a practitioner requires for the purpose of athlete monitoring. They also allow practitioners to visualize their data using graphs. Several resources provide further information on how to get the most value from spreadsheets (24, 42).

Qualitative Analysis

The research techniques discussed in this chapter are mainly quantitative in that they deal with measurements in the form of numbers. However, a range of qualitative techniques are also available to help practitioners analyze their athletes' training and performance (39). Mixed-methods approaches, which combine quantitative and qualitative methods, are also gaining in popularity. It could be argued that magnitude-based inferences are an example of this because they use both numerical data and qualitative descriptors. Mixed methods benefit from the strengths of both quantitative and qualitative approaches to obtain a more complete picture of athlete behavior.

Three types of qualitative data collection can be used for monitoring purposes: interviews, focus groups, and observations. The reality is that these methods are routinely used by practitioners anyway. With some additional planning, practitioners may be able to gain even more useful data from these practices.

Interviews

Athlete interviews can be structured, unstructured, or semistructured. **Structured interviews** present set questions without any deviations based on the athletes' responses. At the other end of the spectrum are **unstructured interviews**, which begin with a general question (e.g., How are you feeling today?) and proceed from there. **Semistructured interviews** are somewhere between these two approaches; practitioners have some questions they would like to ask, but they may change them and the direction of the interview based on the athletes' responses. Semistructured interviews allow practitioners to delve deeper into the responses while also giving athletes leeway to discuss aspects that interest them.

Conducting quality interviews is an important skill and should include recording the sessions. Ideally, this would involve taking notes and getting an audio recording of the interviews for further analysis after completion. Listening is even more critical than asking the questions. A good interviewer needs to know when to stay quiet and just listen to the responses. Data obtained from these interviews can help practitioners determine things such as athlete readiness for training. Solid evidence shows the value of subjective information for athlete monitoring (34). Asking athletes how they feel before the start of a training session can provide important insights into their current states of well-being. Qualitative analysis methods such as finding common themes in the athletes' answers, also known as thematic content analysis, may also be used (30, 40).

Focus Groups

Focus groups are really just extended interviews with a larger number of athletes. Generally, they are conducted with 5 to 10 people and an interviewer acting as a discussion facilitator. Focus groups can be a useful approach for getting detailed information about the opinions and thoughts of athletes in a group. These sessions should also be recorded in some way, and the interviewer should be skilled in the art of facilitating, listening, and asking relevant questions. Qualitative analysis methods can also be used and important themes identified in the athletes' answers (40).

Observations

Observation is a routine part of what most practitioners do with their athletes. Two main types of observations are used in qualitative analysis: participant and nonparticipant observation. With **participant observation**, the practitioner is an active participant in the scene being observed, whereas with **nonparticipant observation**, the practitioner is removed from the group to make objective observations. Whichever approach is used, recording the observations in some way is important (e.g., checklists, field notes). Detailed field notes help practitioners remember important things they have observed. By noting personal aspects such as thoughts, feelings, evaluations, and learnings during training sessions, practitioners also facilitate their own self-reflection (14).

Although some believe that qualitative analysis is a less rigorous, less scientific approach than quantitative analysis, this is not the case. A range of data analysis techniques can be used to analyze the information obtained using qualitative methods (39). Qualitative approaches can provide rich insights into athlete monitoring systems.

Conclusion

Practitioners have a range of monitoring tools available to them. Statistical measures of central tendency, variability, smallest meaningful change, effect size, and standard scores are useful for monitoring the responses of a group of athletes as well as the individuals within the group. Practitioners should always use monitoring tools with the highest reliability and, to improve reliability, always adhere to strict and consistent protocols. Monitoring tools also need to be valid and sensitive to change in the athletes. Although the choice of the monitoring tool is important, the presentation of the results to coaches and athletes is perhaps even more critical. Practitioners should use presentation methods that are meaningful and always consider how the data can be used to affect athlete performance. Graphs can be an effective way to represent the monitoring data and can help identify trends and patterns. Underpinning any analysis method should be the potential for the information to affect decision making. Using a mixed-methods approach to athlete monitoring in conjunction with appropriate data analyses should allow practitioners and coaches to make informed, evidence-based training decisions.

3

Physiological Effects of Training Stress

Fundamental to the understanding of athlete monitoring is an appreciation of the physiological effects of training stress. To optimize their training programs, practitioners need a solid understanding of the **dose–response relationship** and how athlete preparation factors affect this relationship. Optimizing the dose–response relationship is a delicate balance that requires practitioners to accurately titrate the amount of training. An imbalance can result in negative responses, decreased performance, and maladaptations. Athlete monitoring should help practitioners make more accurate adjustments to avoid negative outcomes such as overtraining

and decreased performance. Consensus statements have been written about the overtraining syndrome (71). Researchers have also recently focused on the concept of unexplained underperformance syndrome in elite athletes (10, 63). Effective management of the dose–response relationship is at the heart of what the practitioner is trying to achieve in training; that is, to optimize athletic performance. A clear understanding of how specific training dosages elicit specific responses is a good starting point and should help practitioners improve their training programs.

Several models explain the physiological effects of an acute training stimulus:

the general adaptation syndrome model (101), the fitness-fatigue model (4), and the stimulus-fatigue-recovery-adaptation model (106). These models highlight general and specific factors related to physiological stress monitoring. All three recognize that excessive fatigue without adequate recovery can result in maladaptations, particularly decreased performance. In extreme cases of extended periods of fatigue, functional overreaching and nonfunctional overreaching can occur, as can the most severe condition—overtraining. A good appreciation of these models will help practitioners more fully understand the physiological effects of training stress.

General Adaptation Syndrome Model

The seminal work of Canadian physiologist Hans Selye, the general adaptation syndrome (GAS) model, forms the basis of many discussions regarding the monitoring of physiological stress (100, 101). As outlined in chapter 1, the aim of training is to provide a stimulus that improves performance. Optimizing this relationship requires a solid understanding of the GAS. The model is based on the stages the body, or physiological system, goes through following some type of stimulus. In general, this model proposes that all stressors result in a similar response and that **stress** can be considered a disruption of the body's homeostatic state.

Figure 3.1 outlines the GAS model. Upon the application of a stimulus or stress, the body enters the shock or alarm phase, which results in training fatigue. Acute fatigue is a normal and expected short-term response to the training stress and an important part of the training process. If adequate recovery follows this initial stress, the second phase, known as the resistance phase, occurs, in which the system returns to baseline, or homeostasis. It is during this return to homeostasis that physiological adaptations are made. This ensures that the training stimulus applied in the future does not disrupt the athlete to the same degree (43). For the third phase, known as **supercompensation**, to occur, an adequate recovery period must follow the training stimulus. Supercompensation refers to a return to a level that exceeds the baseline, resulting

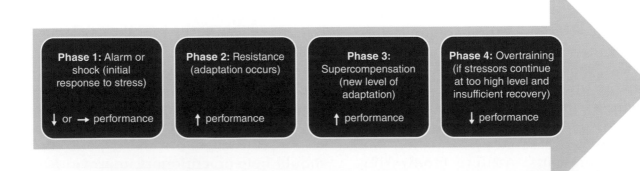

Figure 3.1 Model of the general adaptation syndrome.

in an increased performance capacity. To ensure optimal training adaptations and benefits, the next training stimulus must be imposed during the supercompensation phase. Insufficient recovery can lead to a final phase characterized by decreased performance and eventually overtraining.

Although the GAS model does not cover all aspects of the response to stress, it is useful for explaining the adaptive response to an acute training stimulus. It is worthwhile noting that the GAS model is not a linear response. All athletes experience fluctuations within days, between days, and across microcycles (generally 7-10 days).

Problems can arise in the GAS when a secondary training stimulus is applied too early. The result can be excessive fatigue, which can lead to training maladaptations. This could eventually result in decreased performance and, in severe cases, negative consequences such as overtraining as depicted by phase 4 in figure 3.1. Alternatively, if no secondary training stimulus is applied during the supercompensation phase, any training adaptations may be lost as the athlete returns to pretraining homeostasis levels.

The delicate balance between overload and underload is extremely important for practitioners to manage. An effective athlete monitoring system can inform the practitioner about the training fatigue and adaptations occurring in athletes. Although the GAS model is a simple representation of how training adaptations occur, it provides a good starting point for understanding the effect of acute training stimuli. The problem with oversimplification, though, is that it can cause practitioners to miss several key aspects in their understanding of athlete monitoring. The reality is that the effect of training dosage on training adaptation is very complex. A wide range of factors and interactions occur during training that make it difficult to analyze the training adaptation response. Practitioners must keep in mind that the impacts of stressors are additive and that other factors can affect the athlete's ability to respond and adapt to the stressors that result from the training (5, 66). Traditional concepts of homeostasis need to take into account the multifactorial nature of athlete training. Specifically, practitioners need to understand how athletes perceive the stress and how their training histories affect how they cope with it.

Fitness-Fatigue Model

We have already noted that fatigue is an expected and desired part of the process of training athletes. Although physiologists typically define fatigue as the decline in peak muscle force or power in response to acute exercise (11), this is a rather simplistic definition. Fatigue is actually a holistic phenomenon affected by many factors (11, 57). Practitioners need to consider fatigue in sport performance more holistically given that it affects athletes' physical capacities, technique, decision making, and psychology.

What Is Fatigue?

Fatigue can be categorized as central or peripheral. **Central fatigue** refers to diminished motor drive from the central nervous system (brain and spinal cord); **peripheral fatigue** is due to changes that occur directly in the muscle and impair the contractile processes (11). At the peripheral level, many factors increase or decrease in the body and inhibit physiological processes sufficiently to impair performance. Often referred to as **putative factors** (11), these include adenosine triphosphate (ATP), phosphocreatine (PCr), adenosine diphosphate (ADP), inorganic phosphate (P_i), lactate, hydrogen ions, ammonia, muscle glycogen, blood glucose, potassium, sodium, chloride, changes in calcium handling, magnesium, cytokines, reactive oxygen and nitrogen species, dehydration, serotonin, **hyperthermia** (high core body temperature), and **hypoxia** (decreased oxygen).

The extensive study of central fatigue in recent years has led to the development of the **central governor model**. The basic idea behind this model is that an internal controller manages muscle force and exercise via decreased motor drive (nervous system input to the muscle) and fatigue sensations primarily via perceived exertion (85). In essence, the athlete's central nervous system is responsible for dictating how much force is applied in a given situation. This concept is still widely debated. What is clear is that fatigue in sport is task dependent. For example, the main factors causing fatigue are different during an all-out sprint than during prolonged submaximal exercisc. Fundamentally, much is still not understood about fatigue. Excellent reviews are available that discuss the physiological basis of fatigue in more detail (11, 22, 38, 57).

Measuring Fatigue

Measuring fatigue in sport competition and training can present challenges because of its multifactorial nature. Lab-based studies have provided scientists with some great insights into the mechanisms of fatigue. Although practitioners are commonly less concerned about the underlying mechanisms of fatigue, an increased awareness of them can be useful.

Fatigue can be quantified in sport by using a variety of methods (11). These include mean or peak power output; time or speed; total work; forces applied to force plates, pedals, or oars; and peak forces produced by individual muscles with voluntary effort (**maximal voluntary contractions**). **Low-frequency fatigue**, a type of fatigue often of interest to practitioners, is a result of high-intensity, high-force, repeated stretch–shortening cycles or eccentric contractions (52). The **twitch interpolation technique**, in which an electrical stimulation is superimposed on a maximal voluntary contraction, has also been widely used in research studies to assess low-frequency fatigue (11). Subjective measures such as rating of perceived exertion (RPE) can be used to rate fatigue for the whole body and specific areas or body parts (e.g., the lower body). Modifications of the RPE scale have also been used to rate breathing difficulty. Numerical scales that can be used include the traditional Borg 6-20 scale, a 10-point category ratio scale, a session RPE scale, and a 0-100 RPE scale (see chapter 4).

A negative outcome of athlete monitoring is that practitioners become so focused on the fatigue aspect that they do everything in their power to reduce it as much as possible. This is a mistake because fatigue is a natural and necessary piece of the training puzzle. Overemphasizing recovery strategies can blunt the adaptations to training (27, 94, 95). A complete lack of stress can be a problem similar to overreaching and overtraining in that it results in a lack of adaptation and can lead to decreased performance. This is also a feature of the GAS model discussed previously. Evidence supports this concept; research studies have shown a nonlinear dose–response relationship between training load and stress markers (74, 96). A recent study showed that at both low and high training loads, indicators of stress increased in athletes (74). Some of the responses seen with low loads were similar to those seen with extremely high loads in a group of elite female futsal (a modified form of football) players (74). Athlete monitoring assists in achieving the correct loading balance to optimize adaptations.

Relationship Between Fitness and Fatigue

Fatigue can best be conceptualized as existing on a continuum. Where it falls on the continuum depends on factors including the following (16):

- Cumulative effect of the training load
- Cumulative level of neuromuscular and mental fatigue
- Level of deficit in recovery
- Length of time the fatigue has accumulated
- Severity of the fatigue symptoms

Figure 3.2 shows the relationship between fitness and fatigue that underlies the monitoring of physiological stress in athletes (37, 106). This model depicts how the relationship between fitness and fatigue affects athlete readiness (13, 37). The original idea, based on work from Banister and colleagues, is that athlete performance is related to the difference between fitness and fatigue (4, 12). In this model, the two components are represented as positive (fitness) and negative (fatigue) physiological functions.

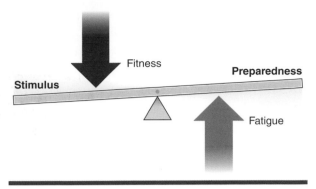

Figure 3.2 Relationship between fitness and fatigue.

The interaction between them results in the change in performance following the stimulus (4). However, multiple aspects (listed at the start of this section) of these fatigue and fitness components ultimately determine the level of athlete preparedness (13). It has been proposed that aspects such as the cumulative effect of load and fatigue, recovery deficit, and the severity of fatigue symptoms explain individual responses in athletes (13, 37). Similar models have been proposed that describe athlete performance as a complex process dictated by individual responses and characterized by a range of factors and their interrelationships (87, 88).

Mechanisms of Fatigue

Neuromuscular fatigue can be a result of changes at the level of muscle (i.e., peripheral fatigue) or of failure of the central nervous system to drive the motor neurons sufficiently (i.e., central fatigue) (34). The parasympathetic and sympathetic nervous systems appear to play a role in fatigue. The **sympathetic nervous system** controls the fight-or-flight response. The **parasympathetic nervous system** is responsible for downregulating the systems of the body. It has been suggested that the fitness effects in the fitness-fatigue model appear to be primarily neural, whereas the fatigue effects are both neural and metabolic (13).

Neural mechanisms are many and varied, but they appear to involve the peripheral nervous system. They can occur via decreased autogenic inhibition (reduced excitability of contracting or stretched muscle), coactivation of intrafusal fibers (muscle spindles that detect the degree and rate of stretch of a muscle), and activation of the neuromuscular complex (13, 34). The sympathetic nervous system, once activated, results in an increased release of stress hormones such as norepinephrine, epinephrine, and cortisol. The activity of the central nervous system increases through upregulation (increased cellular content) of receptors and increased catecholamine (stress hormone) release.

The metabolic component of fatigue is primarily due to decreased storage and use of energy stores such as adenosine triphosphate and phosphocreatine. In addition, increases in the intramuscular levels of inorganic phosphate seem to cause peripheral fatigue by reducing maximal cross-bridge function, the sensitivity of myofibers to calcium, and the release of calcium for the sarcoplasmic reticulum (11). The resulting intramuscular acidosis reduces muscle force and shortening velocity (which decreases power). Lowered muscle glycogen results in less calcium being released from the sarcoplasmic reticulum. It has been proposed that this combined with feedback to the central nervous system contributes to increases in RPE and central fatigue

(11). Downregulation (a decrease) of the various receptors and decreased catecholamine release both decrease nervous system function, which affects the neural aspect of fatigue. Integrative physiological approaches to addressing fatigue are important because multiple mechanisms and systems contribute to the condition.

Lactate is one of the most measured variables in studies of fatigue. However, experts have moved on from the notion that lactate accumulation is responsible for fatigue. The evidence now shows that rather than causing fatigue, lactate is a necessary result of fatigue and actually has some ergogenic effects in terms of helping to restore force (11)—another good example of correlation not meaning causation! One consistent finding is that overtrained athletes have decreased maximal lactate concentrations, whereas submaximal values remain unchanged or are slightly lower (114).

Postactivation Potentiation

Postactivation potentiation (PAP) refers to the short-term enhancement in performance following a specific conditioning activity (e.g., to increase muscular strength, power, or speed). PAP shows how fitness and fatigue interact and some of the underlying mechanisms behind them (47, 99). The two principles that explain the PAP response are the phosphorylation of myosin light chains and the increase in the recruitment of high-threshold motor units (47). A decrease in skeletal muscle pennation angle has also been proposed as a mechanism (65). The classic idea is that the balance between PAP and fatigue results in performance enhancement. That is, the potentiation represents the fitness effect, and there is also the associated fatigue effect. This relationship between fitness and fatigue and the subsequent increase in performance has been observed in several studies with athletes (112). The positive balance between PAP and fatigue is thought to be a result of potentiated muscular contractile activity (93).

An example of using PAP in strength and conditioning practice is to have athletes perform some type of explosive exercise following a heavy set of back squats (99). The practitioner could prescribe three sets at 90% of 1RM for 3 repetitions. At the completion of each set, the athlete rests for several minutes and then performs a set of three vertical countermovement jumps. The PAP response results in greater jump heights and theoretically a greater training response.

A great deal is still not understood about the mechanisms that explain these performance effects and the interaction between the fitness and fatigue components of PAP. Evidence shows that stronger athletes have a greater potentiation response (which is an indicator of the fitness effect) and less fatigue than weaker athletes do (14, 99). This is because stronger athletes have a greater capacity to overcome fatigue because of their ability to tolerate higher loading, and they experience performance enhancement earlier than weaker athletes do (99). Because fatigue has a negative influence on the PAP response, the timing of the recovery period between activities is vital. Practitioners need to consider the protocol used to elicit PAP and the characteristics of the individual athlete (93). Monitoring training and

specific aspects of this part of the program would help to optimize the PAP responses and potential adaptations.

A recent study has cast some doubt on the notion that underlying mechanisms of the central nervous system are responsible for the potentiating effects of acute exercise on subsequent performance (109). Psychological effects could play an important role in performance enhancement, which could be partially explained by the athlete's perceived state of readiness. A detailed understanding of these underlying mechanisms is not important, although it does help in making decisions about critical features of a monitoring system. What is clear is that these fitness and fatigue effects can give some insight into useful monitoring tools for measuring aspects thought to be responsible for fatigue.

Short-term training studies provide further support for the fitness-fatigue model. Differential responses of strength, power, and speed have been shown in studies of overtraining in resistance training, which confirms that there are differences in the responses to stress (13, 31, 32). These studies have not involved athletes completing high volumes of resistance exercise but rather athletes training at near-maximal intensities. One study showed that 3 weeks of high-intensity resistance training of three sessions per week of near-maximal back squats resulted in decreases in speed but no change in strength levels (32). This work also highlights the fact that total work is not the only important factor in acute responses; training load and relative intensity are also critical factors.

Stimulus-Fatigue-Recovery-Adaptation Model

The stimulus-fatigue-recovery-adaptation model describes a general response following the application of a training stimulus (figure 3.3) (37, 106). As with the other models discussed, the application of the training stimulus results in acute fatigue. High perceived fatigue is generally not an issue with athletes as long as it is followed by an adequate period of recovery. In this initial stage, for the 24 to 36 hr following the acute stimulus, often no performance decrement occurs (71). The degree of accumulated fatigue is proportional to the magnitude and duration of the workload experienced by the athlete. A performance supercompensation ensues as long as recovery time has been sufficient. If no new training stimulus is applied during this period after recovery and adaptation are completed, the performance and preparedness of the athlete will continue to decline. In this model this process is sometimes referred to as a state of involution (37).

In the stimulus-fatigue-recovery-adaptation model, the magnitude of the stimulus plays a significant role in determining the length of the recovery-adaptation period. Manipulating the length of the recovery-adaptation period is one of the fundamental tenets of periodization (37, 113). An effective athlete monitoring system should enable the practitioner to gather objective information about an athlete's responses to training and make adjustments accordingly. For example, if the magnitude of a training stimulus is larger than normal, the athlete will experience more fatigue and will need more time for recovery and adaptation (106). Only by having objective measures of an athlete's fatigue will the practitioner know the effect of the load on the ath-

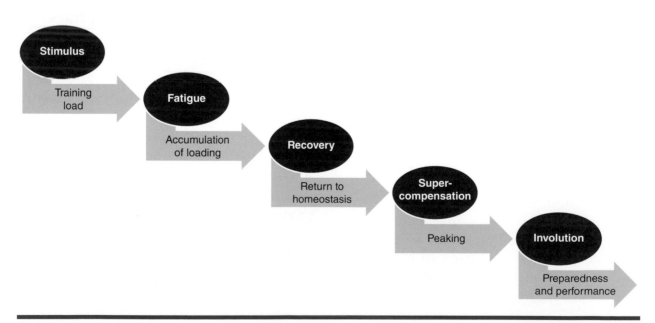

Figure 3.3 Stimulus-fatigue-recovery-adaptation model.

lete. One strategy to address this is to alternate heavy and light training days to offset extended periods of high fatigue and the associated delay in recovery and adaptation. Alternatively, the practitioner can reduce the training stress to cause less fatigue and hasten recovery and adaptation. However, in some periods, such as preseasons, athletes need to be able to tolerate high levels of loading to prepare for competition.

Applications of the Models

The GAS, fitness-fatigue model, and stimulus-fatigue-recovery-adaptation model have some clear applications for practitioners. Fundamental to all of them is the need to achieve a balance between the training stimulus level, the effects of fitness and fatigue, and the degree of adaptation and recovery. The GAS model proposes that the total work alone is responsible for the responses, regardless of the magnitude of the stimulus (13). In the fitness-fatigue model, both the total amount and the magnitude of the stimulus contribute to the postexercise response. As stated previously, multiple factors and fitness-fatigue effects contribute to adaptation (13). The GAS model, which was mainly based on a theory of a general response of the endocrine system to stress, makes a clear distinction between the fitness and fatigue effects (101). However, experts now agree that hormonal responses vary based on the mode of training (19). Resistance training is a good example: Several studies have shown differential effects of hor-

mones such as testosterone, cortisol, and growth hormone to variations in acute training variables and training volume and intensity (19, 59, 60).

The fatigue and fitness effects are independent of each other, but their overall effect is cumulative (see figure 3.2). Of most concern with regard to monitoring are fatigue effects; they result from the training stimulus, but they can also affect a number of systems (13). A good example is the immune system, which can suffer negative consequences as a result of a large cumulative fatigue effect (35).

The manipulation of acute training variables goes a long way in determining athlete adaptation. Practitioners need effective monitoring systems to be confident that they are applying the appropriate training dosages to manage fatigue while optimizing adaptation and recovery. Again, the goal here is not to remove fatigue but to monitor and manage it so that immediate adjustments can be made to the training program.

Fatigue Continuum

Many factors contribute to the acute response to a training stimulus (see figure 1.2 in chapter 1). The athlete's response to the training dosage can be thought of as existing on a continuum with several variables having the potential to make an impact. Practitioners sometimes struggle to distinguish between optimal adaptation due to correct program design and maladaptation due to too much training load and excessive fatigue. If recovery following the acute training stimulus is inadequate, the athlete will move along this continuum to a point where decreased performance or negative consequences such as overreaching and overtraining occur (71). Because no clear point exists at which normal training adaptations meet negative outcomes or maladaptations, it is useful to think of fatigue as occurring on a continuum. The transition from normal adaptation to maladaptation is gradual, and in fact a state of overreaching is necessary to improve performance (figure 3.4). Recognizing these transitions early can help prevent the overtraining syndrome. This is why choosing monitoring tools that are reliable, valid, and sensitive to changes in fatigue is so important.

Chronic stress is another important factor that practitioners need to consider when assessing athletes' physiological responses to training (55, 95). In their conceptual model, Kentta and Hassmen (55) consider the total process of stress and recovery, including critical factors such as the acute magnitude of total stress, the degree of stress the person can tolerate, and the actual total recovery from the stress. People appear to differ greatly in their ability to handle stress. One recent study showed a strong relationship between individual differences in neural responses to stress and stress-induced cortisol release and resting levels of cortisol (46). Stress can affect the body's recovery processes in different ways. For example, during periods of high stress, the body's ability to heal has been shown to be compromised (115).

A body of research evidence suggests that during periods of high stress, athletes have a reduced ability to adapt to training (5, 95, 107, 108). For example, chronic psychological stress results in blunted responses to resistance training; one study revealed that chronic mental stress had an impact on the rate of muscle recovery from heavy resistance training over a 4-day period (108). During periods of high stress (e.g., exam periods for university athletes), practitioners need be mindful of maximizing athlete recovery by adjusting their training programs accordingly.

Increased risk of illness and injury can also occur during periods of high stress (66). A variety of questionnaires are available for monitoring athletes' stress levels (see chapter 4). Factors such as nutrition and athletes' perception of the training stress have also been suggested as having a significant influence on the fatigue continuum (63).

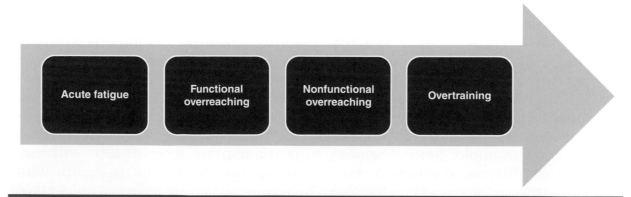

Figure 3.4   Overreaching and overtraining theoretical continuum.

Overreaching and Overtraining

The majority of the research literature supports the concept that overreaching and overtraining exist on a continuum (71). Although the fatigue caused by a stimulus can lead to adaptation, inadequate recovery after the stimulus can result in maladaptation. This maladaptation involves the hypothalamic-pituitary-adrenal axis and all other hypothalamic axes (71, 72). The hypothalamus plays the critical role in the brain of regulating the central responses to stress and training. It also integrates the metabolic, nervous, and hormonal signals. The balance between stimulus and recovery is critical to ensure appropriate adaptations to training.

During periods of overreaching, monitoring can help practitioners avoid decreased performance in their athletes. The terminology used in this area can be inconsistent and confusing, however. Terms such as *staleness, burnout,* and *intensified training* are sometimes used interchangeably with *overreaching* and *overtraining.* When a period of reduced performance as a result of overload training occurs, the athlete has entered a state of **functional overreaching** (3). **Nonfunctional overreaching** is defined as unplanned fatigue and decreased performance following an extended period of overload training with inadequate recovery (83). The **overtraining syndrome** is the final stage of the fatigue continuum and is defined as large decrements in performance and associated psychological disturbances that can last from weeks to months despite extended periods of rest and reductions in training load (see figure 3.4) (71).

Prevalence of Overreaching and Overtraining

Current evidence suggests that the prevalence of overreaching and overtraining can be moderate to high in athletic populations. Matos and colleagues (68) classified athletes as overreached or overtrained based on being fatigued on a daily basis with significant decrements in performance lasting from several weeks to several months. Their study found that 29% of youth athletes experience symptoms of nonfunctional overreaching and overtraining and that athletes competing in individual sports are at greater risk because of the higher volumes of training (37% of individual sport athletes versus 17% of team sport athletes) (68). Higher risk is also seen in those competing at the elite level: 37% of national-level athletes and 45% of international-level athletes experience symptoms. Morgan and colleagues (78) found that 64% of male and 60% of female elite middle-distance runners reported experiencing symptoms during their careers. A study of British athletes (national and Olympic level) reported a prevalence of symptoms of 15% to 35% in men and 4% to 15% in women (58). A small-scale study of elite swimmers monitored for 6 months reported an incidence of 21% (48). The results from all of these investigations show that high-level athletes across a range of sports and ages experience overreaching and overtraining regularly.

Studies of overreaching and overtraining can be difficult to perform in athlete populations. Because of the negative consequences of overtraining in particular, attempting to induce this condition in athletes is unethical. Very few longitudinal overreaching and overtraining studies have been conducted in elite athletes; most of the evidence has been garnered from acute investigations. Another problem with these types of studies is the small number of athletes available (76, 83). Further, the majority of the studies focused only on individual aerobic endurance athletes (48, 61, 62). Some research (18, 97) has been completed with team sport athletes, but very few investigations have been done with purely resistance-trained athletes.

Many descriptive athlete monitoring studies have been conducted across a number of sports (15, 18, 20, 51). These types of investigations can provide practitioners with fascinating insights into how monitoring is occurring in different sporting environments (69, 84). Generally, though, these tend to be observational studies, which can have limited scope and application for scenarios such as overtraining (9, 111).

Functional Overreaching

Functional overreaching can be a planned strategy to increase athletic performance. Practitioners commonly use it to improve the physical capacities of athletes, particularly those with a high training age. Tapering is a good example of how effective monitoring of overreaching can optimize peaking in athletes. The **taper**, a critical part of the periodization plan, involves reducing overall training volume while maintaining the intensity to bring about a peak in performance due to the supercompensation effect (113). A well-designed taper typically results in performance gains of about 3% (range = 0.5-6%) (81), which can mean the difference between winning and losing.

Of the many aspects of designing a training program, the taper causes practitioners the most problems because

so much about tapering and peaking for competition is still not understood. One of the issues with tapering is athletes' highly individualized responses to it. Current research on tapering has, for the most part, used individual aerobic endurance athletes; only a small number of studies have been done on team sport athletes (18, 81, 91). A recent study of elite triathletes demonstrated the importance of monitoring training to avoid negative outcomes as a result of overreaching (3). The athletes in the functionally overreached state performed worse after a 2-week taper than did those defined as "acutely fatigued" as a result of training. This highlights the importance of monitoring the tapering period. For example, an athlete who is fatigued may require a longer tapering duration and greater reductions in training load (81).

Related to tapering are the areas of detraining and reduced training. Buchheit and colleagues (8) studied the effects of a 2-week detraining period in elite Australian rules football players. During this period the players underwent a nonsupervised reduced training program. Various measures of muscular strength and cardiorespiratory endurance revealed either increases or no changes at all. Even longer periods of detraining can result in further improvements in certain physical capacities. Loturco and colleagues (64) investigated the effects of a 28-day taper in four elite pole vaulters. Although this was a small sample size, the study showed significant improvements in the rate of force development and acceleration after the training cessation period. A classic study by Andersen and Aagaard (1) showed that an extended period of detraining resulted in an overshoot of myosin heavy chain IIX isoforms, which could explain the large increases in power and rate of force development that were seen (1, 2). What appears to emerge from this body of research is that typical tapering periods may be quite conservative and that they could be lengthened to maximize athletic performance. However, only by regularly monitoring variables related to performance throughout the program and tapering period can practitioners garner this information from athletes to help them introduce more optimal strategies.

Functional overreaching is generally reversed when an adequate period of recovery of 1 to 3 weeks is provided (62, 71). This allows for the so-called rebound effect, which theoretically allows the athlete to perform at greater capacity. However, issues can arise because functional overreaching can compromise competition performance in the short term. Therefore, the timing and duration of any functional overreaching during a training program is critical.

Functional overreaching strategies are often more effective with advanced and elite athletes, perhaps because they need them to continue making gains in performance. The flip side is that such strategies put athletes at greater risk of moving farther along the fitness-fatigue continuum toward maladaptation. Athletes' tolerance for higher training loads increases throughout their careers, but the need to be closely monitored becomes even more important. With respect to functional overreaching, practitioners need to take a risk–reward approach. Athlete monitoring enables them to make more informed decisions about when to use overreaching approaches during periodization and what to adjust to ensure improved performance occurs while avoiding moving athletes farther along the continuum toward nonfunctional overreaching.

Nonfunctional Overreaching

The time taken to recover from normal performance is the major factor that distinguishes functional overreaching from nonfunctional overreaching (71). Nonfunctional overreaching is associated with periods of reduced performance, psychological distress, and hormonal disturbances. It is often viewed as a precursor to the overtraining syndrome. An athlete who has reached a state of nonfunctional overreaching is generally underperforming and feeling excessively fatigued, and the symptoms last from 2 weeks to 6 months (68).

Research Studies on Nonfunctional Overreaching

The process of nonfunctional overreaching is far from well understood. In addition to research with athletes, research with tactical and military personnel has also provided some interesting insights in this area. A range of monitoring tools can be used for detecting nonfunctional overreaching (16-18, 83). Nederhof and colleagues (83) examined a range of monitoring tools (see chapter 4) in three case studies of elite speedskaters, including the Recovery-Stress Questionnaire for Athletes (RESTQ-Sport), Profile of Mood States (POMS), a reaction time test, and responses of the adrenocorticotropic hormone (ACTH) and cortisol to two bouts of maximal cycling. Clear differences were found between the three athletes (one classified as nonfunctional overreached, one recovering from nonfunctional overreaching, and one healthy). The RESTQ-Sport, reaction time task, and two-exercise protocol appear to be promising tools for diagnosing nonfunctional overreaching.

Coutts and colleagues (18) investigated markers of overreaching in team sport athletes (rugby league) undertaking heavy training loads. A group of players deliberately overreached for 6 weeks followed by a 1-week taper period. The short taper period allowed for supercompensation in running performance, vertical countermovement jump height, and $\dot{V}O_2$max and reduced muscle damage. The glutamine-to-glutamate ratio was the only biochemical marker sensitive enough to distinguish functional from nonfunctional overreaching. Interestingly, the study also showed that nonfunctional overreaching can occur with only relatively small increases in training load above usual levels of training. This highlights the importance of having accurate measures of training load in addition to tools that can identify overreaching.

Exercise and Hormonal Tests for Nonfunctional Overreaching

The two-protocol exercise test has been used in the study of overreaching and overtraining in athletes (71, 72). The theory behind this protocol is that it provides an indirect measure of hypothalamic-pituitary-adrenal reactivity. Typically, two bouts of maximal exercise, separated by 4 hr, are performed, and a variety of hormonal responses are measured. The test can be used to distinguish between functional and nonfunctional overreaching as well as overtraining (73). A nonfunctionally overreached athlete displays a more pronounced neuroendocrine response to the second bout of exercise than does an athlete in a state of functional overreaching (73). An overtrained athlete exhibits an extremely large hormonal response to the first bout of exercise, but this is generally followed by a suppressed response to the second bout (73). This suggests an initial hypersensitivity of the pituitary with exhaustion, downregulation following the second bout of exercise, or both (71).

When considering the hormonal responses to exercise during these tests, practitioners should take into account the variability of these measures. The hormonal axes being monitored need to be considered within the context of their interaction. For example, the hormonal responses during exercise will have an impact on the hormonal responses during recovery (71). Because these hormonal axes function in parallel, it is critical to measure their levels during exercise and after recovery. This is the rationale for using a two-exercise approach. However, it does have its drawbacks, which include logistics, demands on the athlete, and the expense of the hormonal analysis. Using this type of monitoring with a large group of athletes would be challenging; it may be better to reserve it for high-priority athletes identified as at risk of nonfunctional overreaching or overtraining.

Hormone levels related to the hypothalamic-pituitary-adrenal axis have been shown to be disturbed during overreaching (97, 98). Specifically, levels of ACTH, cortisol, and growth hormone have decreased following overreaching (72, 98). The testosterone-to-cortisol ratio has also been proposed to have potential as a marker (see chapter 5 for more details), but the results are less compelling (28-30, 76). The idea is that testosterone represents the athlete's anabolic status and that the cortisol represents the catabolic status. Reports of reduced levels of cortisol with long-term training can be found in the literature (36), although these findings are not consistent (98).

In a study of elite junior football players, athletes who were underperforming showed psychological and hormonal changes consistent with nonfunctional overreaching (98). Levels of resting growth hormone were reduced, and there was a decrease in postexercise ACTH. The suggestion is that the lower levels of growth hormone reflect the reduced anabolic status of the athlete, and under stress, the lower levels of ACTH are a result of disruption to the pituitary-adrenal axis (98). It is common to measure these hormones, both at rest and in response to a bout or bouts of exercise. However, the problem with using these measures is the expense, the logistics of collection, and the challenge of providing real-time feedback to practitioners. Also, a great deal of variability exists with these measures, which limits their usefulness for monitoring athletes for overreaching and overtraining.

Given the importance of mood state in diagnosing overtraining, there has been interest in brain markers such as brain-derived neurotrophic factor (BDNF), which stimulates brain cell growth and repair as well as the development and maintenance of the nervous system. A recent study investigated the relationship between plasma BDNF and mood disturbance as a result of a period of intensified training (89). In a group of eight well-trained cyclists, a 32% increase in mood disturbance occurred after just 1 week of intensified training, and this was accompanied by a decrease in performance. These were both restored after 1 week of recovery, which indicated a state of functional overreaching. Plasma levels of BDNF increased following acute exercise during the intensified period, but there were no clear relationships with the degree of overreaching postexercise or at rest. Resting cortisol was also measured but did not demonstrate any usefulness as a marker of training stress. Mood disturbance, determined using questionnaires such as the POMS, appears to be one of the best markers of nonfunctional overreaching. Halson and colleagues (42) found a 28% increase in mood disturbance in elite cyclists after 2 weeks of intensified training. Mood disturbances, neuroendocrine dysfunction, emotional changes, and disturbed sleep are all associated with nonfunctional overreaching. They are also indicators of disturbance of the regulation and coordination function of the hypothalamus.

Disturbed sleep patterns and increased incidences of illness have been shown in overreached aerobic endurance athletes (45). What is not clear from this work is whether the disturbed sleep is a result of increased training load causing the development of overreaching or a symptom of overreaching. Athletes in a state of nonfunctional overreaching also show deterioration in mood in addition to decreased performance (98). A classic study by Morgan and colleagues (77) showed mood disturbances in female swimmers following 4 weeks of overload training, particularly increased anger and depression. Simple tools for monitoring athletes are invaluable for practitioners, particularly if they can accurately assess athletes' position on the fitness-fatigue continuum and help them avoid moving toward the severe state of overtraining.

Markers of Overtraining

The major difference between nonfunctional overreaching and overtraining is the time it takes to restore normal performance (71). Overtraining can be defined as being excessively fatigued and underperforming for longer than 6 months (68). One of the problems facing practitioners is that, to achieve success, athletes need some periods of heavy training loads (24). Athletes often train multiple times per day to achieve these training loads. When an athlete is suffering from performance fatigue, it is important to determine whether that fatigue is the result of overtraining (71). In a consensus statement, Meeusen and colleagues (71) state that the stress-recovery-adaptation model is too general. They suggest that a diagnosis of overtraining syndrome requires specific exclusion criteria focusing on clinical aspects, followed by nonclinical elements such as training volume, energy balance, nutrition, recovery strategies, and psychology (63, 71). Overtraining is often considered the result of too much training; however, many other factors contribute to it, all of which practitioners need to take into account.

Lewis and colleagues (63) suggested that the term overtraining syndrome may cause practitioners to focus solely on training when the syndrome is multifactorial. Practitioners tend to increase the effort and frequency of training sessions in response to poor results. To avoid this, they need to understand the differences between overreaching and overtraining in athletes. Consistent use and application of terminology may build better relationships between sport coaches and sport scientists. It will also educate practitioners and athletes about the correct application of training load and ensure adequate recovery to optimize performance.

Various methods have been proposed for detecting overtraining in athletes. Ideally, practitioners would identify conditions that can lead to overtraining so they can make adjustments before the syndrome occurs. Several methods

are discussed in more detail in forthcoming chapters. Some symptoms of performance fatigue are unexplained decreases in performance, persistent fatigue, having to make more effort during training, and disordered sleep (including quantity, quality, insomnia, and nap frequency). To determine whether overtraining is the cause of an athlete's fatigue, a practitioner must first eliminate other possible causes. For example, diseases such as anemia, Epstein-Barr virus, Lyme disease, diabetes, and adult-onset asthma can cause performance fatigue, as can muscle damage, cardiac problems, infectious diseases, allergies, injuries, and biological abnormalities. Any recent illnesses and associated symptoms should be noted. Also, practitioners need to look at psychological and social factors and whether the athlete has traveled excessively recently.

Another factor for practitioners to examine to rule out overtraining is training errors. These could be the result of more time spent training, a significant increase in intensity, training monotony, a high number of competitions, or exposure to environmental stressors such as heat, cold, and high altitude. The athlete's training diary or log can be a good source for this type of information.

Decreased athletic performance is a key consideration and should be recorded in terms of the quantity and duration of the decrease. If possible, practitioners should review any recent competition and training data, including perception of effort, heart rate, and global positioning system data. Heart rate measures such as resting heart rate, heart rate response to exercise, and heart rate variability (HRV) can help practitioners monitor for overtraining.

Mood disturbances should also be noted, including stress, anxiety, loss of appetite, lack of libido, and disordered eating. Athletes may report suffering from constant mental fatigue, increased irritability, and difficulty concentrating. With female athletes, menstrual history should be recorded, including menarche, contraception, time of last period, and frequency of periods. Medications and a history of drug use are also worth noting. Nutrition information is vital and can include typical daily food and fluid intake, timing, recent changes in diet, dietary exclusions, and the use of supplements. **Energy homeostasis**, which is clearly important for training and adaptation, refers to the balance between energy intake and energy expenditure. The International Olympic Committee offers guidelines in its consensus statement "Relative Energy Deficiency in Sport" because energy deficiency has been associated with decreased performance in athletes (79, 80). Energy homeostasis is also a particularly important factor in the female athlete triad (79). This refers to the combination of disordered eating and an irregular menstrual cycle, which can lead to decreases in hormones such as estrogen and eventually to losses in bone mineral density (79). Female athletes involved in sports in which a leaner body composition is important for performance can be particularly at risk (79). Energy homeostasis can be monitored using measures of body weight and body composition.

Once medical reasons have been excluded, a diagnosis of overtraining syndrome can be made if the athlete continues to underperform despite continued rest and recovery (63). Diagnosis, however, can be extremely difficult given the wide range of symptoms across individuals (92).

Biochemical, Hematological, and Immunological Markers

Biochemical, hematological, and immunological markers have been proposed for monitoring training that could lead to overreaching or overtraining (see chapter 5 for further details). Biochemical measures proposed include testosterone-to-cortisol ratio, plasma glutamine, creatine kinase, C-reactive protein, serum iron, ferritin, and transferrin. Hematological markers such as red blood cell count, hemoglobin, and hematocrit could also be useful. Immunological markers suggested as valuable for monitoring overtraining are blood leukocyte counts, blood cytokines, salivary immunoglobulin A, and amylase. Cytokines such as interleukin-6 and tumor necrosis factor alpha have potential because of their important roles in immune function and response to exercise (102).

Measures of creatine kinase are good indicators of muscle damage and response to unaccustomed exercise, but no consistent patterns have been noted with respect to overtrained athletes (44). Coutts and colleagues (18) found significant increases in creatine kinase in rugby league players following a 6-week period of intensified training. Following a 1-week taper period, the athletes had a significant return to baseline values that was different from what was seen with the other biochemical markers. This was no doubt a reflection of the reduced amount of muscle damage associated with the reduction in training load. With overtraining, reductions in exercise-induced levels of insulin-like growth factor–binding protein 3 (IGFBP-3) have been reported (21). One study showed relationships between levels of insulin-like growth factor 1 and IGFBP-3 and overtraining as estimated by an overtraining questionnaire (21). Given the role of the sympathetic nervous system, researchers are interested in the potential role of catecholamines in overreaching and overtraining; evidence suggests that they may be a useful marker (48). However, it should be noted that these are not large-scale studies.

Chronic energy deficiency and the resulting glycogen depletion can amplify the stress hormone response, which can be a trigger for overtraining (71). Given the importance of the hypothalamus in regulating energy homeostasis, disruptions in energy balance can affect several key processes. This could indicate inadequate recovery and potential overreaching. Hormones involved with energy balance such as adiponectin and ghrelin have also been put forward as potential markers of overtraining (53).

Cytokines could be a marker of excessive fatigue and illness during nonfunctional overreaching (53). Proinflammatory cytokines have a wide range of roles in the human body and are particularly important in the immune response and signaling the hypothalamus (102, 103). Therefore, it is thought that they could help in distinguishing between functional and nonfunctional overreaching (102, 103). Proinflammatory cytokines have receptors in the hypothalamus and may be responsible for some of the symptoms of overreaching and overtraining seen in athletes (53, 105).

Performance Tests

Overtraining ultimately results in decreased performance. Performance tests are vital for determining the existence of overreaching and overtraining in athletes and can identify recovery from periods of intense training. In a study of elite youth athletes, researchers investigated whether field-based performance tests could make a valid distinction between athletes who were nonfunctionally overreached and controls (97). The field-based performance tests included an interval shuttle run test for football players and the Zoladz test for runners (118). The results showed that with repeated field-based performance tests, performance reduction was associated with different mood profiles, blunted cortisol responses, and decoupling of ACTH and cortisol levels. More research is required with larger cohorts of elite athletes to confirm the efficacy of these types of submaximal performance tests for detecting overreaching and overtraining.

One way to distinguish overreaching from overtraining is to examine physiological and biochemical responses to exercise. One of the features of overtraining is the reduced hormonal response to exercise. As discussed earlier, two maximal exercise tests have been used with some success to distinguish these conditions (72, 73). Given that elite athletes often are required to train twice a day, this model can provide insights into responses to training load. Anecdotally, athletes suffering from nonfunctional overreaching or overtraining have performance decrements during the second session of the day. Meeusen and colleagues showed that the ACTH and prolactin responses to a second bout of exercise and the subsequent time to recover could distinguish between these two points of the continuum (72). In the case of an overtrained athlete, an overshoot of ACTH in the first exercise bout was followed by a complete suppression in the second exercise bout (73). The authors proposed hypersensitivity of the pituitary as an explanation. The use of two maximal exercise bouts appears to have potential for detecting overreaching to prevent overtraining.

The issue with using these biochemical and physiological markers is the time required to analyze and report the results. They can also be somewhat impractical with large groups of athletes. Finding ways to reduce the time and physical demands of the tests would make them more practical. A modification has been to have athletes perform a 30-min bout of exercise, alternating 1 min at 55% of maximal work and 4 min at 80% of maximal work. Two hours later the athlete performs a cycle to fatigue at 70% of maximal work (or for a maximum of 30 min) (49, 50). Hough and colleagues (49) investigated salivary testosterone and cortisol responses, along with RESTQ-Sport scores, following an 11-day intensified training period. They found that the test was sensitive enough to highlight changes in salivary testosterone and cortisol following the intensified training period. Specifically, they noted blunted responses in these hormones following the exercise tests. Performance tests are discussed in more detail in chapter 5.

Heart Rate Measures

Heart rate indices such as HRV are potential tools for monitoring athletes for overreaching and overtraining (6). These measures have the advantage of being very accessible in sport settings. Several studies have suggested some value with this approach (62, 90). In one study a group of highly trained triathletes showed evidence of parasympathetic modulation of heart rate following functional overreaching (62). The use of HRV and other heart rate measures is discussed in more detail in chapter 5.

Heart rate recovery measures have also been investigated as potential markers of overtraining and overreaching. A meta-analysis suggests that heart rate is not uniformly affected by overload training (6). Resting heart rate, HRV, and maximal heart rate may have some utility as markers of short-term fatigue. The moderate degree of alterations in these measures in response to chronic fatigue limits their usefulness. At present, though, the data suggest that these physiological measures have low sensitivity for detecting differences between points on the fatigue continuum. Like other measures, heart rate measures are fully useful only when put in context with other markers of overreaching or overtraining.

Cognitive Tests

The relationship between mental fatigue and physical performance has received attention from researchers (67, 104). In one study, 16 cyclists performed mentally demanding tasks prior to a cycling performance test (67). The group experienced a 15% decrease in the time to exhaustion, and the mentally fatigued cyclists rated their perception of effort during the exercise as higher compared to those in the control condition (67). Another study showed that mental fatigue impaired sport-specific skills such as running, passing, and shooting in football players (104). Practitioners need to be aware of the relationship between physical performance and cognitive effort in athletes because it can have implications for monitoring. Increased perception of effort with training can also be a sign of overtraining (41). Using RPE measures during exercise testing and training can be a simple way to monitor for any signs of overtraining.

Psychomotor speed tests have shown some promise for detecting nonfunctional overreaching and overtraining (82). Advantages of these tests are that they are easy to use and inexpensive.

They are based on the fact that during periods of fatigue, cognitive function and reaction time decrease. Psychomotor slowness has been shown to be consistently present during related conditions such as major depression and chronic fatigue syndrome (82). Psychomotor speed has been impaired following 2 weeks of overload training in trained cyclists and functionally overreached cyclists (82). A variety of apps for assessing attention and reaction time hold some promise for the early detection of overtraining. However, more evidence is needed before any of them can be conclusively recommended in practice.

Monotony

Evidence suggests that athletes undergoing periods of highly monotonous training with little variation in training load are at increased risk of developing overtraining syndrome (23). Interesting research using racehorses showed that alternating hard and easy training days avoided overtraining (7). The horses responded as expected to progressive increases in training load. However, when the recovery days were made less restful and the monotony of the training increased, the horses' running performance decreased and they showed signs of overtraining (e.g., decreased appetite). Results from studies with athletes support this idea (23, 24). The studies by Foster and colleagues showed a strong relationship between certain training indices and overtraining in athletes (23, 24). In a group of 25 athletes comprising primarily speedskaters, a high rate of illnesses resulted when they exceeded thresholds for training **strain** (training load × monotony). A recent study of 32 rugby league players confirmed this

(110). The players were tracked across the preseason and competition period using RPE and wellness questionnaires. Thresholds were identified for training load, monotony (training variation), and strain that were predictors of illness. A reduction in overall well-being also predicted illness. Modeling approaches such as this, along with simple measures of wellness, can provide practitioners with valuable insights into the process of predicting overreaching and overtraining in athletes.

Immune Function

As previously noted, studies of athletes undergoing long-term training with high training loads reveal suppressed immune function, which puts them at greater risk of developing upper respiratory illnesses (117). Research on the immune function of athletes classified as overtrained is lacking. However, anecdotal reports from practitioners suggest that overtraining results in increased rates of infection (102). Other studies suggest the existence of this relationship (92). For example, Reid and colleagues (92) completed a clinical investigation of athletes with persistent fatigue and recurrent infections. Their findings suggest that immune suppression and unresolved viral infections contribute to fatigue, recurring infections, and decreased performance. What is also interesting about their investigation is that the conditions and symptoms were not consistent across the group, again supporting the concept of a multifactorial approach to athlete monitoring. It does seem likely, based on the evidence, that athletes in a state of nonfunctional overreaching or overtraining would be at greater risk of developing upper respiratory tract illnesses.

Sleep

Sleep is consistently mentioned as one of the key elements of recovery for athletes. Monitoring of sleep is believed to be important for preventing overtraining syndrome. Evidence that athletes who do not get sufficient quantities and quality of sleep experience these conditions is lacking (40). One study suggested a relationship between the quantity of sleep and injury rates in adolescent athletes (75). Another recent study revealed that functionally overreached triathletes had a significant decrease in sleep duration (−7.9%), sleep efficiency (−1.6%), and immobile time (−7.6%) during sleep (45). The sleep was monitored each night using wristwatch actigraphy, and these negative sleep patterns were reduced during the subsequent taper phase. Researchers have discovered well-established relationships between sleep deprivation and depressed immune function and decreased work performance (33, 45, 56). In a study by Hausswirth and colleagues (45), of the nine athletes with nonfunctional overreaching, five developed symptoms of upper respiratory tract infection. Also, the highest rate of illness occurred during the final week of the overload period. This agrees with previous research showing a strong relationship between athlete illness and periods of heavy training loads (116). Halson and colleagues (39) reported a greater sleep deficiency in a female sprint cyclist who developed signs of overtraining (persistently feeling fatigued and underperforming for many months). Killer and colleagues (56) found that just 9 days of intensified training in well-trained cyclists decreased sleep quality, mood state, and maximal exercise performance. Approaches for monitoring sleep in athletes have ranged from actigraphy to simple questionnaires in which they rate the amount and quality of their sleep.

Wellness Measures

Psychological and wellness questionnaires can also be used to detect overtraining in athletes (see chapter 4 for more details). Stronger and more consistent relationships with overtraining have been observed with these types of self-report measures. The POMS, Daily Analysis of Life Demands for Athletes, Feeling Scale, Perceived Stress Scale, Total Quality Recovery Scale, Training Distress Scale, and RESTQ-Sport tend to be the most commonly used. These measures generally have good reliability and reflect the dose–response relationship of training load (96). They also appear to be sensitive to the symptoms of overreaching and overtraining. Each questionnaire has strengths and weaknesses, which are discussed more in chapter 4.

Another approach is to use symptom checklists in a training diary or log (48, 77). A simple daily training log is a good starting point for getting detailed information about athletes' training and other aspects of the program. Hooper and colleagues (48) had swimmers complete training logs over a season to detect symptoms of overtraining. The rating scales included subjective ratings of sleep quality, fatigue, stress, and muscle soreness using a scale of 1 to 7; athletes completed them each morning upon waking. The researchers classified the swimmers as "stale" (i.e., overtrained) based on a range of criteria. Blood markers were also measured in the study, including catecholamines, cortisol, creatine kinase, hemoglobin, hematocrit, erythrocytes, and total leukocyte counts. Physiological measures of heart rate, blood pressure, and lactate were also collected.

A recent study showed that a negative life event could have a significant impact on athletes' perceptions of stress and recovery (86). Negative life events include such things as being a victim of crime, serious illness or injury, and the death of a close family member or partner. Sixteen runners were investigated using the RESTQ-Sport; changes were seen during the week of the negative life event and also the week following. Interestingly, changes in performance as measured by running economy supported the link between stress events and subsequent athletic performance.

Environmental factors can also contribute to overtraining (40), including high altitude, heat, and travel (causing jet lag) (25, 26, 40). Overseas training camps are a good example of where these issues could arise. Although such camps are designed with the best of intentions, they can create a perfect storm of factors that could result in an increased incidence of injury, overtraining syndrome, or both. These factors include changes in nutrition, disrupted sleep patterns, and environmental conditions different from what the athlete is used to. Combined with the stress of increased training volume, these factors create challenges in terms of where athletes fall on the fatigue continuum. A solid cost-benefit analysis needs to be conducted before undertaking these types of camps (see the sidebar Individual Responses in a Squad of Athletes in chapter 1). Practitioners can then decide whether they provide enough benefit to justify them.

Another important factor to take into account is the importance of the events or matches taking place. For example, an athlete may be under more pressure in the final year of the Olympic cycle. Therefore, it may be prudent to be even more judicious about monitoring for additional stress and fatigue and make the necessary adjustments. During a competitive team sport season, some matches may be more difficult and place greater demands on the athletes than others. Practitioners may want to predict the difficulty of matches to help them guide the prescription of training loads during the season (54). For example, during weeks in which matches or events are particularly difficult, practitioners may reduce the training loads considerably and incorporate more recovery strategies. In the weeks leading up to key matches, training loads could be reduced in a way similar to the wavelike approach used with tapering. Research studies of the efficacy of these approaches would be enlightening.

Interdisciplinary and Multifactorial Approaches to Avoid Overtraining

What is clear from all this research is that a battery of monitoring tools could help reduce overtraining syndrome in athletes (63). Interdisciplinary teams of support staff are best equipped to help athletes avoid overtraining and guide them back to peak performance following maladaptive conditions. The wide range of symptoms indicates that practitioners need to consider many factors when diagnosing overtraining. Position statements also indicate that physiological responses and symptoms are highly varied and individual (41, 68, 70, 71).

No single monitoring tool can provide a completely accurate diagnosis of overtraining. Thus, practitioners are well advised to use a battery of tests to get a complete picture of the athlete and to help them predict overtraining. A range of long-term monitoring tools will also enable the practitioner to manage the athlete's progression back to full training (40).

Researchers have started to investigate multifactorial approaches to overreaching and overtraining (61). Le Meur and colleagues (61) studied 24 triathletes who were separated into an overload group and a normal training group. They used a multivariate approach that looked at physiological, biochemical, cognitive, and perceptual measures during 3 weeks of training. Following the training period, 11 of the athletes were classified as being overreached based on decrements in performance. Discriminant analysis showed that eight variables could explain the majority of those in the overtrained state based on variations in heart rate and lactate on a maximal incremental test. The study confirmed that a variety of monitoring variables is needed to prevent the transition from overreached to overtrained in aerobic endurance athletes. The authors also proposed that an overreaching index that combines heart rate and blood lactate concentration changes after an intensified training period could be useful for detecting overreaching in athletes.

One multifactorial study monitored 18 elite football players' fitness, fatigue, and running performance during a preseason training camp (9). Several physiological and psychometric measures were collected over 2 weeks. These included training load, wellness ratings, salivary cortisol, and HRV measures prior to training. Regular fitness testing was done using the Yo-Yo intermittent recovery test and global positioning system measures collected from all sessions. Importantly, no injuries were reported during the camp, and all players' fitness levels improved. The HRV and wellness scores were sensitive to subtle changes in training load. The authors concluded that a collection of heart rate, training load, and wellness measures could be used to monitor training-induced changes in fatigue and recovery status.

Hooper and colleagues (48) proposed an interesting multifactorial approach using a range of criteria to determine "staleness," or overtraining, in a group of elite swimmers. The criteria were as follows:

- Failure to increase performance from early in the season to the end of the season
- Failure to increase performance during national trials from previous best times
- Fatigue rating greater than 5 (on a 7-point Likert scale) for more than 7 days
- Comments in training diaries that athletes believed they were not responding well to training
- Noting an illness in the training log that was associated with a normal blood measure such as leukocyte count

Achieving all of these criteria was necessary for a diagnosis of overtraining.

Figure 3.5 shows an example of monitoring for overreaching in a group of athletes; performance measures were taken over 6 weeks during an overload and taper phase. Measures of weekly load, wellness, and performance are shown for both training periods. The graph shows that functional overreaching occurred and that a rebound in performance occurred following the tapering week. By monitoring athletes with a range of monitoring tools, practitioners can track the changes in training load and see how performance and wellness (mood, fatigue, muscle soreness, sleep, and stress) are affected.

Using a multifactorial approach with a battery of monitoring tools is a sound way to establish whether an athlete is susceptible to overtraining. Because no single measure can accurately predict the existence of overreaching or overtraining, practitioners should investigate and use a range of monitoring tools.

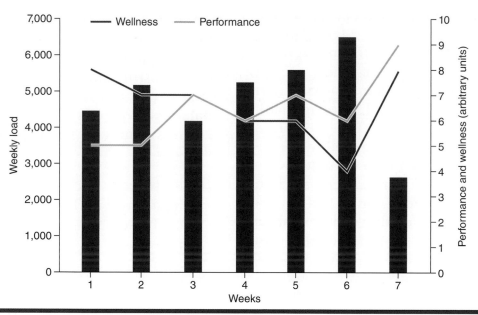

Figure 3.5   Monitoring overreaching in athletes with performance and wellness measures over time (7 weeks) during an overload and taper phase.

GUIDELINES FOR AVOIDING OVERTRAINING

Practitioners can use a variety of strategies to avoid overtraining syndrome and decreased performance in athletes (70). Prevention is the most important consideration because the most viable strategy for addressing full-blown overtraining syndrome is complete rest and recovery. Athlete monitoring, correctly embedded in a training program, will go a long way in keeping athletes from developing overtraining syndrome.

The following strategies can help practitioners prevent overtraining in their athletes:

- Have regular conversations with athletes and ask them how they feel.
- Keep a training diary to record the details of all training sessions and competitions.
- Make adjustments to training loads when performance declines.
- Progressively increase the training load using carefully planned periodization to avoid large changes from week to week.
- Avoid excessive monotony in training by alternating heavy and light days.
- Consider the intelligent use of rest days and training variety to avoid boredom and monotony.
- Individualize training loads for each athlete based on tolerance level.
- Understand stressors that can be adding to the stress of training for the athlete (e.g., life load events such as exams and relationships).
- Consider the role of environmental conditions such as heat, high altitude, and jet lag with travel.
- Optimize recovery.
- Optimize sleep and rest strategies.
- Ensure adequate and balanced nutrition.
- Use wellness questionnaires to record athletes' psychological and emotional states.
- Make adjustments to training loads and frequency when an athlete exhibits excessive fatigue.
- Make a note of any illnesses, and be prepared to stop or reduce training to aid recovery.
- Gradually transition the athlete back to full training loads after any periods of no training.
- Use objective criteria for return to sport that takes into account the athlete's tolerance for loading.
- Perform regular health checks with an interdisciplinary team that includes a physician, a physiotherapist, a nutritionist, and a sport psychologist.

Conclusion

Several models attempt to explain the acute response of athletes to training. The GAS model, fitness-fatigue model, and stimulus-fatigue-recovery-adaptation model are all important to understand. Traditional concepts of homeostasis in relation to stress should be modified to take into account the multifactorial nature of the acute physiological stress of training. The fatigue continuum provides an overview of the progression of fatigue to functional overreaching to nonfunctional overreaching to overtraining. All of these states are characterized by decreases in performance but are defined by the degree of recovery required. Early detection of signs of nonfunctional overreaching is important because it allows the practitioner to adjust the training program before the athlete progresses to overtraining syndrome. No single marker can detect the progression from functional overreaching to nonfunctional overreaching to overtraining. Therefore, practitioners should consider a range of monitoring tools to create a full picture of athletes' fatigue levels.

4

Quantifying Training Stress

To optimize an athlete's adaptation to a training program, practitioners must initially quantify the level of training stress and the physiological responses to that stress. Many subjective and objective research-based measurement tools are available to guide training program design and optimize training sessions. Coaches, sport scientists, and strength and conditioning practitioners need a good understanding of these measurement tools to avoid using a tool just for the sake of using it. Ultimately, the measurement tool needs to help a practitioner make decisions about the athlete's program. This chapter provides an overview of the common measurement tools used to assess external and internal training load for athlete monitoring.

Measurement Tools

Athlete training programs can be quantified in numerous ways. The training sessions within the training program can be measured in terms of **frequency** (how often), **intensity** (how hard), **duration** (how long), and **mode** (type of exercise). **Training load** can be quantified as a measure of external load or internal load. At its simplest, training load is the product of session intensity and duration, as follows:

Training load = intensity × duration

Measures of **external load** look at factors such as distance covered, athlete speed, and session duration. The increasing use of microtechnology in sport (e.g., power meters, global positioning system [GPS] devices, accelerometers) has allowed practitioners to monitor external load in athletes during training and competition with accuracy and in real time.

Internal load refers to the physiological stress on the athlete during training, which is what largely determines the adaptation to the training program. Heart rate, rating of perceived exertion (RPE), and lactate are examples of measures of internal load. When monitoring athletes, practitioners need to consider both external and internal load. Traditionally, training has been prescribed using external measures despite individual differences in response to external load (66, 76). For example, an athlete may generate the same number of watts during two cycling tests (external load) performed during two sessions but report different perceptions of effort or have different heart rate responses (internal load) in the two tests. Research also suggests that athletes can experience different internal responses to the same external workload (66). Issues can arise when a practitioner prescribes external loads for a group of athletes without considering the individual differences in internal load, which can indicate fatigue and ultimately adaptation. Practitioners need to understand the difference between external and internal load and how they interact in athlete monitoring.

External Load

External load measures are commonly used for quantifying training in aerobic endurance sports and team sports. The increasing use of wearable technologies has allowed for more systematic and detailed information on the external load measures such as distance covered and athlete speed (129). An example of a measure of external load is a football player covering 9,725 m during a match.

EXTERNAL MEASURES FOR MONITORING TRAINING LOAD

External training load refers to things such as weight lifted, total distance run, and the number of sprints, impacts, and jumps performed in a training session. Without this information, the practitioner cannot assign appropriate loads. Technology such as GPS, accelerometry, and power meters are now used widely to provide objective measures of external load. Practitioners without access to this type of technology can note what the athlete does in the training session (e.g., sets, repetitions, load, number of intervals, distance, time, length and number of recovery periods). However, these measures do not provide information on how the athlete is responding to the training load. This is why measures of internal load are also important to monitor.

Time–Motion Analysis

Tracking sport performance and training is a popular way to monitor athlete fatigue and recovery (169). A range of methods and technologies can be used to perform time–motion analysis in athletes, and wearable technologies are now an integral part of many professional sport environments. Simple **pedometers** record the number of steps the person takes by recording each time the force sensitivity threshold exceeds vertical acceleration. However, because pedometers cannot measure factors such as change of direction and energy expenditure, they have low applicability for athlete monitoring.

Simple **accelerometers** are now used widely for monitoring in training programs. Devices such as the Fitbit (www.fitbit.com), Jawbone UP (www.jawbone.com/up), Microsoft Band (www.microsoft.com/microsoft-band), and Garmin Vivosmart (www.garmin.com) provide data on heart rate, step count, energy expenditure, and sleep, although research suggests a wide variation in reported data (156). The small devices are often wristbands and can be integrated with custom software for further analysis (156). Currently, research on their use and application for athlete monitoring is lacking, particularly in terms of their reliability and validity. Research comparing these devices or validating them against accepted research methods is particularly limited (52, 156).

Global Positioning Systems

The use of GPS and accelerometry technology is becoming increasingly widespread because it allows practitioners to measure a wide range of metrics in athletes during both training and competition. These navigational systems consist of a series of satellites that send continuous signals to GPS receivers, which can then be used to calculate the distance to the satellites (106). By integrating the signals of the four satellites, the devices can calculate accurate distances and velocities. GPS devices used in sport provide information on distance and speed; the **inertial sensors** (accelerometers, gyroscopes, magnetometers) embedded in the units provide additional detail on activities such as jumps and collisions. GPS units can provide quantitative information on athlete performance, differences in position demands, and player movements during training and competition (162). Several reviews are available on GPS and its reliability and validity (7, 42, 106, 162).

Inertial Sensor Technology Inertial sensors can be worn or attached to equipment in a range of sports, including swimming (129), team sports such as rugby league (78) and American football (183), and running (29). This area of research is relatively new and expanding all the time, resulting in many types of technology and processing procedures that make comparisons across studies difficult. The technology has huge potential to provide real-time feedback on key variables for athlete monitoring, and it has application for coaching. For example, inertial sensors could provide a swimming coach with information about a swimmer's velocities and accelerations during starts and turns (129). Inertial sensors can also be attached to sporting equipment such as boats, oars, and paddles to provide information about the mechanical characteristics of performance during training and competition. Devices attached to a barbell during resistance training, for example, can be used to determine barbell velocity (158).

Practitioners using inertial sensors need to consider key issues such as measurement range, sampling frequency, signal filtering, data storage and transfer, and battery life. The placement of the sensor is also important (11, 12); researchers have compared the results of sensors placed on the upper back and near the hip and discovered significant differences in some variables (11). Issues can also arise with athlete compliance; some athletes dislike wearing these devices, particularly on the upper back. The development of smaller devices that can be incorporated into footwear and be completely nonobtrusive would help alleviate these issues.

GPS Systems   In a survey of high-performance sport practitioners, 43% of respondents indicated that they used GPS as part of their athlete monitoring system (169). Another survey of professional football clubs from Australia, Europe, and the United States (soccer) found that 40 out of 41 clubs surveyed collected GPS data from every player during every training session (1). Time–motion analysis systems such as GPS and movement pattern analysis from digital video (e.g., Stats, http://stats.com) are becoming increasingly embedded in elite sport programs. The modern GPS and accelerometry units are small and light, which makes them easy to wear, noninvasive, and useful for monitoring athletes during training sessions. In addition, many sports are now allowing athletes to wear these devices during competition. As a result, a large amount of research on athletes' external load measures from GPS and accelerometry has emerged in recent years (7, 42).

The evolution of GPS devices from simply measuring distance covered to more sophisticated measures such as accelerations and impacts has provided practitioners with more information for athlete monitoring. Measures that appear to be most commonly used for athlete monitoring are **work rate** (e.g., meters covered per minute), load (usually some derivative of other variables such as acceleration that are collected by the technology), time spent in high-intensity work ranges, and total distance covered (169). The survey of professional football clubs found the most common variables used for monitoring to be acceleration variables, total distance, distance covered at speeds greater than 5.5 m/s, and metabolic power (1). Other widely used measures are the number of accelerations and decelerations (92), impacts (41), and metabolic power (39).

The information obtained from GPS devices can be used for a variety of purposes. In terms of sport performance, practitioners are often interested in fatigue over the course of training and competition and athletes' pacing strategies. Another common approach has been to assess athletes across levels of performance (e.g., elite, subelite, youth). Position-specific information helps practitioners more accurately design training programs that reflect the demands of the sport. Effective use of GPS data may help with the transition of youth athletes to higher levels of competition. For example, by knowing the running demands of a position in a sport at the elite level, the practitioner can set specific targets to progressively overload an athlete safely to reach those levels.

Given the widespread use of GPS devices, it is critical that practitioners understand the benefits and limitations of this technology. Microsensor devices such as accelerometers, magnetometers, and gyroscopes have provided more accurate measurements of the physical demands and activity profiles of sports.

These allow practitioners to calculate variables such as collisions and impact (41), metabolic power (39, 97), and accelerometer load (61). The accumulated mechanical stress on the athlete, which is calculated from the vector magnitude of accelerations, decelerations, changes of direction, and impacts, can be provided by scores of metrics. These accumulated load metrics are a feature of most commercial systems. For example, metrics such as Player Load (Catapult, www.catapultsports.com) and New Body Load (GPSports, http://gpsports.com) are generated (37). Impacts can be determined from the summed accelerations from three planes (i.e., forward–backward, left–right, and up–down). These take into account impacts generated during running, tackling, jumping, and colliding. These measures have been shown to have moderate to strong relationships with internal load such as session RPE in sports such as football (69), Australian rules football (66, 93), and rugby league (111). Measures of g-forces can then be categorized according to zones (e.g., impacts ranging from light to heavy).

High-speed running is also a measure that often interests practitioners. For example, a practitioner may define the threshold for high-speed running as >14.5 km/hr (9 mph or >4 m/s) and the threshold for very high-speed running as >19.1 km/hr (12 mph or 5.3 m/s). The speed zones used by researchers and practitioners can vary greatly and appear to be sport specific (46, 78). Zones can also be determined for movement activities such as walking (e.g., <2.0 m/s or 0.45 mph [0.72 km/hr]), jogging (e.g., 2.1-3.5 m/s or 4.70-7.83 mph [7.61-12.6 km/hr]), running (e.g., 3.6-5.5 m/s or 8.05-12.30 mph [13-19.8 km/hr]), and sprinting (e.g., >5.5 m/s or 12.30 mph [19.8 km/hr]). Maximal accelerations can also be defined using thresholds (e.g., >2.78 m/s^{-2}).

Repeated bouts of high-intensity running in quick succession also interest practitioners involved with team sports (94). This could be defined as three or more high accelerations (e.g., >2.79 m/s^{-2}), high speed (5 m/s), or contacts with less than 21 s of recovery between efforts (9, 64).

Metabolic power is typically measured as total energy expenditure (in joules) and average relative metabolic power (in watts per kilogram) (39, 68). These measures can be indicators of high-intensity distance covered and give an estimation of energy cost (68). The measures obtained from GPS devices can be expressed as absolute numbers or relative to the time of the training or competition.

Reliability and Validity of GPS Devices Many studies have investigated the reliability and validity of GPS devices in sport for a range of measures such as distance, velocity, accelerations, and decelerations (92, 162). Research has been conducted to establish player profiles in a range of sports such as American football (183), rugby union (117), rugby sevens (157, 178), rugby league (41), Australian rules football (93), field hockey (90), netball (37), cricket (120), and football (177). By monitoring an athlete's performance, a practitioner gains clearer insight about the sport's demands and valuable information to use when designing the athlete's training program. For example, because running demands vary by position in a team sport, practitioners can use the GPS data of each athlete to design position-specific training programs.

The reliability of a GPS device appears to decrease as the speed of the activity increases (88). Reliability is affected by factors such as the sampling rate, velocity, duration, and type of activity (7, 27). The sampling rate refers to how many pieces of data the GPS device collects per second. For high-speed movements such as sprinting and impacts, high sampling rates are necessary. For example, a GPS device with a rate of 10 samples per second (or 10 Hz) may be sufficient for measuring slower speeds, but a sampling rate of 100 Hz might be needed to measure faster speeds. Practitioners working in team sports in particular need to take many variables into account when their athletes are using GPS devices in competition. Factors such as team tactics, the quality of the opposition, environmental conditions, and team cohesion can greatly affect the data (76). The intensity of match play might be higher against a challenging competitor, which may be reflected in the amount of high-speed running. Also, a playing style that emphasizes defensive or attacking aspects could result in differences in total load on the players.

Given that a number of companies produce devices with GPS technology, studies have used different types of systems, which can make comparisons difficult. Issues can also arise when athletes in a single squad use different GPS devices. To avoid between-device errors, athletes should consistently wear the same type of GPS device, as well as the same device from session to session (89, 95). Also, practitioners need to be wary of comparing different types of GPS technology (147). Research comparing different types of devices has found significant differences (95, 147). One study compared 5 Hz and 10 Hz units and found the 10 Hz units to be more accurate with less error for total distance, high-speed running, and very high-speed running (147). The coefficients of variation for very high-speed running were still high, however. In general, the accuracy of GPS devices increases as the sampling rate increases. However, as the speed of the movement increases, the reliability decreases.

Issues with validity and reliability also exist concerning impacts and collisions using the accelerometry data from GPS devices (41). Being able to accurately quantify the impacts associated with the sport and monitor these during both competition and training would greatly benefit practitioners, but more research is required in this area.

The validity of metabolic power measures derived from accelerometry has yet to be fully confirmed (39, 143). Changes of direction and acceleration increase the energy cost of sport activities and so need to be taken into account when assessing sport demands (143).

Application of GPS and Accelerometry Data

One of the most important considerations with GPS and accelerometry technology is the sheer number of variables that can be obtained. Akenhead and Nassis (1) identified 44 variables (not including RPE and heart rate measures) collected by practitioners. The fact that many of these variables can be reported as absolute measures (total amount of change or quantity) or relative measures (amount of change or quantity based on another factor such as time or body weight) increases the complexity of data interpretation. This raises the important question of which variables to measure. Practitioners sometimes become enamored with variables such as distance covered or running speed, but the reality is that the value of some measures is questionable. For example, in many team sports, more-skilled teams run less than less-skilled teams (85, 148).

GPS REPORT FROM A TRAINING SESSION

GPS devices are very helpful for monitoring training load. A great deal of data can be collected in real time to make sure athletes achieve training targets and make needed adjustments during the workout. Practitioners need to determine the optimal way to collect real-time data and then feed it back to the coach and athlete. Commercial GPS devices typically come with their own reporting tools that practitioners may be able to modify to report the most pertinent information. Reports should focus on three to five measures that are most important to the coach and athlete so as to not overwhelm them with unnecessary information. Another layer of data with other measures can be gathered to obtain an overview of the external load for the training session. This combined with internal load measures such as heart rate and perceived exertion reveals a complete picture of the effect of the training load on the athlete.

Player name: Athlete A
Position: Center (netball)
Session type: Team training

Measure (units)	Target	Result
Duration (minutes)	60	63
Distance at speed >5 m/s (meters)	500	577
External load metric (arbitrary units)	700	719
Accelerations (number)	50	57
Heart rate at 85-96% (% of session duration)	80	84

Comments: All targets achieved for the training session. No extra work required.

GPS devices have a potential role in injury prevention. Using GPS data, Murray and colleagues (134) found that injury rates in rugby league players were affected by the amount of recovery between matches. Gabbett and colleagues (60, 62, 63, 65) investigated the relationship between training load and injury in rugby league players using GPS data. Excessive preseason and in-season training loads were shown to increase the risk of soft tissue injury (60). By establishing thresholds for individual athletes, practitioners can more effectively monitor them for increased risk of injury. In a study of American football players at the Division I college level, Wilkerson and colleagues (185) found that inertial sensors provided information on injury risk by tracking load degree and variability.

Using time–motion analysis data in conjunction with speed thresholds based on maximal testing is becoming increasingly common (110). One of the limitations of GPS is the use of arbitrary or generalized speed zones when assigning a target running speed to an athlete, which is generally not recommended. Prescribing an individualized speed threshold is better because it provides valuable information

For example, an athlete performs 2 sets of 10 repetitions with 50 kg in exercise A and 3 sets of 5 repetitions with 80 kg in exercise B.

$$\text{Volume load (kg) for exercise A} = (2 \times 10 \times 50 \text{ kg}) = 1,000 \text{ kg}$$

$$\text{Volume load (kg) for exercise B} = (3 \times 5 \times 80 \text{ kg}) = 1,200 \text{ kg}$$

$$\text{Total repetitions} = (2 \times 10) + (3 \times 5) = 35 \text{ repetitions}$$

$$\text{Training intensity} = (1,000 \text{ kg} + 1,200 \text{ kg}) \div 35 \text{ repetitions} = 62.9 \text{ kg/repetition}$$

When monitoring resistance training, practitioners must keep records of the sets, repetitions, and loads lifted. They must also use one method consistently.

Internal Load

Measurements of external load may not provide an accurate description of the physiological stress on the athlete during training and competition. Fitness outcomes are related to the internal load, which includes both the psychological and physiological load imposed on the athlete. Monitoring internal load provides important information on how the athlete is adapting to training. Measures such as heart rate and RPE are the most common methods of monitoring internal load (76); practitioners also use subjective ratings of wellness (160). Blood markers such as lactate and physiological measures such as $\dot{V}O_2$ are also considered internal load measures.

Rating of Perceived Exertion

Perception of effort is commonly used to monitor training in athletes and can be used to determine exercise intensity (22, 51). Many factors contribute to the perception of effort during exercise, including hormone concentrations, neurotransmitter release, muscle mass recruited, substrate concentrations, psychological characteristics, environmental conditions, and personality traits (22). The RPE scale was designed by Gunnar Borg to measure interindividual differences in perceived exertion (22).

INDIVIDUALIZATION OF INTERNAL MEASURES

Athletes' internal responses are determined by a range of factors, including age, training history, physical capacity, genetics, and injury history. As such, they are unique.

We have already noted that the same external load can result in very different internal responses for different athletes. For example, a defensive lineman in American football and a marathon runner will have different perceptual and physiological responses to performing a 315-lb (143 kg) squat. Also, different internal responses can be found in the same athlete. For example, a middle-distance runner just returning from an injury will have different internal responses to running a 1,500-m time trial than she would have had before becoming injured.

It provides an overall subjective measure of perception of effort by integrating the information from the muscles and joints (the periphery) with the information from the cardiovascular and respiratory systems and the central nervous system (22). A variety of scales can be used to measure RPE; one of the most common is the **Borg 6-20 scale** (21, 51). This scale is linked to exercise heart rate; by adding a zero to each number, it represents the relative intensity of the heart rate in beats per minute.

The **category ratio (CR)-RPE scale** is also widely used in athlete monitoring (19, 51). The CR-10 uses values ranging from 0 to 10 to measure RPE on a nonlinear scale (20). The verbal statements are placed on the ratio scale in such a way that each represents twice the intensity of the preceding statement (e.g., *strong* and *very strong*). On the CR-10 scale, 0 represents nothing at all and 10 represents maximal exertion.

Research has consistently shown a strong correlation between the CR-RPE scale and physiological measures such as heart rate and lactate (20, 138). However, evidence shows that this relationship is not as strong as previously thought: A meta-analysis indicates the validity of RPE as $r = .62$, .57, and .64 for heart rate, blood lactate, and $\dot{V}O_2max$, respectively (33). The CR-RPE scales may be better for high-intensity exercise in which fatigue involves nonlinear responses (e.g., team sports). RPE is often combined with other physiological measures such as heart rate, lactate, and session duration to provide a complete picture of internal load.

Another CR-RPE scale, with values ranging from 0 to 100 (CR-100), has become increasingly used by practitioners (16, 53). The **Borg CR-100** scale is also known as the centiMax scale and, like the CR-10 scale, also uses a set of verbal anchors and numbers but with a greater range (0-100) (16). Some suggest that it is a more sensitive measure because of the wider range of numbers, which results in less clustering around the verbal anchors (53). The CR-100 scale also equates to a percentage, which may make it more intuitively appealing to coaches and athletes (18, 53).

When using RPE for the first time, practitioners should familiarize athletes with the scale. This can involve explaining what is meant by perceived exertion and then anchoring the perceptual range for the athlete. Verbal anchors gives the athlete a reference point for what the values on the scale represent in terms of intensity. Given that athletes are used to a range of exercise intensities, explaining the perceptual range should be relatively straightforward. For example, when using the CR-10 scale, the athlete could be asked to recall exercising at maximal exertion (RPE = 10) compared to being at complete rest (RPE = 0).

Modifications of classic RPE scales have also been developed with potential application for athlete monitoring. For example, scales have been used to assess perceived exertion in various regions of the body (e.g., legs, lungs) (17). Also, the increased interest in velocity-based training in strength and conditioning has resulted in attempts to develop scales of perceived velocity (13, 14). This would benefit practitioners who do not have access to technology such as linear position transducers. Another approach has been to investigate RPE as an overall measure of exertion and of the active muscles during a particular bout of exercise (184). Perceived level of exertion for respiratory effort has also been used (5, 17, 70, 184). Weston and colleagues (184) investigated the application of differential RPE during Australian rules

10 is equal to 0 RIR, indicating that no more repetitions can be performed (i.e., maximal effort); an RPE of 9 is equal to 1 RIR, indicating that one more repetition could be performed; an RPE of 8 is equal to 2 RIR, indicating that two more repetitions could be performed; down to an RPE of 1, which indicates that the set required little to no effort (186). More research is required to confirm the efficacy of these approaches.

Session RPE could be used to prescribe training by revealing to practitioners how athletes are perceiving the training stimulus. For example, consistently high session RPEs during a period of training could indicate the need to change the training program. Lockie and colleagues (109) investigated the use of session RPE for monitoring sprint and plyometric training. The progressive overload used in the training program was reflected in the session RPE values, supporting the usefulness of the measure. Zones of training intensity could also be used as a rough guide to training. Zones for session RPE such as low (≤3), moderate (4-6), and high (≥7) have been used in research and practice (111, 130). Although the limitations of session RPE do need to be acknowledged, its practical value and ease of use strongly support its use as part of athlete monitoring programs. However, its application for guiding training prescription requires further study.

Monotony and Strain

The session RPE measure of session load (duration × session RPE) is the most common way to use this metric. However, other measures such as training monotony and strain can provide valuable information about athletes (54). Weekly load is calculated by summing the session loads for the individual training sessions for the entire week. **Training monotony** is the variation of session load over the week. It is calculated by taking daily mean load and dividing it by the standard deviation of daily load. This standard deviation can be calculated over the course of a microcycle from 7 to 10 days. It could also be thought of as a measure of the sameness of the training. For example, if very little variation occurs in the training load from day to day, the monotony would be high. This could be a case of low loads or high loads because it refers simply to the variation or sameness of the training.

Training strain is the product of monotony and the weekly load. Research has shown that during periods of high strain and monotony, athletes are at greater risk of illness and injury (15, 54, 145). High strain is the product of high training load and high training monotony. By monitoring the variables of load, monotony, and strain over a period of time, practitioners can determine individual thresholds of risk for overreaching and overtraining. As explained in chapter 3, athletes generally tolerate and adapt to high training loads when recovery is sufficient. One study found that RPE alone effectively monitored training load in elite Australian rules football players (179). Interestingly, the authors found that the session RPE method did not increase the ability to predict illness or injury. The study also showed the importance of taking into account all aspects of training: Monitoring just the field-based running activities was not as effective at predicting illness or injury (179). The majority of research suggests that using session load is a robust method for determining training load in athletes (69, 111).

Relationships Between Session RPE and Other Measures

Research has shown that session RPE provides essentially the same information as more objective physiological measures such as heart rate (54, 56). Research by Foster (54) has shown strong relationships between session RPE and summated heart rate zone scores ($r = .75$-$.90$). In football players there were also very strong correlations between session RPE and heart rate zones ($r = .50$-$.85$) (87). Another advantage of this method is that collecting the information is easy and inexpensive. Session RPE may be a more valid measure than heart rate for high-intensity activities such as resistance training.

It has been reported that 80% to 90% of athletes give a single number from the session RPE scale (56). A small number of athletes insist on breaking up the session and rating each part. This highlights the importance of educating athletes on the purpose of the session RPE method.

Session RPE as a measure of internal load has been used across a wide range of sports. Team sports such as cricket (120), Australian rules football (126, 130, 155), rugby league (111, 173), football (soccer in the United States) (3, 69, 87), basketball (131, 132), wheelchair rugby (141), and rugby union (40, 117) have used session RPE. Individual sports such as marathon running (113), cycling (154), tennis (71), diving (125), martial arts (73, 140), and swimming (180) have also used this method, and it has been shown to be reliable and valid in most cases. Wallace and colleagues (180) found a strong relationship between session RPE and distance covered (113) ($r = .65$) during training in a group of elite swimmers. In fact, research has shown that a combination of internal and external load factors predicts session RPE in team sports better than individual measures alone (69, 111). A study by Gallo and colleagues (66) showed that factors such as years of competitive experience, playing position, and fitness level mediate the relationship between external load and session RPE load. This also highlights that athletes' characteristics influence their individual responses to training and should be considered with athlete monitoring. Research provides further support for the concept of session RPE as a valid indicator of training intensity (66, 87, 180).

Implementation of Session RPE

Some practitioners have attempted to apply session RPE to parts of the training session and remove the warm-up and cool-down from the calculations. Although taking into account only the parts of a session in which the athlete is actually training might improve the relationship with other measures of external and internal load, doing so may be challenging with large groups of athletes in team sport settings. Although this segmented approach to session RPE has been used by researchers (75), the session RPE measure is designed as a global rating of intensity. As such, practitioners are encouraged not to leave the warm-up and cool-down portions of the workout out of the session RPE calculations.

Researchers have also been interested in how session RPE relates to match performance (8). Looking at acute training load thresholds can be useful for practitioners, but it can be more informative to look at session RPE relative to chronic training over a previous mesocycle (e.g., the previous 4 weeks). This approach has been used to measure the **training stress**

balance by comparing the weekly load and strain to the average monthly load. Something like a 4-week rolling average can be useful (84). Training stress would be negative when the current training week exceeds the preceding 4 weeks' training load or strain and positive if it is lower than the average of the preceding 4 weeks (84). Research has shown that a positive training stress balance for strain is a strong discriminator of match results in Australian rules football (8). This further supports the importance of measuring strain as part of any load monitoring system (54).

Context is crucial when looking at internal and external load measures. A combination of measures should be used to accurately quantify training stress across the range of activities performed by athletes. The within-athlete differences and relationships between internal and external loads should be determined for each athlete prior to implementing the monitoring program. Practitioners should also establish baselines for session RPE for each training activity and intensity to add value to the monitoring. Weaving and colleagues (182) completed a **principal component analysis** (a statistical technique that reduces data to a set of primary variables) on measures of training load in rugby league players performing different training activities. During skill training, external load measures (e.g., total impacts and body load) explained the largest proportion of training load variation. During speed training, internal load measures (training impulse and session RPE) explained the greatest amount of variance. This highlights the importance of considering the external load within the context of the environment the athlete is training in and of using a mixture of internal and external load measures to monitor training.

OMNI RPE Scale

Pictorial representations of RPE have also been developed for a variety of modes of exercise (151-153, 176). Specific scales have been developed for running and cycling exercise as well as for resistance training (151). These **OMNI RPE** scales can be a useful alternative for monitoring RPE in athletes (see figure 4.2). The OMNI RPE scales have both verbal and exercise mode–specific pictures along the 0-10 scale. Linking pictures with verbal and numeric scales has been shown to improve the reliability of the tool (151).

Heart Rate

Taking measures of heart rate is one of the most common ways to monitor exercise intensity. Akenhead and Nassis (1) reported that 40 out of 41 professional football clubs collected heart rate data (in addition to GPS) from every player at every training session. Heart rate monitoring enables practitioners and athletes to accurately measure the relative intensity of each bout of exercise and any associated recovery periods. Also, practitioners commonly use heart rate to prescribe training intensities based on the linear relationship between heart rate and $\dot{V}O_2$ across a range of submaximal steady-state exercise workloads (115). Limitations exist, however, when using heart rate to determine intensities for intermittent exercise involving short bursts of high-intensity maximal activity (38).

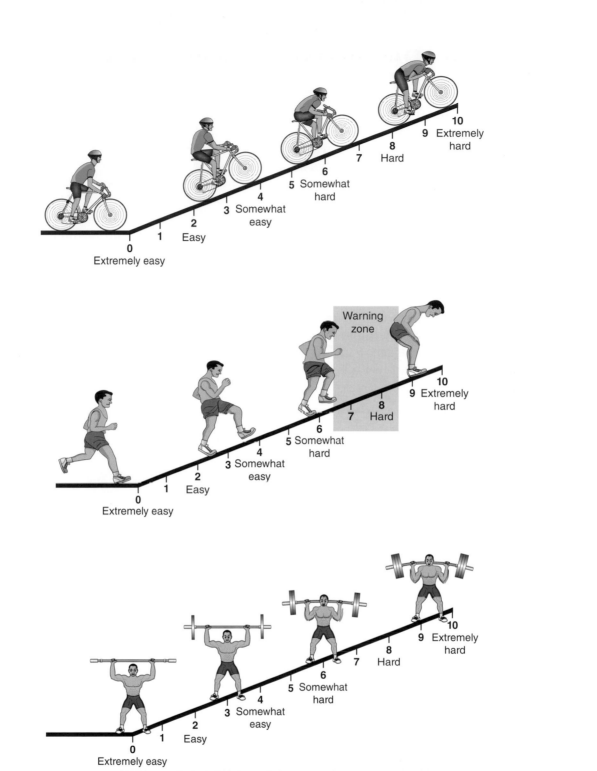

Figure 4.2 Pictorial representations for the OMNI RPE scales for cycling, running, and resistance training.

Reprinted, by permission, from R.J. Robertson, 2004, *Perceived exertion for practitioners* (Champaign, IL: Human Kinetics), 11.

SESSION LOAD, MONOTONY, AND STRAIN CALCULATION

Practitioners need to be mindful of how calculation methods affect the results of their load calculations. Traditionally, they have relied on session load or RPE alone for monitoring; adding in measures of strain and monotony can develop a full picture of what is happening with the athlete across the training cycle.

Figure 4.3 shows how the training load, monotony, and strain are calculated using the session RPE method. It is important to note that the way these calculations are performed can have a significant impact on the results. Practitioners need to decide how to approach rest days and be aware that most high-performance athletes are training more than once a day (a factor that needs to be included in the calculations). The practitioner can also include calculations of rolling averages across the days and weeks to look at patterns emerging from the monitoring data (chapter 2). Also, practitioners need to be aware of the methods of calculation used when comparing the results of the monitoring data to published research. Good practice involves collecting information over a period of time, becoming familiar with the scales, and using the same tool or tools consistently. Figure 4.4 shows a plot of training load, monotony, and strain for an elite athlete over the course of a year.

Figure 4.3 Training load, monotony, and strain calculations in an elite athlete.

Day	Session type	Duration (min)	RPE	Session load	Daily average
Monday	Gym	60	6	360	360
Tuesday	Field	120	7	840	
	Field	75	6	450	645
Wednesday	Gym	60	7	420	
	Field	120	8	960	690
Thursday	Track	60	8	480	
	Field	120	6	720	600
Friday	Gym	75	6	450	
	Field	150	7	1,050	750
Saturday	Gym	90	7	6 30	630
Sunday	Recovery	30	1	30	30
Total weekly load				6,390	
Daily mean load				529.29	
Daily standard deviation				252.00	
Monotony				2.10	
Strain				13,419	

The total weekly load is calculated as the sum of all the session loads. Daily mean load is then calculated by taking the average of all the daily averages. Daily standard deviation is the standard deviation of those daily averages. Monotony is calculated as daily mean load divided by daily standard deviation. Strain is calculated as total weekly load multiplied by monotony.

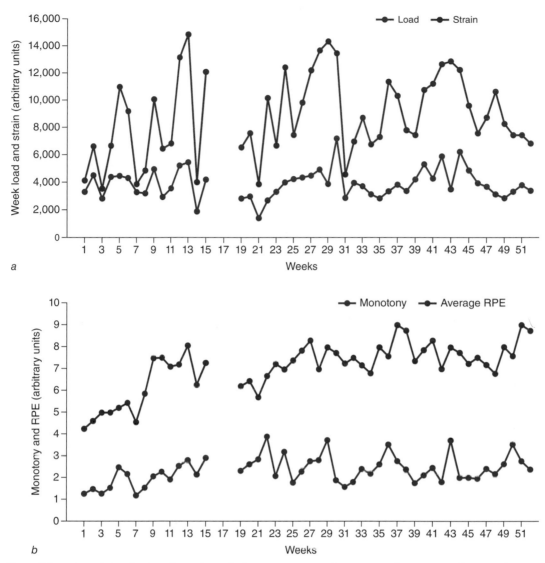

Figure 4.4 *(a)* Training load and strain and *(b)* monotony and RPE over the course of 1 year for an elite athlete.

A range of heart rate monitors are available for use in athlete monitoring. Standard heart rate monitors consist of a transducer worn around the chest that transmits wirelessly to a display. Others use sensors on a wristband, fingertip meter, or smartphone. Monitors that use a chest band, however, are more accurate and valid (170). Heart rate monitors are available from companies such as Polar Electro (www.polar.com) and Suunto (www.suunto.com).

Resting heart rate has been a popular method for assessing training status for many years (103). Given that longitudinal studies have reported a large amount of variability in resting heart rate (26), it appears to have a somewhat limited use for athlete monitoring. Heart rate recovery and heart rate variability are two common heart rate–based methods for athlete monitoring. These are discussed in more detail in chapter 5.

Lactate

As discussed in chapter 3, lactate is one of the most widely measured physiological markers and can be an indication of internal load. Portable systems and the use of finger prick samples have increased the utility of this measure. Issues still exist with obtaining regular samples from athletes during exercise to enable accurate monitoring and training prescription. Moreover, large intra- and interindividual differences occur with lactate concentrations depending on factors such as glycogen availability, environmental conditions, hydration, type of exercise, and sampling techniques (26). Recently developed systems that do not require taking blood samples appear to have good validity (23). In addition, near-infrared spectroscopy technology has the potential to monitor lactate levels. The portable and noninvasive nature of all of these technologies means that they can be used in the field for athlete monitoring.

Training Impulse

Practitioners are always looking for ways to quantify and reduce training to a single metric. A range of heart rate measures can be used to quantify the **training impulse (TRIMP)**. Practitioners can think of TRIMP as the total training load imposed on the athlete during the exercise bout (10, 31). It is based on a systems model approach that integrates all the components of training into a single value. This mathematical model can be used to describe and estimate the effects of a training session or program on an athlete's performance (26), but the practitioner must know the athlete's resting heart rate and maximal heart rate. TRIMP is calculated using the following equation:

$$TRIMP = D \times (\Delta \text{ heart rate ratio}) \times e^{(b \times \Delta \text{ heart rate ratio})}$$

where D = session duration, the constant $e = 2.718$, and the weighting factor $b = 1.67$ for women and 1.92 for men (133) and where Δ heart rate ratio = (average heart rate during exercise − resting heart rate) ÷ (maximal heart rate during exercise − resting heart rate).

The weighting factor b is used to emphasize the greater stress of higher-intensity training and reflects the generalized curve of exercise intensity and blood lactate (which is different for men and women) (133).

Consider a male athlete who completes a 60-min training session. During the workout, his average heart rate was 150 beats/min and his maximal heart rate was 180 beats/min. At rest, his heart rate is 45 beats/min.

$$\Delta \text{ heart rate ratio} = (150 \text{ beats/min} - 45 \text{ beats/min}) \div (180 \text{ beats/min} - 45 \text{ beats/min}) = 105 \div 135 = 0.78$$

$$D = 60 \text{ min}, e = 2.718, \text{ and } b = 1.92$$

$$TRIMP = 60 \times 0.78 \times 2.718^{(1.92 \times 0.78)} = 60 \times 0.78 \times 4.47 = 209.20$$

An alternative approach to TRIMP involves calculating an exercise score for each training session (47, 57). Sometimes referred to as the Edwards method (47), it involves multiplying the duration of the session by a multiplier determined by the intensity band or zone; the heart rate is expressed as a percentage of peak heart rate. For example:

$$\text{zone 1} = 50\text{-}60\% \ HR_{peak}$$

$$\text{zone 2} = 60\text{-}70\% \ HR_{peak}$$

$$\text{zone 3} = 70\text{-}80\% \ HR_{peak}$$

zone 4 = 80-90% HR_{peak}

zone 5 = 90-100% HR_{peak}

This summated heart rate zone method can be calculated as

TRIMP = (duration in zone 1 × 1) +
(duration in zone 2 × 2) +
(duration in zone 3 × 3) +
(duration in zone 4 × 4) +
(duration in zone 5 × 5)

Consider a female athlete who completes a 90-min training session. During the workout she spends the following durations in each zone: 1 = 14 min, 2 = 10 min, 3 = 49 min, 4 = 11 min, and 5 = 6 min.

TRIMP = (14 × 1) + (10 × 2) + (49 × 3) +
(11 × 4) + (6 × 5) = 14 + 20 + 147 +
44 + 30 = 255

Borresen and Lambert (25) investigated the relationship between the Edwards method and session RPE for quantifying training load. The results showed that in athletes who spent a greater amount of their training time performing higher-intensity activities, the heart rate–based methods overestimated training load; in athletes who spent more time doing lower-intensity activities, the session RPE method overestimated training load. Limitations of the equations that use a weighting factor are due to the range of heart rates within an intensity band and the fact that a difference of 1 to 2 beats/min can greatly affect the result (25).

Another option developed by Lucia and colleagues (112) is to use heart rate zones that are below the ventilatory threshold (low intensity), between the ventilatory threshold and the respiratory compensation point (moderate intensity), and above the respiratory compen-

sation point (high intensity). **Ventilatory threshold** refers to the break point in the respiratory rate during incremental exercise relative to $\dot{V}O_2$ (i.e., when breathing suddenly begins to increase at a faster rate) (101). The respiratory compensation point is reached at a higher $\dot{V}O_2$ than the ventilatory threshold when hyperventilation occurs (101). The method of Busso and colleagues (30) simplifies the TRIMP equation by multiplying the session duration by the average fraction of maximal aerobic power throughout the exercise bout.

Limitations of Heart Rate–Based Methods

Heart rate–based methods have several limitations when used for determining internal load. First, they require practitioners to measure and monitor an athlete consistently, which is impractical when working with a large number of athletes. Also, athletes must wear heart rate monitors during exercise. Further, heart rate–based methods are not ideal for modes of exercise such as resistance training and interval training. Busso and colleagues (30) attempted to use a TRIMP measure with weightlifters by incorporating the percentage of 1RM and the number of repetitions rather than duration. Traditionally, though, TRIMP measures have been used with aerobic endurance activities. Practitioners also require a level of technical ability to accurately analyze and interpret heart rate data. Moreover, issues such as technology failure can result in missing data, which limits the usefulness of the information.

Despite these limitations, heart rate–based methods can be valuable for monitoring training load in aerobic endurance activities. As a result, calculating

TRIMP and session RPE are now popular methods of quantifying training load in athletes. However, practitioners who are prescribing training sessions based on these measures need to ensure that they accurately quantify internal load. This provides further support for the recommendation to use multiple methods when monitoring athletes.

Wellness Assessments

Practitioners and athletes commonly use questionnaires and training diaries to quantify training (82). Because of the subjective nature of these tools, it is important to evaluate their effectiveness. Borresen and Lambert (24) found that 24% of athletes overestimated and 17% underestimated training duration in training diaries. Only 59% of the athletes accurately reported the average training duration for the week. Foster and colleagues noted a moderate relationship between the coach-prescribed training load ($r = .72$), training duration ($r = .65$), and training intensity ($r = .75$) and what the athletes actually did (58). As mentioned in chapter 1, coaches and athletes differ in their perceptions of what occurs in training and how hard the sessions are (28, 58, 146, 180). Thus, practitioners should be somewhat cautious about relying on athletes' self-reported information to guide training prescription.

Because each athlete's response to training stress is unique, a variety of wellness measures have been developed. Typically, they ask athletes about their levels of stress, muscle soreness, mood, fatigue, motivation, coping, and sleep. Questions about recovery and nutrition are often included as well. As discussed in chapter 3, athletes who experience overreaching or overtraining have higher mood disturbances. Therefore, wellness assessments can be very useful for determining athletes' levels of stress (82) and identifying when they are at greater risk of becoming ill or injured (160). Similar to session RPE, the biggest advantage of wellness assessments is that they are easy to implement and inexpensive. They should, however, be used in conjunction with other monitoring metrics such as performance tests, physiological measures, and training load.

Many wellness questionnaires have been studied in a range of athlete populations (76, 160). Questionnaires that assess mood state, training distress, muscle soreness, life demands, recovery, and other aspects of athlete wellness can be found in the literature (76, 160). Practitioners often use their own questionnaires because published questionnaires have too many items and thus take too much time to complete and analyze and because they lack sport specificity (169). Unfortunately, research into the effectiveness of these custom-designed questionnaires is limited.

Mood State Questionnaires

Mood state tools such as the Profile of Mood States (POMS) and the **Brunel Mood Scale (BRUMS)** (www.mood profiling.com) are questionnaires that provide information about an athlete's overall disposition and look at factors such as tension, vigor, anger, depression, and fatigue. The POMS questionnaire has 65 items that measure six moods, or feelings: tension–anxiety, depression–dejection, anger–hostility, vigor–activity, fatigue–inertia, and confusion–bewilderment (119). The athlete rates each item on a 5-point Likert scale from 0 = *not at all* to 4 = *extremely* in terms of what best describes how they feel right now. Research has shown relationships between training load and mood state measured using the POMS questionnaire (77, 150).

Practitioners should not rely on a single questionnaire to determine mood state because many factors can affect the results. The advantages of the POMS questionnaire, particularly the short version, are that it is easy to administer to a group of athletes and a solid foundation of research supports its use (119, 160). Also, the POMS questionnaire is robust enough that it is possible to examine how an athlete answers a subset of the questions. For example, a practitioner might be interested only in the responses related to fatigue–inertia when monitoring an athlete's fatigue level. Figure 4.5 shows a variety of internal load meas-

ures, including a POMS measure, using line graphs (see chapter 2).

The BRUMS questionnaire, derived from the POMS questionnaire, was developed to provide a quick assessment of mood state in adolescents and adults (171, 172). This 24-item questionnaire uses the same 5-point Likert scale as the POMS questionnaire, which has 65 items. Because the average completion time for the BRUMS is only 1 to 2 min, it has good practical application (105). It could be used, for example, prior to training sessions or as a quick assessment of athlete mood state.

Training Distress

The **Training Distress Scale (TDS)** assesses training-related distress and readiness

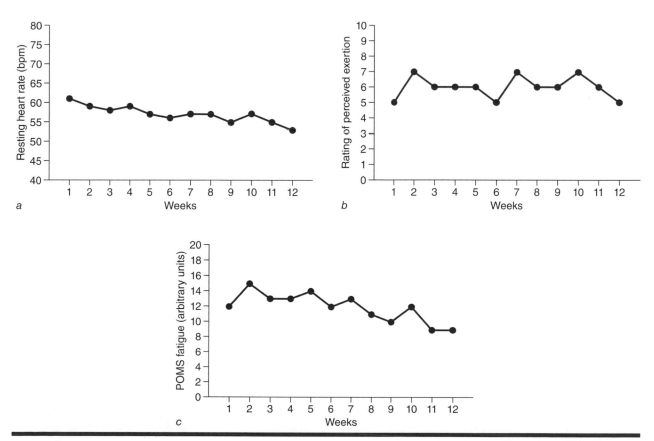

Figure 4.5　Measures of (a) heart rate, (b) RPE, and (c) wellness in runners over a 12-week training block.

to perform (72). An advantage of this short (22 questions) scale is that it includes mood disturbance, stress, and behavioral subscales. Plus, it assesses distress symptoms such as general fatigue, difficulties with concentration, sleep disturbance, changes in appetite, and physical discomfort (59). Athletes rate the extent to which they have experienced the symptoms in the previous 24 hours on a 5-point Likert scale with 0 = *not at all* and 4 = *extreme*. The laboratory and field-based validation studies on a range of athletes by Grove and colleagues (72) showed that the TDS is a valid measure of training and performance readiness in athletes.

Muscle Soreness

Delayed-onset muscle soreness (DOMS), which occurs 24 to 48 hours following a hard training session, is a natural and expected response in athletes. The large body of research about the causes of DOMS points to inflammation as the cause (83). Issues can arise when DOMS limits the athlete's training; there is evidence that training with sore muscles while trying to sustain a high training load can lead to overreaching (121). Therefore, it is important to monitor the degree of muscle soreness in athletes. **Visual analog scales (VAS)** are a common method used to measure DOMS (107, 139) and can also be used to assess training intensity (124, 135, 149).

Figure 4.6 shows a VAS scale for pain. On this 100-mm scale, the 0 represents no pain and 100 represents extreme, or unbearable, pain. A pain rating index can then be calculated and the intensity of pain determined by the distance (in mm) of the athlete's mark on the scale from the left-hand side. A CR-10 scale for pain has also been used, which rates the pain from 0 for no pain to 10 for maximal pain.

Practitioners are often interested in muscle soreness in a particular region or regions of the body (e.g., the quadriceps or the whole lower body) and ask athletes to rate soreness or pain in those areas. More complex questionnaires investigate the multidimensional aspects of pain such as sensory and emotional aspects. The **McGill Pain Questionnaire** consists of 78 words from which athletes select those that best describe their pain (122). Cleather and Guthrie (36) compared the McGill Pain Questionnaire and the VAS for the pain rating of DOMS. They found no significant differences in the ratings of DOMS following resistance training, suggesting no great advantage for using the McGill Pain Questionnaire.

Practitioners using the VAS for rating the intensity of training sessions can replace the terms in figure 4.6 with *not intense at all* and *extremely intense*. Research suggests that the VAS and CR-10 scale can be used interchangeably for measuring the intensity of training

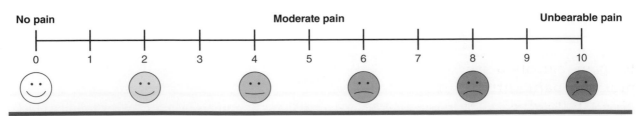

Figure 4.6 VAS for muscle soreness.

(135). Neely and colleagues (135) found that the CR-10 and VAS scale could be used to measure the degree of leg exertion during cycling exercise in young men. The CR-10 appeared to be more sensitive, although particularly at higher levels of intensity possibly because of its ability to discriminate between the levels with the use of the verbal anchors. The session RPE scale has been compared to the CR-10 and VAS and shown to provide the same information (124, 125). Rebelo and colleagues (149) studied a modification of the VAS scale to assess training load in football players. Two scales were used that ranged from *no effort at all* to *maximal effort* and *not demanding at all* to *maximally demanding*. They used this to calculate session load by multiplying the VAS score by the duration of the session. This method obtained the same information as the TRIMP calculation using the Banister (see chapter 3) and Edwards methods.

Palpation is also used to assess the degree of DOMS because athletes may not notice muscle soreness without some type of mechanical stimulus. It is possible to measure the pain objectively by using a specially designed pressure probe to standardize palpation; this is commonly used in research studies (107). Studies have shown that using a subjective pain assessment scale that ranges from 0 to 10 (0 = *no pain*, 10 = *maximal pain*) is as accurate as using a probe (104, 164), however. It is possible to use ratings of different regions of the body to obtain an accurate picture of where the DOMS is occurring (107).

Lau and colleagues (107) compared different methods of measuring muscle soreness, including a VAS, a CR-10 scale for pain, palpation at various sites, and pressure-pain thresholds (pain mapping), following eccentric exercise of the elbow flexors. This comprehensive analysis showed that the VAS was preferable over the CR-10 scale for rating pain (107). The VAS appears to be more sensitive and provides better resolution for measuring pain, but the CR-10 scale more effectively rates perceived exertion (135).

Wellness Inventory

Wellness inventories can be used to monitor athletes. Most gather ratings of perceived muscle soreness, general well-being, fatigue, stress, and sleep; some also incorporate questions about nutrition and recovery. An example is the **Hooper index**, which uses ratings of fatigue, stress, muscle soreness, and sleep on a scale from 1 (*very, very low, or good*) to 7 (*very, very high, or bad*) (81). Questionnaires may also include aspects of illness by asking athletes whether they are currently sick and listing some common symptoms (e.g., runny nose, sore throat, cough) (173). Further, specific regions of the body (e.g., low back, quadriceps, hamstrings, calves, groin, upper body) can be rated for the degree of muscle soreness. The inventories often use Likert scales (e.g., 0 = *a complete absence of soreness* to 6 = *severe pain*) (86).

Most practitioners use self-designed questionnaires; a survey of high-performance sport practitioners suggests that 80% use their own questionnaires (169). Research has shown that these questionnaires are sensitive to detecting changes in measures of stress and fatigue in elite athletes (118, 126, 160). Table 4.1 shows an example of a wellness questionnaire (118) for rating sleep quality, muscle soreness, stress, and fatigue; the scores are summed to obtain an overall wellness score. Lower scores indicate a better perception of overall well-being, and higher scores indicate a worse sense of well-being. Z-scores or standard difference scores can then be calculated

TABLE 4.1   Wellness Questionnaire for Sleep Quality, Muscle Soreness, Stress Levels, and Fatigue

	1	2	3	4	5	Score
Sleep quality	Very poor	Poor	Average	Good	Very good	
Muscle soreness	Very sore	High	Average	Low	Very low	
Stress level	Very stressed	High	Average	Low	Very low	
Fatigue level	Very fatigued	High	Average	Low	Very low	
Total						

(chapter 2). Custom-designed forms typically have 4 to 12 items that are measured using either 1-5 or 0-6 Likert scales (169). Questionnaires are easy to administer, are inexpensive, and provide quick feedback to practitioners and athletes.

Several modifications of wellness questionnaires are available. A questionnaire by Chatard and colleagues (32) includes eight items, and each question is assessed on a 7-point scale from 1 = *not at all* to 7 = *very much*. The items are training exertion, sleep quality, muscle soreness, illness, concentration, training efficiency, anxiety or irritability, and general stress (32). This questionnaire was developed as a sensitive measure of training load and performance in swimmers (6). The English translation of the **French Society for Sports Medicine questionnaire** (50) consists of 54 items that require a *yes* or *no* response. A total of more than 20 *yes* answers suggests excessive training load or overtraining (114). It also contains six items in which athletes rate their physical states on a VAS.

Given the importance of sleep for athletes, questionnaires are available that can determine this aspect of athlete recovery (100). One questionnaire asks athletes to record aspects of sleep in the morning upon waking (100). They record how long it took them to go to sleep (sleep latency) and whether and for how long they woke up (referred to as sleep fragmentation and wake after sleep onset). The quality of sleep can also be rated using a Likert scale in which 1 indicates very poor sleep and 5 indicates very good sleep. Activity monitors such as actigraphs and wearable devices can be used to provide more objective measures of sleep, although their validity has been questioned (156).

Daily Analysis of Life Demands for Athletes

The Daily Analysis of Life Demands for Athletes (**DALDA**) questionnaire assesses athletes' daily levels of stress (figure 4.7), thereby providing a record of their psychological well-being and response to training. Part A includes questions about general stresses, and part B covers stress-reaction symptoms. Each item is scored by marking *worse than normal, normal,* or *better than normal.*

Figure 4.7   DALDA questionnaire.

Initials _____ Trial day _____ Date _____

Circle the correct response for this moment: 1 = worse than normal; 2 = normal; 3 = better than normal.

PART A							
1. Diet	1	2	3	6. Climate	1	2	3
2. Home life	1	2	3	7. Sleep	1	2	3
3. School/college/ work	1	2	3	8. Recreation	1	2	3
4. Friends	1	2	3	9. Health	1	2	3
5. Sport training	1	2	3				
				Total			
PART B							
1. Muscle pains	1	2	3	14. Enough sleep	1	2	3
2. Techniques	1	2	3	15. Recovery between sessions	1	2	3
3. Tiredness	1	2	3	16. General weakness	1	2	3
4. Need for a rest	1	2	3	17. Interest	1	2	3
5. Supplementary work	1	2	3	18. Arguments	1	2	3
6. Boredom	1	2	3	19. Skin rashes	1	2	3
7. Recovery time	1	2	3	20. Congestion	1	2	3
8. Irritability	1	2	3	21. Training effort	1	2	3
9. Weight	1	2	3	22. Temper	1	2	3
10. Throat	1	2	3	23. Swellings	1	2	3
11. Internal	1	2	3	24. Likeability	1	2	3
12. Unexplained aches	1	2	3	25. Runny nose	1	2	3
13. Technique strength	1	2	3				
				Total			

"A tool for measuring stress tolerance in elite athletes," B.S. Bushall, *Journal of Applied Sport Psychology* 2(1): 51-66, 1990 Taylor and Francis, reprinted by permission of the publisher (Taylor & Francis Ltd, http://www.tandfonline.com).

The DALDA questionnaire can be administered during the training year and is easily scored by the practitioner. The results are best interpreted using graphs and can show trends in the athlete's ability to cope with training and stress levels. Practitioners can use this information to plan subsequent training sessions. The DALDA questionnaire is not designed for comparing athletes; rather, it is for tracking individual athletes over the course of a year or season.

Recovery Stress Questionnaire for Athletes

The Recovery Stress Questionnaire for Athletes (**RESTQ-Sport**), which provides a measure of perceived stress and recovery in athletes (96), is one of the most widely used questionnaires in athlete monitoring (160, 169). It is comprises 76 questions divided into 19 scales; 7 scales relate to general stress, 5 relate to general recovery, 3 relate to stress in sport, and 4 relate to specific recovery in sport. The items are rated on a Likert scale ranging from 0 (*never*) to 6 (*always*). The sum of the stress and recovery scales is calculated along with the differences between them. Table 4.2 shows an overview of the RESTQ-Sport scale.

The RESTQ-Sport has been found to be sensitive to both acute and chronic training load (160). Saw and colleagues (160) found the fatigue subscale and three recovery subscales to respond to both acute and chronic training load. Collapsing the subscales into a single score for stress and recovery seems to provide different information. This highlights for practitioners the importance of considering the subscales as well as the overall score when analyzing the results from this questionnaire.

Given practitioners' concerns regarding the time required to complete questionnaires, using shortened versions of the RESTQ-Sport might be worth considering (169). The original RESTQ-Sport is probably more suitable for weekly application, but practitioners should also obtain more regular insight into the wellness of their athletes. The Short RESTQ-Sport has 32 items that cover physical, mental, emotional, and overall aspects of stress and recovery (99). Subscales of particular interest to practitioners (e.g., injury or fatigue) may also be available. The Short RESTQ-Sport has been developed with eight items: physical performance capability, mental performance capability, emotional balance, overall recovery, muscular stress, lack of activation, negative emotional state, and overall stress. Each item is rated on a scale from 0 (*does not apply at all*) to 6 (*fully applies*). The validity of these questionnaires has been confirmed in the literature (99). The results are best viewed in a figure to see the trends and differences in the scales (figure 4.8).

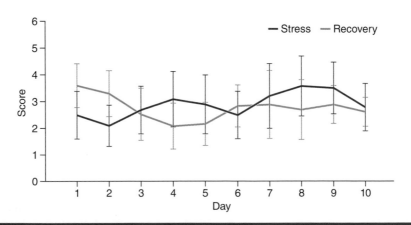

Figure 4.8   Athlete RESTQ-Sport scores over a preseason training phase.

TABLE 4.2 RESTQ-Sport Scale

Scale		Scale summary
1	**General stress**	Subjects with high values describe themselves as being frequently mentally stressed, depressed, unbalanced, and listless.
2	**Emotional stress**	Subjects with high values experience frequent irritation, aggression, anxiety, and inhibition.
3	**Social stress**	High values match subjects with frequent arguments, fights, irritation concerning others, general upset, and lack of humor.
4	**Conflicts/pressure**	High values are reached if in the preceding few days conflicts were unsettled, unpleasant things had to be done, goals could not be reached, and certain thoughts could not be dismissed.
5	**Fatigue**	Time pressure in job, training, school, and life; being constantly disturbed during important work; overfatigue; and lack of sleep characterize this area of stress.
6	**Lack of energy**	This scale matches ineffective work behavior such as inability to concentrate and lack of energy and decision making.
7	**Physical complaints**	Physical indisposition and physical complaints related to the whole body are characterized by this scale.
8	**Success**	Success, pleasure at work, and creativity during the past few days are assessed in this area.
9	**Social recovery**	High values are shown by athletes who have frequent pleasurable social contacts and change combined with relaxation and amusement.
10	**Physical recovery**	Physical recovery, physical well-being, and fitness are characterized in this area.
11	**General well-being**	Besides frequent good moods and high well-being, general relaxation and contentment are also in this scale.
12	**Sleep quality**	Enough recovering sleep, an absence of sleeping disorders while falling asleep, and sleeping through the night characterize recovery sleep.
13	**Disturbed breaks**	This scale deals with recovery deficits, interrupted recovery, and situational aspects that get in the way during periods of rest (e.g., teammates, coaches).
14	**Burnout/emotional exhaustion**	High scores are shown by athletes who feel burned out and want to quit their sport.
15	**Fitness/injury**	High scores signal an acute injury or vulnerability to injuries.
16	**Fitness/being in shape**	Athletes with high scores describe themselves as fit, physically efficient, and vital.
17	**Burnout/personal accomplishment**	High scores are reached by athletes who feel integrated in their team, communicate well with their teammates, and enjoy their sport.
18	**Self-efficacy**	This scale is characterized by how convinced the athlete is that he/she has trained well and is optimally prepared.
19	**Self-regulation**	The use of mental skills for athletes to prepare, push, motivate, and set goals for themselves are assessed by this scale.

Reprinted, by permission, from M. Kellmann and K.W. Kallus, 2001, *Recovery-stress questionnaire for athletes: User manual* (Champaign, IL: Human Kinetics), 6-7.

Total Quality Recovery Scale

Given the importance of recovery, monitoring this aspect of the athlete's program may be useful (98). The **Total Quality Recovery** scale is based on the Borg 6-20 scale. According to Kentta and Hassmen (98), the primary aspects of this assessment are perceived recovery and action recovery. Athletes rate their recovery over the previous 24 hours using the question "What is your condition now?" The scale can also be adapted to the 0-10 scale, as follows:

Modified Total Quality Recovery Scale

  0 Very, very poor recovery

  1 Very poor recovery

  2

  3 Poor recovery

  4

  5 Reasonable recovery

  6

  7 Good recovery

  8

  9 Very good recovery

10 Very, very good recovery

To measure recovery, athletes score themselves in four main categories over the previous 24 hours: nutrition and hydration, sleep and rest, relaxation and emotional support, and stretching and active rest. Points are given for each aspect of questionnaire (20 points maximum). A score of less than 13 indicates incomplete recovery from training (98). This system has been modified widely and is used in many high-performance programs. All systems award points for various recovery strategies and set a target for each day or week. Very little research exists on the effectiveness of this approach (103). However, the system is easy to implement and has practical application.

Another recovery tool is the **Perceived Recovery Status Scale**, which assesses changes in performance (108). The scale ranges from 0 (*very poorly recovered and extremely tired*) to 10 (*very well recovered and highly energetic*). One study showed that this scale has the potential for monitoring recovery following heavy resistance training (165). Scores of 0 to 2 may indicate underperformance, which makes this scale potentially useful as a marker of training readiness. However, more research is needed in athletic populations to confirm this (35).

Guidelines for Wellness Measures

The implementation of wellness measures determines whether the results will positively affect an athlete's training program (160). Saw and colleagues completed a study of the factors that influence the implementation of wellness measures in sport (159). The study involved semistructured interviews with a range of athletes (*n* = 8), coaches (*n* = 7), and sport science and medical staff (*n* = 15) from a national sport institute in Australia representing 20 sports. The authors found the social environment to be critical for helping with athlete buy-in and coordinating those involved in the monitoring. The perceived connection of the questionnaire to athletes' goals and its contribution to their training were particularly important motivators (159).

Practitioners must educate coaches and athletes about the need for honest and accurate answers in wellness questionnaires. This will help alleviate coaches' concerns that athletes may give false responses to either avoid training or hide illness or injury from the coaching staff. Practitioners should never rely on a single questionnaire as the basis of their monitoring programs. The results from any questionnaire need to be considered in context with the results of other measures. Questionnaires that cover a wide range of self-report measures but ask a smaller number of questions are ideal (67, 160). Ultimately, practitioners need to consider the design of the questionnaire and the factors that could influence the data (159). It is also important that the wellness measures be taken at the same time of day (103).

The most useful measures appear to be perceived muscle soreness, fatigue, wellness, and sleep duration and quality. Measures can be collected on a regular basis; one study reported that 55% of practitioners collect this information daily (169). However, athletes required to answer the same questions every day can develop questionnaire fatigue. Wellness measures collected during a period of a regular training load to determine the athlete's normal variation can help practitioners determine appropriate thresholds. It may not be appropriate to determine these thresholds during periods of low loading or high loading because these periods have been associated with mood disturbances and potential maladaptations (123).

The time needed to analyze the questionnaires and provide feedback to athletes and coaches is another important consideration. Well-designed questionnaires should result in quality information without placing great demands on athletes and practitioners. Before designing their own questionnaires, practitioners should consider the many validated questionnaires available. They should be aware, however, that just because a questionnaire has been designed and implemented does not mean that it is reliable

and valid. Also, athletes responding to questionnaires are influenced by the wording of the question and its context and format (159, 161).

Technology can help with the implementation of questionnaires (159). Many practitioners have their athletes complete questionnaires on smartphones or tablets (1). Research conducted in the area of injury prevention and monitoring shows the value of using technology in this way (48, 49). Using apps and incorporating social media may also increase athlete buy-in and compliance.

Analysis of Wellness Questionnaires

A variety of methods can be used to analyze the results of wellness questionnaires (see chapter 2). Likert scales are commonly used, and higher scores generally indicate greater well-being. The usual practice is to code the responses as numbers and then perform calculations. Because of the categorical nature of these types of questionnaires, the types of calculations that can be used are limited. Analysis methods more meaningful than simply calculating the mean are suggested. A survey by Taylor and colleagues (169) revealed that the most commonly used method was to observe trends in an athlete's data over successive days and sessions.

Some practitioners identify red flags that indicate meaningful changes in performance (e.g., ±1.5 standard deviation away from the mean) (118). Others use a traffic light system with red, yellow, and green lights signifying set thresholds that indicate required actions. A red light might indicate the need for a certain intervention, a yellow light might indicate the need for a closer inspection of all monitoring data, and a green light might signify that everything is fine and the athlete can train as normal. For muscle soreness, practitioners can use intraindividual standard deviation values to identify changes outside of the athlete's normal variation.

The lack of research on practically meaningful changes in wellness questionnaires limits practitioners' ability to make informed decisions about important thresholds and appropriate actions. They generally use wellness questionnaires to highlight potential problems with fatigue and recovery (169). Practitioners would likely benefit from applying some of the statistical approaches covered in chapter 2. Guidance on appropriate analysis methods is particularly limited in high-performance sport settings (159). A threshold value of ±1 can be used for wellness scales as a rough guide for the smallest meaningful change

(174). Figure 4.9 shows z-scores over the course of a training camp for a team sport athlete. A steady decline occurred in the wellness scores as a result of high training loads. Using the criteria of 1.5 standard deviations, this threshold was exceeded on days 8 and 9.

A fundamental consideration for practitioners is what intervention to implement once they have identified irregularities in athlete monitoring data. This is discussed in more detail in chapters 7 through 9. Using the example in figure 4.9, the practitioner could decide to reduce the training load after day 8 of the training camp for this athlete. What is clear is that a practical application of these monitoring strategies should be undertaken on a daily and weekly basis using a range of methods.

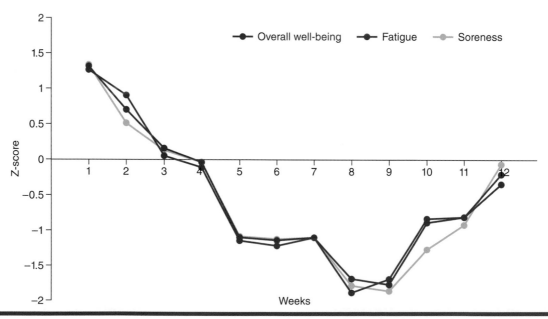

Figure 4.9 Tracking wellness in a training camp using composite wellness scores and identifying red flags.

Conclusion

Practitioners monitoring athlete training should consider both external and internal measures of load and accurately quantify the training stress. GPS, accelerometry, and power meters can be used to measure external load. When designing training programs, practitioners must understand the effect external training load has on the internal responses of their athletes. Measures of internal load such as heart rate, RPE, and TRIMP provide critical information about the athlete's response to stress. The subjective responses from wellness questionnaires can provide valuable information on the stress levels of athletes and their responses to training load. This can then be useful for detecting early signs of overreaching or overtraining. In particular, measures of mood disturbance (POMS, BRUMS), symptoms of stress (DALDA, TDS), and perceived stress and recovery (RESTQ-Sport, Total Quality Recovery, Perceived Recovery Status Scale) are useful. However, practitioners should use a combination of internal and external methods of monitoring training load to quantify the physiological stress of training and competition. They also need to consider how to analyze, interpret, and use this information to optimize athlete monitoring.

5

Measures of Fitness and Fatigue

Practitioners require objective tests to help them evaluate their training programs, assess their athletes' training and competition workloads, and monitor their fatigue. However, no single marker or test can do all of these things. Practitioners must therefore include a range of measures of fitness and fatigue (e.g., neuromuscular and wellness) in their athlete monitoring programs.

Many monitoring tests are used to assess athletes' physical performance. Several types are also widely used in research studies with athletes (91, 97, 194). However, many of these are not suitable for regular monitoring because of their low portability into the field, expense, unsuitability for testing large groups of athletes, lack of sensitivity, and poor reliability. An isokinetic dynamometer, for example, would be beyond the budget of most sport programs and may be logistically difficult to use to regularly monitor a squad of athletes. Monitoring tests must objectively measure fitness and fatigue while being practically viable. This chapter outlines measures of fitness and fatigue that can be used for athlete monitoring—specifically, neuromuscular fatigue; heart rate; biochemical, hormonal, and immunological markers; and performance tests.

Neuromuscular Fatigue

Tests to detect neuromuscular fatigue are widely used in high-performance sport (1, 91, 194). **Neuromuscular fatigue** refers to the reduction in maximal voluntary contractile force. As discussed in chapter 3, it is a result of deficits within the central nervous system, in the neural drive to the muscle, or within the muscle itself. A large body of research addresses the use of neuromuscular fatigue tests in sport (29, 38, 74, 91, 124, 210). However, because most were conducted in laboratory settings, their reliability and validity have not been established in sport settings.

Low-frequency fatigue is often of interest to practitioners (67). It is a result of high-intensity, high-force, repeated stretch–shortening cycles or eccentric (lengthening) muscle actions (104). It can be directly assessed with muscle or percutaneous (through the skin) stimulation using the **interpolated twitch technique**, which determines the activation level of skeletal muscle during a voluntary contraction (27, 156). However, because this method is not suited for regular athlete monitoring in most settings, other methods have been developed to indirectly assess low-frequency fatigue in activities such as running and jumping (41). These activities involve the stretch–shortening cycle in which the muscle acts like a spring: Absorbed energy is stored as elastic energy during the stretching phase and then recovered during the shortening contraction. Both slow (long) and fast (short) stretch–shortening cycle activities are found in sports. Slow stretch–shortening cycles (>0.25 s) occur in jumps performed in volleyball (long ground contact times and high displacements); fast stretch–shortening cycles (<0.25 s) occur in sprinting (short ground contact times and low displacements).

Vertical Jumps

Using vertical jumps to assess neuromuscular fatigue in athletes is a common approach, and good evidence now supports its efficacy (194). Taylor and colleagues (194) found that 54% of respondents to a survey on athlete monitoring in high-performance sport used some type of vertical jump test. The advantages of these tests are that they are easy and not fatiguing; athletes generally do not take issue with performing two or three jumps before a training session. Technological devices such as force plates, linear position transducers, accelerometers, and contact mats can be used for these tests. Jump height can also be assessed using a vertical jump apparatus or a tape measure. Smartphone apps that provide information during jumps are also available (5). Variables that can be measured using this technology include force, velocity, and displacement (73). Specific measures such as jump height, mean and peak power, mean and peak velocity, and peak force are popular with practitioners (194). Other measures such as the ratio of **flight time to contraction time** can also be useful for athlete monitoring (39). Flight time represents the time from takeoff to landing, and contraction time is measured as the time from the start of the vertical jump to takeoff (38). The ratio of flight time to contraction time gives the practitioner insights into the movement strategies athletes use during jumps. Gathercole and colleagues (73) suggested that relying solely on output measures from jump analyses such as jump height and power has limitations and that time-related variables are more sensitive to fatigue. Therefore, practitioners are encouraged to use more valid measures of fatigue such as flight time to contraction time.

Figure 5.1 shows a vertical countermovement jump performed by an athlete on a force plate. The athlete stands on the force plate (or contact mat) with hands on hips and is instructed to jump as high as possible with maximal effort. The depth of the vertical phase of the jump is self-selected. Alternatively, the test can be conducted using a measuring stick. It is also possible to measure jump height via smartphone apps (5). Having athletes perform the test next to a wall and mark with chalk the spots they reach is another alternative.

Reliability and Validity

Many research studies have been conducted to establish the validity and reliability of jumps as indicators of neuromuscular fatigue in athletes (38, 40, 72, 78, 100, 161). The general approach has been to gather the measures from matches and then track the variables over the course of the year—especially during the competitive season—to see how they change during periods of loading and unloading (68). Cormack and colleagues studied the effects of Australian rules football matches on neuromuscular fatigue (39) and also across a competitive season (40). This was done after establishing the reliability of the measures during single and repeat jump

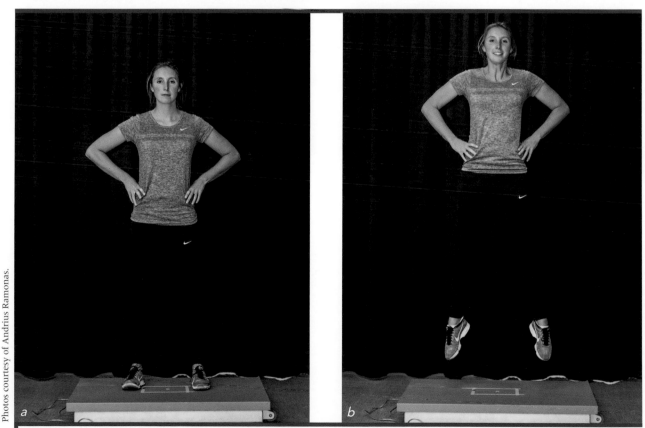

Photos courtesy of Andrius Ramonas.

Figure 5.1   Vertical countermovement jump of an athlete measured on a force plate: (*a*) starting position and (*b*) jump phase.

tests (41). Following match play, force plate testing revealed that the measures of 6 of 18 variables declined and the main performance measure (jump height) remained stable. The time courses of the changes in these variables following the match were also very different.

The lack of sensitivity of jump height is interesting given that it is commonly used in jump tests (46, 137). Studies have found no changes in measures such as jump height during periods of heavy training (31, 46). In many other studies, researchers have examined the use of jumps for detecting neuromuscular fatigue across a range of sports (40, 72, 75, 78, 100). Findings have been mixed, and little consensus currently exists about which variables are the most sensitive to fatigue. In a study of elite female rugby sevens players, Gathercole and colleagues (72) showed that variables such as flight time and jump height decreased with increasing fatigue. They also noted alterations in the jumping mechanics as indicated by changes in the time-dependent variables. The disparity of the findings is most likely due to the wide range of equipment, testing protocols, sports, and athlete levels used in these studies.

Practitioners have tended to focus on concentric aspects of jump performance. However, the eccentric phase of the vertical jump can also provide critical information (42, 43). Given the importance of the eccentric phase in stretch–shortening cycle activities, this should not be ignored by practitioners (42, 43). Looking at the force–time curve in its entirety provides a more complete picture of how the athlete is performing (42).

Jump Testing Protocols

A variety of jump testing protocols can be used in athlete monitoring. Single jumps are more time efficient than repeated jumps and therefore are typically recommended (137). Repeat jump testing also tends to be less reliable in athletes (41). Loaded jumps can also provide a measure of the athlete's ability to tolerate external load (137). Practitioners have the option of using an absolute (total) load or a relative (percentage of body weight or percentage of maximal strength) load with this type of monitoring (137). Laboratory-based studies of the relationship between low-frequency fatigue and changes in jump performance are not conclusive, so practitioners should not rely on these measures alone for athlete monitoring (67).

Monitoring jump height during vertical countermovement jumps may indicate the athlete's 1RM in the squat (103). Jimenez-Reyes and colleagues (103) tested track and field athletes and established regression equations to use with jump height to determine their 1-repetition maximum (1RM) squat. Other studies have determined that estimating 1RM from submaximal loads in various exercises is possible (102). Attempts have also been made to use rating of perceived exertion (RPE) to estimate variables such as power output during exercises (6). However, more research is needed to clearly establish the relationship between perceived exertion and training loads. As a guide for training, however, it can be useful.

Comparisons between bilateral and unilateral jumps can provide additional information on asymmetries (137). Awareness of an athlete's asymmetries may be important from both an injury prevention standpoint and a performance standpoint. In terms of performance, Bailey and colleagues (3) found a significant negative relationship between the degree of asymmetry and jumping performance in university athletes. Technology that allows for the assessment of jumps performed bilaterally but measured unilaterally with dual force plate systems can reveal asymmetries (105). Specific asymmetries can be measured without requiring the athlete to perform single-leg jumps. Athletes undergoing rehabilitation, for example, can benefit from performing bilateral jumps because they are less stressful than single-leg jumps.

The ratio of vertical jump height with countermovement to **static jump** height can be calculated as the **eccentric utilization ratio** (138). Vertical static jumps are performed using a similar protocol to vertical jumps, but the athlete pauses at the bottom of the jump for 2 to 3 s to remove the stretch–shortening cycle enhancement. The eccentric utilization ratio is calculated as follows:

Eccentric utilization ratio =
vertical countermovement jump
height ÷ vertical static jump height

Consider an athlete who jumps 48 cm (18.9 in.) on a vertical countermovement jump and 45 cm (17.7 in.) on a vertical static jump:

Eccentric utilization ratio =
48 ÷ 45 = 1.07

Variables such as jump height and peak power can be used in the calculation. A higher ratio represents a greater contribution of the stretch–shortening cycle (137). A low ratio could indicate that the athlete needs to perform more stretch–shortening cycle work such as plyometrics.

Technological devices such as linear position transducers provide information on displacement and velocity and give real-time feedback during a set and during individual repetitions of an exercise (95). A study by Randell and colleagues showed that athletes receiving real-time feedback using this type of technology achieved greater training gains (175). Several reviews provide an overview of the technology that can be used for athlete monitoring during resistance training (10, 95).

When monitoring jumps and performance tests, practitioners tend to focus on the numbers. However, examining and recording the athlete's technique can provide useful insights (72). This can be achieved by using measures that indicate the jump mechanics such as time to peak force and ratio of flight time to contraction time.

Practitioners should consider conducting their own research to establish which measures are most worth monitoring (see chapter 7). Common analysis methods rely on the visual analysis of trends or arbitrary thresholds (e.g., a 10% decrement) to identify fatigue (194). Methods outlined in chapter 2 are effective for analyzing this type of monitoring data.

Attempts have been made to assess training readiness with vertical countermovement jumps (32). In a study of recreationally trained men, Claudino and colleagues (32) used pretraining vertical countermovement jump testing to modify the subsequent plyometric session. They used **minimal individual difference** in jump height, which refers to the maximal variation of random error (212). If the participants were identified as fatigued or their performance had improved, adjustments were made to the training program. If they were fatigued, one set was removed from each exercise; if they had improved, one set was added. Although the results were not conclusive and the participants were relatively untrained, evidence suggested that this approach had resulted in performance

Drop Jumps

Drop jumps, which are also used to monitor neuromuscular fatigue, have been found to have adequate reliability (140). Because of the more reactive nature of drop jumps, they may be more sensitive to fatigue (94). For testing, the athlete stands in an upright position on a box with hands on hips (figure 5.2), steps (not jumps) off the box with the dominant leg, drops onto the force plate or contact mat on both feet, and immediately does a vertical jump with maximal effort.

The instructions given to the athlete should be standardized as much as possible (125). Asking the athlete to keep ground contact time as brief as possible and to jump as high as possible is a good strategy. The athlete can be told to think of the ground surface as a hot plate to ensure a short contact time. The height of the box used for this test can vary, but an intermediate height of 30 cm (12 in.) seems to be sufficient for monitoring purposes with team sport athletes (94). A range of jump heights can be used to develop a profile of the athlete and to determine the athlete's stretch tolerance profile. The **stretch tolerance profile** is a series of measures from drop jumps from increasing heights resulting in greater stretch. It provides another way of quantifying the athlete's reactive ability.

The **reactive strength index** can be determined from drop jump testing and has been proposed as a measure of explosiveness (155). It can be calculated in several ways, but typically it involves measuring the ratio of jump height to contact time (155). A force plate, contact mat, or device that measures jump height and contact time can be used. It is also possible to calculate the index as the ratio of flight time to contact time (139).

$$\text{Reactive strength index} = \text{jump height (m)} \div \text{contact time (s)}$$

Consider an athlete who performs a drop jump from a 40-cm (15.7 in.) box and achieves a jump height of 0.45 m (17.7 in.); the contact time was 0.298 s.

$$\text{Reactive strength index} = 0.45 \text{ m} \div 0.298 \text{ s} = 1.51$$

In a modified version of the reactive strength index, the ratio is calculated between the jump height and the contact time during a vertical countermovement jump rather than a drop jump (112, 191). Suchomel and colleagues used a loaded (20 kg, or 44 lb) and an unloaded vertical countermovement jump to calculate a modified reactive strength index (191, 192). The modified reactive strength index was found to be reliable for discriminating between athletes from different sports (192). Performing the test without boxes is an advantage because it removes the need for extra equipment. Whichever calculation is used for the reactive strength index, the practitioner must use the same protocol. It is also critical to be mindful of the testing protocol used in research studies in cases in which practitioners are comparing their results to published findings.

Muscle Stiffness

Muscle stiffness can also be used for athlete monitoring. At its simplest, stiffness refers to the relationship between force and the degree of deformation and is related to stretch–shortening cycle activities (143, 215). High levels of muscle stiffness have been shown to be related to increased soft tissue injury and repetitive stress (172, 209). Methods

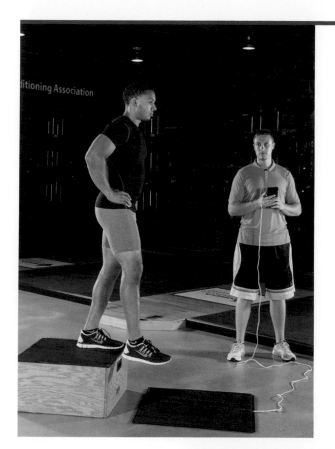
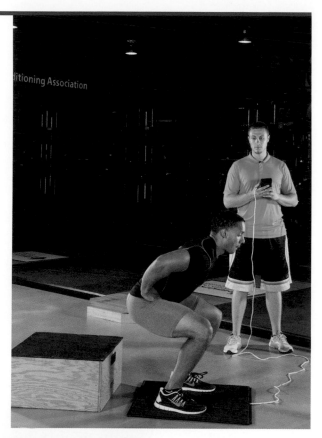
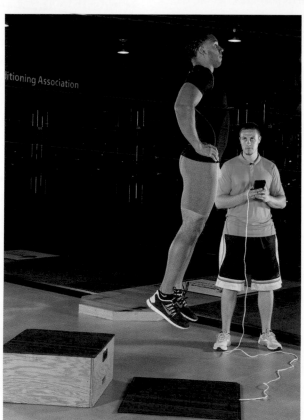

Figure 5.2 Drop jump on a contact mat.

for assessing muscle stiffness include the vertical hop, broad jump, and drop jump tests (144, 170). Vertical pogos and jumping bilaterally with straight legs are other possible methods. The vertical hop test (unilateral) can provide an overall measure of lower-body stiffness. The bilateral and unilateral tests can be performed on a contact mat or force plate. Often, they are performed using repeated jumps (e.g., five in succession) (143). Unilateral testing can reveal differences between the limbs and stiffness imbalances. In a repeat jump test, athletes are instructed to perform the jumps in time with a metronome or to maintain a steady frequency. The test generally has adequate reliability but is not as reliable as other types of jump tests (127, 171).

A common approach for calculating muscle stiffness is the Dalleau method (57). Alternatively, muscle stiffness can be calculated more simply as ground reaction force divided by displacement of the center of mass (126).

Force Production

Monitoring measures of muscular strength and power can help with exercise prescription, provide sensitive and immediate feedback to practitioners, and determine whether an athlete's training adaptations have plateaued (140). Strength assessments include isometric tests, repetition maximum tests, and dynamometry (139).

Isometric tests such as the isometric mid-thigh pull (86), isometric squat (7), and isometric bench press (216, 217) can help with the regular assessment of athletes' strength. Isometric tests have several advantages. First, they are highly reliable, particularly for variables such as peak force. Peak force measures from isometric tests have been shown to be very reliable; Coefficient of variation greater than 2% have consistently been reported (110, 197). Another advantage is that they also enable practitioners to test large groups of athletes in a more time-efficient manner than that provided by traditional 1RM testing. Maximal isometric testing correlates very well with 1RM for exercises such as the back squat, deadlift, and power clean (7). Finally, isometric testing is also relatively less fatiguing than 1RM testing, so it can theoretically be done more regularly.

The isometric mid-thigh pull test is typically performed on a force plate with a fixed bar at mid-thigh height; two or three trials are performed. Weightlifting straps and tape can be used to help with grip, and the athlete should be instructed to push as hard and as fast into the ground as possible for 3 to 5 s. Instructions are important for this type of testing; research shows differences in force production depending on the type of instruction (90). Providing 3 to 5 min of rest between trials is also recommended. However, evidence suggests that shorter rest periods do not affect maximal force-producing capability (131). Peak force can be expressed in absolute terms or relative to body weight, which is known as ratio scaling.

Allometric scaling (53) takes into account the body size of the athlete and can be used to compare across a range of body sizes. Allometric scaling equations, which describe the relationship between body mass and other aspects such as muscular strength (53), use an exponential factor in the calculation. The most commonly used scaling equation uses a simple power law function:

$$\text{Performance variable} = a \times \text{body mass}^b$$

where a is the scaling coefficient and b is the exponent term, and both are estimated from the data using regression.

To simplify the process for practitioners, the following formula can be used. Appropriate estimated exponent terms can be found in the literature, such as the article by Crewther and colleagues (53).

$$\text{Allometric scaled peak force} = \text{peak force} \div (\text{body mass}^{0.67})$$

For example, an athlete with a body mass of 90.5 kg (199.5 lb) generates a peak force of 4,218 N during the isometric mid-thigh pull test. The equation is as follows:

$$\text{Allometric scaled peak force} = 4218 \div (90.5^{0.67}) = 206.1 \text{ N}$$

Rate of force development can also be assessed as part of the isometric mid-thigh pull test. The **rate of force development** refers to the rate of change in the force–time curve and can be used as a measure of explosiveness in the athlete (87). Obtaining reliable and valid measures of an athlete's rate of force development requires very strict control of the testing conditions (e.g., straps improve reliability). The method used to analyze the rate of force development can make a large difference in the result (87). Predetermined time bands can be used (e.g., 0-50 ms and 0-200 ms) in addition to calculating the average rate of force development, but the reliability of these measures is questionable (87). Instead, practitioners should use peak force rather than rate of force development for athlete monitoring because it has the highest reliability. The test sensi-

tivity is another important consideration (see chapter 2). The research findings are somewhat inconsistent; no clear evidence shows that peak force changes significantly in responses to acute training load and fatigue (39).

Bilateral Versus Unilateral Assessment

Grip dynamometry has been proposed as a unilateral strength assessment for athlete monitoring (166). Grip strength assessments can be performed regularly because they are less fatiguing than other types of strength assessments. Whether this test can be used as a direct measure of training readiness is less clear, and no definitive studies show this to be the case.

Unilateral testing allows for the assessment of imbalances between the right and left sides of the body. **Bilateral asymmetry** can be calculated as a ratio as follows:

$$\text{Bilateral asymmetry} = \text{strength of the right side} \div \text{strength of the left side}$$

For example, an athlete has the following results on the unilateral leg press: right leg = 1,973 N; left leg = 1,730 N.

$$\text{Bilateral asymmetry} = 1,973 \text{ N} \div 1,730 \text{ N} = 1.14$$

The following equation can be used to express the imbalance as a percentage:

$$\text{Bilateral asymmetry} = [(\text{right leg} - \text{left leg}) \div \text{stronger leg}] \times 100$$

Using the preceding example,

$$\text{Bilateral asymmetry} = [(1,973 - 1,730) \div 1,973] \times 100 = 12.3\%$$

Bilateral asymmetry assessments can also allow practitioners to calculate the degree of the **bilateral deficit** (137). The bilateral deficit can be calculated as follows:

Bilateral deficit = [(strength of the right side + strength of the left side) ÷ bilateral strength] × 100

For example, an athlete has the following results on the unilateral leg press: right leg =1,973 N; left leg = 1,730 N; bilateral = 3,598 N.

Bilateral deficit = [(1,973 + 1,730) ÷ 3,598 N] × 100 = 102.9%

Force Measures for Rehabilitation Monitoring

Various force assessments have been used as potential predictors of injury. Tests such as the **groin (adductor) squeeze test** are used to monitor athletes (44, 150, 179). The groin squeeze test is conducted in a supine position using a sphygmomanometer between the legs, which are positioned at 45° (58). The athlete squeezes the device as hard as possible for several trials, and the maximal pressure achieved is recorded (58). A relationship between groin pain and lower-body strength levels on the adductor squeeze test has been found in athletes (150). Roe and colleagues (179) found decreases in adductor strength in youth rugby union players following match play. As a monitoring tool this test appears to be reliable and sensitive to fatigue.

Recently, assessments that look at the strength of the hamstrings have been used (22, 132, 163). McCall and colleagues (132) investigated the reliability and sensitivity of an isometric lower-limb hamstrings test in elite football players. The athletes performed the task in a supine position with the leg raised onto the force plate. The sensitivity of the test was determined by measuring the isometric strength following match play and by measuring muscle soreness (132).

Dynamic Strength Index

Combining measures from a variety of monitoring tests can provide interesting information on athletes' neuromuscular status. For example, the **dynamic strength index** has received attention from researchers (197, 216, 217). Practitioners have compared the isometric and dynamic force-producing capacities of athletes to determine which aspect needs priority in training programs. The dynamic strength index is calculated as the ratio of ballistic peak force from a static jump to isometric peak force (186), as follows:

Dynamic strength index = ballistic peak force (N) ÷ isometric peak force (N)

Consider an athlete who has the following results during a static jump and isometric mid-thigh pull, respectively (2,042 and 2,811 N):

Dynamic strength index = 2,042 N ÷ 2,811 N = 0.73

The dynamic strength index has been shown to be a highly reliable measure of strength qualities in athletes, and it can be used as a guide for training emphasis (197). A ratio of <0.6 could be an indication that the practitioner should increase the amount of ballistic training. A ratio of >0.8 could mean that the amount of maximal strength training needs to be increased. Ratios can be useful, but practitioners also need to take into account the magnitude of the result (186). By tracking the strength values from week to week across a season, they can observe trends in the results of individual athletes and compare them to the smallest meaningful change (see figure 5.3).

Considerations for Neuromuscular Fatigue Monitoring

The measures used to track athlete fatigue demonstrate a diurnal rhythm (195, 196). A study by Teo and colleagues (196) showed clear changes in measures of peak force and rate of force development during the isometric mid-thigh pull across the day, and maximal values were found later in the day. Taylor and colleagues (195) demonstrated that warming up extensively could remove some of the diurnal effects, but they still existed for most measures during vertical counter-movement jumps. These monitoring tests should be conducted at the same time of day to control for these effects. As outlined in chapter 3, it is important to attempt to control as many of these factors as possible when testing. Because neuromuscular fatigue is just one type of fatigue in athletes, practitioners should not rely on this measure alone for obtaining the full picture of how athletes are tracking.

Heart Rate

Physiological markers such as heart rate can be used as objective markers of fatigue (see chapter 4). Submaximal exercise protocols and measures of heart rate can provide valuable insights for athlete monitoring. These approaches are increasingly used in both team and individual sports (20, 23, 119). Heart rate variability and heart rate recovery can both be used to monitor fitness and fatigue.

Heart Rate Variability

Heart Rate Variability (**HRV**) is widely used in sport to provide insight into an athlete's readiness to train (169). HRV is a measure of the normal variation in beat-to-beat intervals, and it can be determined using several indices. One of the more reliable is the natural logarithm of the square root of the mean sum of squared differences between adjacent normal RR intervals (Ln rMSSD) (168). Very simply, this is a measure calculated over a period of time (e.g., 60 s), and the data are used to mathematically determine the beat-to-beat difference. The increased use of HRV for monitoring is

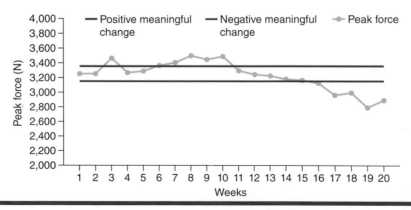

Figure 5.3 Maximal force measures over the course of a competitive season.

due to the improvements in the analysis software and heart rate monitor hardware as well as smartphone apps (see chapter 6).

As discussed in chapter 3, the autonomic nervous system controls physiological functions such as heart rate via the interaction between the sympathetic and parasympathetic nervous systems. During training, heart rate responds to periods of stress and rest in a nonlinear manner. That is, heart rate increases during high-intensity work (sympathetic response) and then decreases during periods of lower-intensity work or recovery (parasympathetic response). Low HRV is an indicator of the sympathetic system driving the heart rate response, which suggests that the athlete is not tolerating the training load (20). Because the research on athletes is somewhat inconsistent, practitioners should not rely on this single marker for athlete monitoring (169).

As discussed in chapter 3, findings from investigations of HRV as a marker of overreaching and overtraining are not clear (20). Indices such as Ln rMSSD have been shown to have better reliability and can be used for assessments over a short period of time (2, 64). This requires 10 to 60 s of measurement with the athlete lying in a supine position and can be calculated using a spreadsheet (20). It is important to establish a baseline of typical values for athletes in addition to collecting the information under consistent conditions (e.g., when the athlete wakes up). Practitioners should be aware that assessing HRV when an athlete is standing will yield different results than when the athlete is supine (185).

Single measures of HRV have not been shown to be useful for tracking fatigue in handball players and triathletes because of the high day-to-day variation in the measures (21, 169). For example, the monthly changes in HRV measurements were not sensitive to performance changes in handball athletes (21). Using a 7-day rolling average with elite triathletes was shown to be more sensitive than single measurements (167). In a study of Australian rules football players, in which training loads changed substantially, measures of HRV did not change (23).

For these measures to be useful for athlete monitoring, many assessment points are needed to get a complete picture of the athlete's ability to cope with the training load. For monitoring purposes experts have recommended measuring HRV for a minimum of 3 days per week, taking a weekly average, or using a rolling 7-day average (169). This should be done over a longer period to obtain a full picture of the athlete's response to training. An increase in chronic HRV is associated with a positive response to training, and a decreased HRV indicates a negative response to training (169). The HRV findings should be put in context with the training history of the athlete and the current phase of training (20).

Figure 5.4 shows average HRV results for an athlete over a 12-week period leading up to an important event.

Heart Rate Recovery

The recovery period after a bout of exercise can be used as a monitoring tool (118). Immediately after exercise, the parasympathetic nervous system causes a rapid decrease in heart rate (20); decrements in heart rate recovery have been suggested as an indicator of fatigue, detraining, or an inability to cope with the assigned training load (14). Conversely, improvements in heart rate recovery can be an indicator of fitness

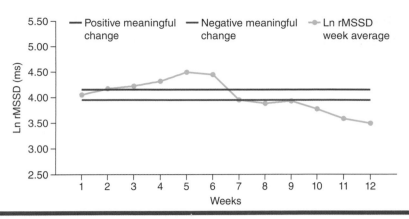

Figure 5.4   Morning resting weekly HRV results for an athlete over a 12-week period.

improvements (13, 56). Researchers have also found some evidence that heart rate recovery is a marker of overreaching (14); however, the findings are not consistent. Some research suggested that faster heart rate recovery is associated with worsening performance in athletes (198). Thomson and colleagues (198) found this to be the case with trained cyclists and triathletes. Another study revealed faster heart rate recovery and increases in RPE in the days following an ultramarathon (129). This again highlights the need for practitioners to avoid relying on one measure for athlete monitoring. Those using heart recovery as a monitoring tool should also use other measures such as RPE.

One of the issues with heart rate recovery is the impracticality of using it daily because it requires an exercise performance test. The magnitude of the technical error in these types of tests has also been shown to be quite high (118, 200). Also, the test conditions need to be as consistent as possible to increase the utility of this test.

Heart rate recovery can be calculated over varying periods of time (20)—for example, a submaximal 5-min cycle followed by 5 min of recovery (200).

Athletes cycle at a fixed intensity of 130 watts at 85 rpm for 5 min and then sit quietly for 5 min while heart rate is monitored continuously. Heart rate is averaged during the final 30 s of the exercise bout. Heart rate recovery can be expressed as the absolute heart rate recovery (number of beats recovered in a given time) and the relative difference between the average heart rate in the final 30 s of the exercise and the heart rate 60 s after the completion of the exercise (120). This protocol can also be used for determining HRV measures. Its advantage is that it can be used as part of the warm-up during training sessions and thus facilitate monitoring athletes regularly.

Researchers have also used the heart rate interval monitoring system (118). One protocol consists of four running stages (8.4, 9.6, 10.8, and 12 km/hr, or 5.22, 5.97, 6.71, and 7.46 mph) of 2 min interspersed with 1-min rest intervals (118). These can be preset by recording an auditory signal. This test could be used in the warm-up because of its submaximal nature and short duration (13 min). Heart rate is recorded 1 min after the final running stage.

$$\text{Heart rate recovery (\%)} =$$
$$(\text{heart rate at 1 min recovery} \div$$
$$\text{heart rate at end of stage 4}) \times 100$$

or

$$\text{Heart rate recovery (\%)} =$$
$$[(\text{heart rate 60 s postexercise} -$$
$$\text{heart rate average during exercise}) \div$$
$$\text{heart rate 60 s postexercise}] \times 100$$

Consider an athlete whose average exercise heart rate is 173 beats/min; after 1 min of recovery, it is 136 beats/min.

$$\text{Heart rate recovery (\%)} =$$
$$[(173 - 136) \div 173] \times 100 = 21.4\%$$

Considerations for Heart Rate Monitoring

Monitoring heart rate is convenient and useful for practitioners. Measures of heart rate such as heart rate recovery and HRV can provide insights into factors such as athlete fatigue and adaptation to training (20). However, practitioners should be aware of the limitations of these methods and their inability to provide information on all aspects of the training process. Therefore, practitioners should use them in conjunction with other monitoring tools such as RPE. Several excellent reviews are available on the use of heart rate as a monitoring tool (11, 14, 20, 169).

Hormonal and Biochemical Markers

A variety of hormonal and biochemical measures have been used in athlete monitoring as markers of training stress (203, 208); they provide information about how athletes are adapting to training load (85). Practitioners considering these markers need to understand their functions and exercise responses and their limitations. Hormonal and biochemical measures need to be made frequently (at least weekly) to be of greatest value. Because many involve complicated and expensive assays and expertise to analyze the information, slow turnaround of the results limits their usefulness in most athletic environments. Thus, they are not often used in high-performance sport (1, 194). The survey by Taylor and colleagues (194) indicated that less than 8% of practitioners use any form of biochemical or hormonal monitoring. Akenhead and Nassis (1) found slightly higher usage in their survey of practitioners in football: 24% had used blood analysis, and 24% had used saliva analysis.

Research findings obtained in laboratories have limited applicability to elite sport. They do, however, provide an important platform for the understanding of hormonal responses to exercise. Many researchers have attempted to overcome the limitations associated with laboratory-based studies by investigating hormone and biochemical responses in sport settings (39, 40, 47, 71, 99, 130, 148, 154, 158). Even though many studies have been conducted, the responses of hormonal and biochemical measures to various types of exercise and sport vary greatly. The responses of these markers are directly influenced by regulatory elements such as training program design, environmental factors (e.g., temperature, age, gender), nutritional status, and psychology (e.g., arousal level) (117).

Measurement Methods

Mediums such as blood, saliva, and urine can be used for analyzing hormones and other biochemical markers.

Because measures of blood and saliva are often strongly related, practitioners often prefer saliva measures because they are easier to obtain. For example, the correlation between saliva and serum measures of testosterone and cortisol has consistently been shown to be high (122, 153, 159, 204). These findings have been confirmed in research reporting a strong relationship between salivary and serum cortisol at rest (r = .93) and during exercise (r = .90) (159). Lane and Hackney (122) investigated the association between serum and saliva analysis of testosterone in aerobic endurance athletes performing varying intensities of exercise. Their data showed strong correlations, particularly at moderate and high exercise intensities (r > .89). The main advantage of collecting saliva for athlete monitoring is its noninvasiveness compared to blood collection. Many athletes find blood collection stressful, which results in elevated levels of stress hormones. Saliva samples also allow for analyzing biologically active free hormone levels (50).

Urine analysis is another relatively noninvasive method for measuring certain hormonal and biochemical markers. Specific adaptations in the hypothalamic-pituitary-adrenal axis can be investigated by analyzing urinary cortisol and cortisone levels (82). It is important to remember, however, that urine analyses provide only a general indication of hormone levels, and they can be time consuming.

Whichever analysis method they use, practitioners need to consider how they will store the samples. Hormones are affected by temperature and should be stored in cool conditions as soon as possible. Certain types of blood analysis require the separation of plasma and serum. It is also important to avoid the repeated freezing and thawing of samples.

Hormone Monitoring

Although limitations exist with blood and saliva measures of hormones, they can provide information on athletes' health status (178). Hormones such as cortisol, testosterone, and catecholamines can provide insight into the functioning of the hypothalamic-pituitary-adrenal axis, which has implications for the early detection of overreaching and overtraining (see chapter 3). Examining hormonal responses to exercise can provide a clearer picture of athletes' adaptive states than looking only at resting (basal) hormonal levels (208). However, resting salivary hormone levels may give some insight into workout performance by individual athletes, with some research suggesting that these levels potentially moderate training adaptations (48). The acute responses of the endocrine system during training and following training sessions are related to the intensity and duration of the exercise stimulus and to the athlete's physical condition (187). Hormones also appear to play a critical role in mediating adaptations in elite athletes (88, 89). However, more research is required to determine these relationships and establish the role of hormone monitoring for both predicting and tracking the effects of training programs.

Practitioners need to be mindful of issues that can arise with variability in the assays. Variation can occur between the samples in the same assay (intra-assay variability) and between the assays (interassay variability). For example, hormones such as cortisol and testosterone exhibit a circadian rhythm: Levels typically peak around 1 hr after waking and then progressively decrease throughout the day (196) (see figure 5.5).

Testosterone

Testosterone is an anabolic hormone responsible for many functions in the body, including growth, development, and protein synthesis (208). The synthesis and secretion of testosterone increases as a result of the effects of catecholamines, and the levels of testosterone increase following an acute bout of moderate- to high-intensity exercise (116, 117). Levels of resting testosterone are highly individual and can vary greatly across the competitive season in athletes (40). Therefore, practitioners need to consider individual differences and establish a baseline when assessing the usefulness of testosterone as a marker for athlete monitoring.

An emerging body of evidence suggests that testosterone responses can be used to assess training and competition readiness. Although traditionally it was believed that acute increases in anabolic markers such as testosterone are important for muscle hypertrophy and performance gains, this has not been consistently demonstrated in the literature (213, 214). Part of testosterone's role is as a driver of motivation to contribute to performance increases. Crewther and colleagues (54) found that the testosterone response to a midweek workout in rugby league players could be somewhat predictive of the match result on the weekend. A study by Beaven and colleagues (8) showed a relationship between salivary levels of testosterone and strength gains in rugby union players. In female athletes, a relationship has been found between self-selected training load and levels of testosterone, which suggests that testosterone levels are important in women (36). Resting salivary testosterone concentrations have been shown to have a relationship with strength and power performance in weightlifters (49). Because saliva reflects the biologically active hormone, this finding could be attributed to individual differences in the target tissue response to hormones, the result of training, and genetic factors such as muscle fiber type distribution, the target tissues' capacity to bind to the hormones, and the number of hormone receptors.

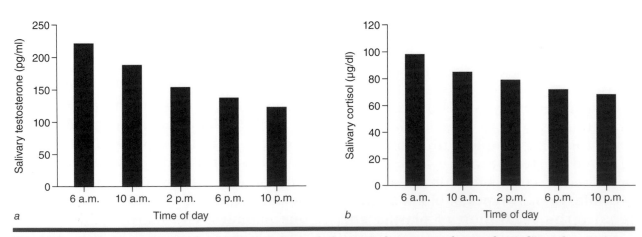

Figure 5.5 Multiple measures of *(a)* testosterone and *(b)* cortisol over one day to show diurnal variation.

Taken together, the findings suggest that monitoring testosterone levels in athletes could help guide training prescription. For example, how the athlete responds to a particular type of workout may identify optimal sessions (9). Beaven and colleagues (9) identified the hormonal responses of rugby union players to four different workouts. They discovered maximal gains when the athletes trained using the protocol that maximized their testosterone response.

Relationships between testosterone levels and match outcomes in sport have also been found (54, 76, 77). Testosterone seems to play important roles in psychological aspects such as motivation, which highlights its role in athletic performance (52). The use of priming workouts on the day of competition is speculated to aid performance by increasing levels of circulating hormones. Although performance increases have been shown with these types of approaches, the clear impact on match outcomes has yet to be demonstrated conclusively. Identifying workouts and approaches to training that optimize adaptations to training could be aided by monitoring these hormone levels in athletes.

Testosterone levels in athletes can be affected by a number of factors. In elite female athletes, oral contraceptive use has been shown to affect levels of resting testosterone (51). This study also provided some evidence of a reduced testosterone and cortisol response to exercise and competition in elite hockey players taking oral contraceptives (51). These findings could have implications for athletes' responses to explosive exercise (28) and training loads (36). Menstrual cycle effects on athlete hormonal responses are less clear, but taking them into account in athlete monitoring does appear to be important (123). Certain stages of the cycle may provide windows in which to maximize the response to training. A study by Nakamura and colleagues (152) showed different acute responses to resistance training depending on the phase of the menstrual cycle. Sung and colleagues (193) investigated the effects of strength training during different phases of the menstrual cycle. The results showed differential responses depending on how the loading was distributed across the menstrual cycle. Specifically, follicular phase–based training resulted in greater increases in muscular strength and hypertrophy (193). It should be noted that the majority of these studies have used untrained or recreationally trained participants rather than elite athletes. Monitoring athletes' menstrual cycles as well as the medications they are taking would provide practitioners a picture of how this aspect of physiology responds to training.

Cortisol

Cortisol, a glucocorticoid that is released from the adrenal cortex in response to stress, has important roles in metabolism and immune function (117). It is also considered a marker of catabolic status. Levels of cortisol are higher following an acute bout of exercise and competition (60, 117). The release of cortisol is stimulated by adrenocorticotropic hormone (**ACTH**), which is secreted by the hypothalamic-pituitary axis in response to stress. The increase in cortisol occurs approximately 15 to 30 min after adrenocorticotropic hormone release (12). Cortisol has many important functions, including stimulating **gluconeogenesis** (a metabolic process that makes glucose from noncarbohydrate sources), which results in sparing blood glucose and protein stores in the body. During metabolism, cortisol increases protein

MENSTRUAL CYCLE MONITORING

Practitioners working with female athletes should take into consideration the menstrual cycle and its potential role in performance. Fluctuations in several hormones (estrogen, progesterone, follicle-stimulating hormone, and luteinizing hormone) occur over the course of a normal menstrual cycle (162). Research has shown that exercise performance can vary during the menstrual cycle, although the findings have not been consistent (152, 162, 180). Experts have suggested taking these variations into account when designing training programs, but it would need to be done on an individual basis (180, 193). This may prove too time intensive in team sports, but it may be possible in individual sports. The starting point would be to track the menstrual cycle of the athlete using a training diary and analyze the information relative to the subsequent performance in training and competition. Of particular importance would be any menstrual cycle disturbances, because these can have negative effects on overall health and performance (19).

breakdown in skeletal muscle and connective tissue, amino acid transport into the liver, glycogen synthesis in the liver, and **lipolysis** (breakdown of lipids) (12). The cortisol response is related to the intensity, duration, and mode of exercise (117). One study showed a decrease in resting levels of cortisol after 24 weeks of aerobic endurance training (83). Interestingly, the degree of the decrease in resting cortisol was related to physical function improvements in the participants.

Like testosterone, cortisol has also been shown to be related to athletic performance (37). Several research studies have been conducted with respect to cortisol levels in athletes (59-62, 83, 160). Given its importance as a stress hormone, it is one of the most commonly measured markers in athlete monitoring. A study by Cook and colleagues (37) showed differences in the levels of cortisol and testosterone in elite compared to nonelite female athletes. The higher levels could indicate elite athletes' greater capacity to handle high training loads.

Testosterone-to-Cortisol Ratio

Given that testosterone is an anabolic hormone and cortisol is a catabolic hormone, the ratio between them is intuitively appealing as a monitoring tool in sport. The research findings, however, are mixed, no doubt because of the high degree of variability in these hormones in athletes (183) and because the interaction between them appears to be complex (59). High levels of both **interindividual** (between individuals) and **intraindividual** (within a single individual from sample to sample) variability are found with most biochemical markers, which can limit their usefulness for athlete monitoring.

Some have suggested that a high ratio indicates a more anabolic status in athletes, whereas a ratio reduced by more than 30% indicates a state of catabolism (203). A low ratio is also believed to be indicative of reduced adaptation to training. A study by Edwards and Casto (60) showed that the resting level of cortisol in female university-level athletes appeared to modulate the change in testosterone level in competition. Monitoring both cortisol and testosterone prior to training and competition could give some indication of athletes' readiness to perform.

Epinephrine and Norepinephrine

The catecholamines **epinephrine** and **norepinephrine** (sometimes referred to as adrenaline and noradrenaline) are released in response to stress and reflect the acute demands of exercise (12). Catecholamine levels have potential as a monitoring tool because they have important roles in force production, energy availability, and muscle contraction (117). They also appear to be important for augmenting the effects of hormones such as testosterone (117). An increase in catecholamine levels during exercise appears to be related to intensity (25). However, less is known about the chronic responses to exercise. Epinephrine and norepinephrine have properties that regulate homeostasis to meet the increased demands of muscle force production, both before and during resistance exercise (69). In one study, athletes who maintained force production throughout the exercise protocol had higher catecholamine concentrations than those whose performances decreased (69).

Growth Hormone

The response of the growth hormone–insulin-like growth factor 1 axis is potentially useful for athlete monitoring (117). **Growth hormone** has important physiological functions, including stimulating muscle hypertrophy by facilitating amino acid transport and stimulating lipolysis (12). Exercise acutely stimulates growth hormone secretion; resistance training has been shown to acutely increase growth hormone levels (117). An important issue in monitoring growth hormone levels is the type of assay used (115). Many commercially available assays detect circulating growth hormone concentrations. Growth hormone (and most hormones) exists as a family of related proteins of different molecular weights and structures. Most traditional commercial assays measure one form and therefore neglect many others. More than 100 molecular isoforms of circulating growth hormone exist, but the traditional measurement approach in the exercise literature has focused on the primary one, 22-kDa isoform (115). The relationships between growth hormone concentrations in the serum, growth hormone signaling pathways, and long-term changes in performance and body composition are not well understood. As these relationships become clearer, the role of exercise-induced growth hormone release may become defined, and its use in biochemical monitoring could be more useful.

Insulin-Like Growth Factors

Hormones such as **insulin-like growth factor 1 (IGF-1)** and **insulin-like growth factor binding protein 3 (IGFBP-3)** have been studied as markers of stress and shown to increase with acute exercise (63). Growth factors are important for regulating many of the body's processes involved with the anabolism of bone and skeletal muscle (12). IGF-1, a polypeptide produced by the liver, has an important role in mediating metabolic and anabolic responses (117). The IGFBPs act as carriers of IGF in circulation and help to regulate their biological actions. It has been proposed that a reduction in resting IGFBP-3 can be used as a marker of overreaching and overtraining (63).

The evaluation of alterations in the levels of total IGF-1 and its binding proteins may be of interest because they may affect performance and reflect physical overload in athletes (63, 117).

The response of IGF-1 to long-term training is not clear from the available research (208). Short-term resistance training studies have reported no change in the resting concentration of IGF-1 (133), whereas other studies have shown significant elevations in resting IGF-1 (114). Overreaching resulting from an increase in training volume and intensity has been shown to reduce IGF-1 concentrations but return them to baseline when normal training resumed over the next cycle (174).

Glutamine and Glutamate

Plasma **glutamine** and **glutamate** may be useful markers of high training loads (46). These amino acids have several functions, including protein synthesis and acid–base balance regulation. Similar to testosterone and cortisol, the ratio of these two markers may provide a measure of training adaptation. Some research evidence suggests that the levels change with training load and could suggest immune status (46, 93). Studies have shown decreases in glutamine during periods of high training loads, but findings with respect to this marker's ability to detect overtraining have been inconsistent (109, 145). Evidence suggests that the glutamine-to-glutamate ratio may be sensitive enough to identify nonfunctional overreaching (46).

Leptin

Leptin, a protein hormone, relays signals to the hypothalamus to regulate appetite and energy balance, and it has roles in metabolism (208). Simsch and colleagues (187) reported decreases in resting levels of leptin in rowers following high-intensity resistance training. A study by Nindl and colleagues (157) revealed no decrease in leptin concentration following high-volume resistance exercise, but a delayed decrease may have reflected the large disruption in metabolic homeostasis caused by training. Jurimae and colleagues (107) have shown a relationship between training volume and plasma leptin.

As with all hormone measures, it is important to control for nutrient intake and diurnal variations; these factors may account for the differences seen in studies. Leptin has been shown to decrease under conditions similar to overtraining when training volumes have been high (107, 187). Resting levels of leptin are also reduced in aerobic endurance athletes and decreased in postexercise periods when levels of training stress are high (108). This suggests that measuring leptin levels may be useful in monitoring training.

Adiponectin and Ghrelin

Adiponectin and **ghrelin** are both important hormones in the regulation of energy homeostasis, but no strong evidence can be found for their utility in monitoring. Jurimae and colleagues (108) suggested that decreased levels of adiponectin postexercise during periods of high training volumes could indicate heavy training stress.

Considerations for Hormone Monitoring

Hormone monitoring has several advantages. Many measures can be obtained noninvasively using saliva and urine. Regular monitoring of hormones may help practitioners implement appropriate interventions such as reduced training loads or periods of rest aimed at recovering hormonal status. However, they need to be mindful of several limitations of hormone monitoring. Factors that can affect hormone concentrations include sampling conditions and sample storage. Nutritional intake can modify significantly either the resting concentration of some hormones or their concentration change in response to exercise (117). In female athletes the hormonal response depends on the phase of the menstrual cycle. Hormone concentrations at rest and following exercise are different. Practitioners should also be aware of diurnal variations in hormone levels and obtain samples at approximately the same time of day. Also, the reproducibility of some hormone analyses can be poor. Finally, hormone analyses can be time consuming and expensive, which presents challenges for regularly monitoring these measures.

Biochemical Monitoring

Many substances involved in the metabolic process (called **metabolites**) have been studied with the aim of establishing their usefulness for monitoring training and performance (208). The following sections discuss some of these biochemical metabolites, specifically looking at measures using blood assays. As with hormone monitoring, practitioners need a basic understanding of the role of metabolites and their significance when considering them as monitoring tools.

Creatine Kinase

Exercise-induced muscle damage is a normal response to heavy training loads. Practitioners are therefore often interested in measuring the degree of muscle damage; subjective ratings of muscle soreness are one way to do this (see chapter 4). In response to unaccus-

tomed heavy exercise, various enzymes and blood markers increase, including **creatine kinase**. Measures of creatine kinase are the most commonly reported in the literature (182). The enzyme is located inside muscle cells, but after heavy exercise it can be released into the blood. Thus, creatine kinase levels can reflect the degree of muscle damage. However, although these levels are a good measure of muscle damage and response to unaccustomed exercise, no consistent patterns have been noted in overtrained athletes. Coutts and colleagues (46) found significant increases in creatine kinase in rugby league players following a 6-week period of intensified training. A 1-week taper period resulted in a significant return to baseline values, which was not the case with the other biochemical markers. This was likely due to the reduced amount of muscle damage associated with the reduction in training load.

Creatine kinase can be used to assess muscle damage in athletes, but with generally large amounts of variability (85). However, because a clear relationship does not always occur between levels of creatine kinase and performance, practitioners should use caution when interpreting the results. In general, the level of creatine kinase increases in response to acute training load (208). Others have recommended using levels of creatine kinase to assess recovery of muscle damage in the short term following training or competition (45). Measures of this marker may be of greater value during the preseason and training camps, when training loads are particularly high. However, the response of creatine kinase to long-term training is not consistent, most likely because athletes have become accustomed to the chronic training stress (17). With this measure it is important to establish a clear baseline from a large number of samples. Ideally, this should be done over several days to establish the degree of variability in the athletes.

Other Measures of Muscle Damage

Other measures of muscle damage have been investigated and have potential use in athlete monitoring. Those that can indicate the degree of muscle damage include myoglobin, ammonia, uric acid, urea, and troponin (16). Measures such as C-reactive protein and creatinine have also been investigated (208). Redox homeostasis and adaptation to training may be an important part of the stress–adaptation response; some suggest the existence of an optimal dose of exercise and production of reactive oxygen and nitrogen species (27).

Alpha-Amylase

Alpha-amylase is another potential stress marker that is released along with catecholamines and certain neuroendocrine secretory proteins (chromogranin A) in response to acute physiological stress (85). These are considered useful markers of autonomic nervous system activity. In a study of elite track and field athletes, the levels of chromogranin A decreased over the course of the preseason period, but no changes in alpha-amylase were seen (85).

Hypoxanthine

Research has shown that hypoxanthine may be a useful indicator of training status during some training phases (219). **Hypoxanthine** is a marker of anaerobic metabolism and reflects the exercise-induced degradation and resynthesis of protein in the muscle. Long-term training causes declines in plasma hypoxanthine concentrations; the extent of the change relates to the amount of high-intensity anaerobic exercise (219). Because the levels of hypoxanthine indicate metabolism in skeletal muscle under anaerobic conditions, this metabolite may provide insights into training adaptation (208, 219).

Red Blood Cell Function

Markers of red blood cell function from a standard blood panel count may have a role in monitoring. They include leukocyte, hematocrit, hemoglobin, and blood cell counts. Hematological changes have been reported in overreached and overtrained athletes (92, 93, 177), although some studies have not shown any changes (47). Hooper and colleagues (101) found that neutrophil number gave some indication of training staleness in elite swimmers during the early part of the season. The body of research suggests that blood parameters such as blood count, C-reactive protein, urea, creatinine, liver enzymes, glucose, ferritin, sodium, and potassium are not capable of indicating overreaching or overtraining in athletes (177). Many of these markers do not accurately represent physiological changes before and after training (145). Despite these limitations, these markers do provide information on athletes' health status (145).

Considerations for Biochemical Monitoring

Practitioners would be wise to take into account many of the considerations mentioned for hormone monitoring. Many metabolites can be measured in a variety of mediums such as blood and saliva and, as discussed in chapter 6, sweat and tears. As with hormones, large individual responses to training exist in athletes, which can make interpreting monitoring results difficult. Practitioners also need to consider the logistics of these measures, especially cost and the time needed to analyze the results. Table 5.1 provides a summary of the primary hormonal and biochemical markers that have potential in athlete monitoring.

Practitioners considering a hormonal and biochemical monitoring program need to do the following:

- Compare exercise-induced measures with baseline measures from the same person.
- Take diurnal variation into account; collect samples at the same time of day.

TABLE 5.1   Functions, Advantages, and Disadvantages of Primary Hormonal and Biochemical Markers

Marker	Function	Advantages	Disadvantages
Testosterone and cortisol	May indicate anabolic and catabolic balance.	Can be measured in saliva and blood. One of the simplest assays.	Analysis is costly. Variability is high.
Epinephrine and norepinephrine	Have important roles in force production, energy availability, and muscle contraction.	Indicate response to stress and reflect acute demands of exercise.	Require blood samples. Analysis is complicated and expensive.
Growth hormone	Has a role in anabolic status and a wide range of metabolic functions.	Can indicate differential response to forms of exercise.	Requires blood sample. Analysis is complicated and expensive.
IGF-1 and IGFBP-3	Involved with anabolism of bone and skeletal muscle.	Can be measured in saliva and blood. IGFBP-3 may be reflective of training load.	Analysis is complicated and expensive.
Glutamine and glutamate	Glutamine-to-glutamate ratio indicates excessive training stress.	Are potential biochemical markers of overreaching.	Require blood samples. Analysis is costly and time consuming.
Creatine kinase	Provides information on muscle damage.	Has been widely researched, and evidence exists for its utility during periods of heavy training loads.	Requires a blood sample. Analysis is costly and time consuming. Degree of variability is high.
Hematological measures	Are standard clinical tests of red blood cell count, hemoglobin, and leukocyte count.	Are useful for determining health status.	Require a blood test. Have low utility for determining overreaching and overtraining.

Data from Gleeson et al. (80); Meeusen et al. (145); Urhausen et al. (203); Viru and Viru (208).

- Exercise caution when comparing results to previously published results because assays can produce very different data. Growth hormone is a good example of this.

- Analyze hormones and biochemical markers in combination with other physiological and psychological measures such as RPE, wellness questionnaires, and exercise performance tests.

- Keep in mind that circulating levels of hormones and other markers in blood and saliva, particularly at rest, are not always good indicators of molecular and cellular responses.

- Take into account the effects of other factors such as nutrition, training status, stress, menstrual cycle, and medications. Single measures of a hormone or biochemical marker do not necessarily provide accurate information about an athlete's training status.

- Most important, use hormonal and biochemical monitoring to make objective decisions about athlete training.

Despite previous studies of biochemical and endocrine responses in athletes, weekly variations in elite-level athletes are poorly understood. Changes in the biochemical and hormonal status of athletes happen during a sport season (33, 40). Various magnitudes of suppression or elevation can occur independently or in parallel. It is possible that changes in these variables are related to workload or performance and, in the case of hormone measures, may reflect modifications to total-body anabolic and catabolic balance.

Immunological Markers

Immune system measures can be used as an index of physiological stress in response to training load. As discussed in chapter 2, excessive training loads can result in the suppression of the immune system and put athletes at risk of getting sick (80). Several markers can provide insight into the immune status of athletes. The most commonly used and researched are immunoglobulin A and cytokines.

Immunoglobulin A

Antimicrobial proteins such as **immunoglobulin A (IgA)** have been widely researched as markers of immune status in athletes because of their potential role in upper respiratory tract infections (URTIs) (202). IgA is the most abundant immunoglobulin in the mucosal fluids and is the first line of defense against microorganisms that cause URTIs (79). Several studies have shown that salivary IgA levels are associated with the incidence of these infections (55, 79, 146, 154). In a 50-week study of America's Cup sailors, researchers analyzed weekly saliva samples for IgA levels (154); the level of IgA was found to be associated with an increased risk of developing an URTI. A decline in IgA levels over 3 weeks seemed to predict the onset of illness. Interestingly, the fatigue rating scale used in the study was also related to relative IgA levels, which highlights the value of subjective questionnaires when IgA analyses are not available.

A dose–response relationship also appears to occur between levels of IgA in the saliva and training load (33, 34, 164). Following heavy periods of training and up to 36 hr following match play, suppression of IgA levels occurs (33). The findings are not consistent, though, and a high degree of individual variability in the response has been noted (80, 148).

Weekly monitoring of salivary IgA offers a way to assess athletes' immune status. The measures typically used are IgA concentration, saliva flow rate (determined by timing the collection of the saliva for analysis), and IgA secretion rate. Being able to predict the onset of illness is very useful for maximizing training time and avoiding missed sessions. Putlur and colleagues (173) examined changes in IgA levels in female university football players over 9 weeks during the season. They reported that illness occurred at a higher rate among the players compared to active controls, and the incidence of illness was lowest in weeks with reduced training loads (173). In the players, 82% of illnesses occurred following a decrease in IgA levels, and 55% were preceded by a spike in training load. These findings were similar to those of Foster (66), who noted that 84% of athlete illnesses could be explained by a preceding increase in training load. This provides evidence that an increase in training load can lead to an increase in illness and that monitoring athletes' immune status is useful for avoiding lost training and competition time. Figure 5.6 shows an example of salivary IgA and training load tracked over the course of a training camp in athletes.

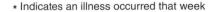

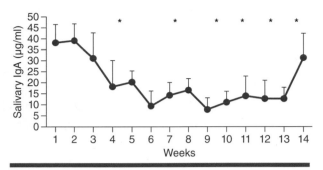

Figure 5.6 Time course of salivary IgA over a season in a squad of athletes and incidence of illness.

Cytokines

Proinflammatory **cytokines** such as interleukin-6, interleukin-8, interleukin-10, interleukin-1ß, and tumor necrosis factor alpha have been shown to be important in the acute and chronic exercise response in athletes (188). The main role of cytokines appears to be as cell-to-cell communicators, and they have important roles in skeletal muscle. Periods of excessive training stress accompanied by inadequate rest and recovery can induce inflammatory responses in skeletal muscle, which leads to chronic inflammation (190). Cytokines play a significant role in this process, and large increases in these markers occur following acute bouts of exercise (79, 188). It has been suggested that these cytokines could provide information about inflammation and stress in the body (188, 189).

Of the various types of cytokines, **interleukin-6** has received the most attention because of its release from skeletal muscle during and after exercise. Because it induces lipolysis and fat oxidation and is involved in glucose homeostasis during exercise, interleukin-6 could be used as an indicator of heavy training loads.

Postexercise levels of **tumor necrosis factor alpha** could also indicate increased training load and inadequate recovery (188, 189). However, this has yet to be directly determined in elite athlete populations.

A disadvantage of using cytokine measures in athlete monitoring is that all of these cytokines respond to exercise and are related to each other. Like many other markers, expense and the time-consuming nature of the analysis are also limitations for many monitoring programs. Because new cytokines are being discovered all the time, further investigations will no doubt determine their utility for athlete monitoring. Table 5.2 provides a summary of the primary immunological markers that have potential in athlete monitoring.

Considerations for Immune System Monitoring

The current information regarding the immune system and training suggests that periods of intensified training result in depressed immune cell function (80). However, these changes do not appear to distinguish between athletes who adapt successfully to high training loads and those that develop overtraining syndrome. Other measures, such the antimicrobial peptide lysozyme, can be measured in saliva (55). A study of rugby union athletes revealed who both salivary IgA and lysozyme had potential as monitoring measures, although there was a great deal of variability (55). Methods for monitoring immune status are particularly appealing for practitioners because of their potential to reduce lost training time and increase athletes' availability to compete. However, the

TABLE 5.2   Functions, Advantages, and Disadvantages of Primary Immunological Markers

Marker	Function	Advantages	Disadvantages
IgA	IgA and other antimicrobial proteins are an important first line of defense against URTI.	Can be measured in saliva. Relative decline in athlete's salivary IgA over the 2- to 3-week period before a URTI appears to precede and contribute to risk	Variability of measures is high. Analysis is time-consuming and expensive.
Cytokines	Important in the acute and chronic inflammatory exercise response in athletes.	A number of analyses are possible from single blood samples. Assays are being developed for saliva.	Analysis is extremely costly and complicated.

Data from Gleeson et al. (80); Meeusen et al. (145); Viru and Viru (208).

implementation of these markers needs to be weighed against the financial cost and complex analysis required.

Performance Tests

Given that sport is ultimately about performance, tests that directly measure performance can be useful for monitoring athletes. A key initial decision is whether to use a maximal or submaximal test. Maximal performance testing can be challenging to implement on a regular basis because of the resulting fatigue. Typically, performance tests are performed in conjunction with other physiological, perceptual, or biochemical tests. Ideally, baseline values for measures such as resting and exercise heart rate, RPE, lactate, and hormone levels are available for comparison (using the statistical tools from chapter 2). As discussed in chapter 3, performance tests can provide information on overreaching and overtraining. Rather than relying on repeated bouts of maximal performance tests, practitioners could use field-based performance tests to determine the potential for overreaching and overtraining in their athletes.

A variety of performance tests have been used and studied by researchers (91). A survey of high-performance sport practitioners revealed that 61% used some type of performance test monthly (30%), weekly (33%), or more often than weekly (36%) (194). Tests included submaximal cycling and running tests, maximal strength and jump tests, sprints, and sport-specific tests. The challenge for practitioners is finding a test they can use on a regular basis (i.e., daily or weekly).

Submaximal Testing

Maximal tests have often been used to assess overtraining in athletes, but practitioners are also interested in using reliable and valid submaximal performance tests to monitor training. The advantage of these tests is that they can be performed more frequently than maximal tests. For example, the Lamberts and Lambert submaximal cycle test requires the athlete to cycle at a fixed predetermined heart rate while power output, RPE, and heart rate recovery data are collected (121). Training-induced acute and chronic fatigue are reflected differently in this submaximal test, which has important practical applications for monitoring. A case study of an elite cyclo-cross athlete showed that the test detected changes in the athlete's training status and could indicate the occurrence of acute fatigue that could lead to performance impairments (119). Athletes identified as suffering from reduced performance based on heart rate responses following a submaximal running test also demonstrated hormonal changes and mood state responses typical of athletes experiencing nonfunctional overreaching (184).

Submaximal running tests can be used for athlete monitoring (206, 207). Vesterinen and colleagues' (206) submaximal running test was modified from the Lamberts and Lambert submaximal cycle test (121). The test involves three stages of running at 70% (6 min), 80% (6 min), and 90% (3 min) of maximal heart rate. RPE using the CR-10 scale is measured after the final stage. Running speed and heart rate are measured over the final 5 min of each of the first two stages and for the final 2 min of the third stage. Heart rate recovery can also be calculated using 60 s of recovery at the end of the test. Research has shown that the changes in running speed during the final two stages can reflect changes in training load and be used to monitor adaptations to aerobic endurance training (205, 206). Other field-based performance tests are an interval shuttle run test for football players and the Zoladz test for runners (220).

Sprint Testing

Sprint testing can also be used for monitoring athletes (74, 96). Because sprinting is an important determinant of sport performance, particularly in team sports, practitioners are interested in regularly monitoring aspects of it (149). Measuring sprint performance via time is the most common method (218).

Sprint tests can be conducted over a set distance such as 30 m. Measuring time alone can provide helpful monitoring information because preliminary data show that speed slows following a fatiguing training session in team sports (151). Sophisticated timing devices are not always necessary; handheld devices have been reliable for experienced testers (128). Moreover, sprint testing is highly reliable in athletes (74). Researchers have compared 20-m sprints to jump testing and found that jump testing was more sensitive for monitoring fatigue in team sport athletes (74). Other technology for measuring running speed is discussed in chapter 6.

Cycle-based ergometer sprint tests appear to have potential for athlete monitoring (142, 210, 211). These tests have advantages for practitioners working with non-body-weight-support sports such as cycling and rowing and for athletes restricted from running such as during rehabilitation. The Wingate anaerobic test is one of the most commonly used cycle ergometer tests, but it is highly fatiguing. An ergometer with adjustable resistance measures the rate of pedal revolutions. Typical protocols involve a warm-up followed by a set test time such as 30 s. The amount of work performed is determined from the resistance value and the number of pedal revolutions. Power is generally calculated as work divided by time for each 5-s time interval. Parameters such as peak power, average power, and fatigue can be calculated.

Other protocols are more suited for monitoring athletes, such as a protocol for elite Australian rules football players that involves two 6-s maximal sprints separated by 1 min of recovery (210, 211). The test has been shown to be reliable and sensitive to neuromuscular fatigue in elite team sport athletes (210, 211). One advantage of this test is than it takes very little time to complete and is less fatiguing that the standard Wingate protocol.

Velocity Testing

Velocity-based testing (106), which has been studied for many years (15, 201), provides objective information about the quality of velocity-based resistance training (175). Studies have shown that exercise velocity can be used to estimate an athlete's 1RM (35, 81). As a result, barbell or jump velocity can be a useful monitoring measure. Sanchez-Medina and Gonzalez-Badillo (181) studied the loss of velocity and determined that it indicates neuromuscular fatigue during resistance training. Their results indicated that by monitoring the velocity of repetitions during a training session, it was possible to estimate the degree of metabolic stress (lactate and ammonia levels) and neuromuscular fatigue. Baker and Newton also showed that power and velocity decreased after a certain number of repetitions in elite rugby league players (4). Practitioners can use this information to set velocity thresholds to ensure an optimal training stimulus. This would avoid the need for athletes to perform unnecessary repetitions in training, thus increasing session efficiency.

Movement Screening and Flexibility Testing

Movement screenings and flexibility tests can be used to assess athletes' flexibility, mobility, body posture, and general movement competency as well as to monitor the risk of injury (70, 97). No consensus on which screening is best has emerged, and there are no clear links between the results of a screening and an athlete's risk of injury (111, 134, 136, 165), which raises questions about their usefulness.

Simple movements such as the overhead squat can be performed to assess bilateral mobility of the hips, knees, ankles, shoulders, and thoracic spine (26). Scoring systems can then be used to rate the movements qualitatively. For example, numerical rating scales can be used to rate the movements of the squat, single-leg squat, lunge, or push-up, but validation studies regarding these approaches are minimal (70, 97). Most of these scales have set criteria for what constitutes good or poor movement patterns, and practitioners use various adaptations (134, 141, 165). Similar to wellness questionnaires, practitioners seem to prefer modifications of existing tools for their particular sport settings. Good practitioners perform performance and postural screening routinely by viewing athletes' performances during warm-up and training and use this information to guide their choice of modifications to the session's load assignments.

Flexibility measures include goniometers, which measure joint angle, and sit-and-reach boxes, which measure a combination of low back and hip flexibility. During a flexibility test, the athlete should move slowly into the fully

WEEKLY SUBMAXIMAL RUNNING TESTS FOR TRACKING TEAM SPORT ATHLETES

Submaximal running tests avoid the need for expensive and time-consuming laboratory-based tests. For practitioners working in team sports that involve significant amounts of running, submaximal running tests can provide important information about athletes' current fitness and fatigue levels. This type of testing can be incorporated into the warm-up, but a heart rate monitor or some other means of measuring heart rate is needed to capture the data. RPE scales are a good alternative and can be used to complement other aspects of the monitoring system. One simple test is a 5-min run at a set running speed (e.g., 9 km/hr, or 5.6 mph) followed by a seated 5-min recovery (24). The practitioner can measure heart rate and RPE at each minute during exercise and recovery and use this information to determine heart rate recovery.

stretched position and hold the position while the result is measured in centimeters or inches. The knee-to-wall test involves comparing right and left sides and calculating the difference in dorsiflexion range of motion while performing a weight-bearing lunge (113).

Balance and Stability Testing

Balance is the ability to maintain static and dynamic equilibrium, or the ability to maintain the body's center of gravity over its base of support (147). **Stability** is a measure of the ability to return to a desired position following a disturbance to the system (147). Commonly used tests of balance and stability are timed static standing tests (eyes closed and standing on one or both legs) (18), balance tests using unstable surfaces (135), and tests using specialized balance testing equipment (176). Tests are also available for evaluating aspects of balance and stability such as postural sway. Clarke and colleagues (30) found that postural sway can be an indicator of neuromuscular fatigue in athletes.

Two tests with good reliability that have been widely researched are the **balance error scoring system** and the **star excursion balance test** (18, 84, 199). The balance error scoring system test is conducted using a variety of positions on a firm surface and on a soft surface (figure 5.7). The positions are held for 20 s with eyes closed and hands on hips. Athletes are told to remain as steady as possible, and if they lose their balance, they attempt to regain their initial position as quickly as possible. The error scores from the balance error scoring

system test are summed into a single score.

In the star excursion balance test, the athlete stands in the center of a grid with eight 120-cm (47 in.) lines extending out at 45° increments. The athlete maintains a single-leg stance facing in one direction while reaching with the contralateral leg as far as possible for each taped line, touches the farthest point possible, and then returns to the bilateral position. Within a single trial, the athlete remains facing in the initial direction and the stance leg remains the same; the other leg does all of the reaching. The distance from the center of the star to the touch position is measured. Some have suggested that testing the front, side, and rear positions is sufficient (98).

Performance Ratings

Although practitioner and athlete ratings of performance are subjective, they can be useful for monitoring an athlete during competition and training (38). A common approach is to use a wellness questionnaire and have athletes rate their performance on a Likert scale from 1 (*extremely poor*) to 10 (*excellent*) (65). Practitioners can rate the athlete's performance using a similar scale. In a study by Cormack and colleagues (38), practitioners were asked to rate athlete performance using the following scale: 1 = *poor performance*, 2 = *moderate performance*, 3 = *good performance*, 4 = *very good performance*, 5 = *excellent performance*. Ideally, measures would be obtained from a range of practitioners. Interestingly, in Cormack and colleagues' study, the athletes with higher levels of neuromuscular fatigue during play were rated as performing more poorly by the practitioners.

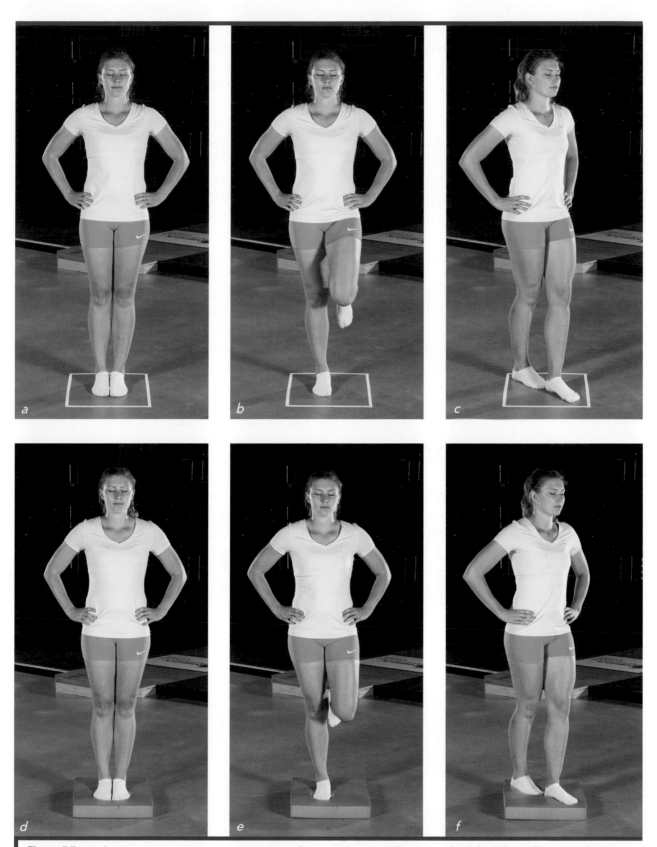

Figure 5.7 Balance error scoring system: (*a-c*) firm surface condition and (*d-f*) soft surface condition.

In summary, a performance test can be used for athlete monitoring if it meets these criteria:

- Is reliable and valid and sensitive to change
- Can be performed on a regular basis (weekly testing appears to be standard, but some may require more frequent assessments)
- Is easy to administer
- Can be performed in a variety of settings
- Does not take too long to perform and, ideally, can be included in the warm-up
- Does not require specialized equipment (a tape measure and a stopwatch can be sufficient)

Conclusion

Many methods can be used to assess fitness and fatigue. However, decisions about the training readiness of athletes should not be made on the basis of one monitoring tool. Jump tests such as the vertical countermovement, static jump, and drop jump tests are sensitive to neuromuscular fatigue and easy to administer with athletes. Force production tests can also be used to monitor fatigue in athletes. Measures such as heart rate variability and heart rate recovery can provide insights into the athlete's preparedness to train. Athletes' variability in hormonal and biochemical responses suggests the importance of analyzing the results individually. Various markers can indicate immune function in athletes. Several are sensitive to training load, but responses have been highly variable. Although the evidence supports the use of certain hormonal and biochemical markers, they have limited practical application because of high cost and logistical issues. Performance tests can be useful for tracking fitness and fatigue, but no single measure can provide a complete picture. However, enough evidence is available to suggest that a combination of several measures can provide useful information about athletes' training status, adaptation to workload, and fatigue levels.

6

Current Monitoring Practices and Technologies

Previous chapters make it clear that many practitioners are using athlete monitoring. Because technology forms the basis of many monitoring practices, awareness of its benefits and limitations is important. Technology is constantly developing, and new products have potential applications for athlete monitoring. Practitioners need to make sound decisions about whether, how, and when to implement technology into their athlete monitoring programs. Current and emerging technologies that can be applied to monitoring athletes are described in this chapter to provide a solid rationale and guidelines for using technology.

Monitoring Practices in Sport

Several reports have described monitoring practices used by practitioners (3, 94, 127, 128, 141). In a survey, Taylor and colleagues (141) divided training monitoring into quantifying training load and measuring fatigue responses to training or competition. Of the 55 respondents working in high-performance sport programs, 91% reported using some type of monitoring. Self-reporting questionnaires were particularly popular with respondents; 55% reporting using them to monitor fatigue on a daily basis. Saw and colleagues (127) demonstrated the value of these subjective measures and summarized the literature in this area, indicating that they are widely used in practice (see chapter 4).

Monitoring with global positioning systems (GPS) and accelerometry devices is popular in high-performance sport; 43% of high-performance sport practitioners responding to the Taylor and colleagues survey reported that they use this technology (141). Respondents worked in team sports as well as individual sports such as rowing and cycling. Wearable technologies are also used increasingly for monitoring sport and the general public (62). This technology is ranked consistently as one of the most important trends in exercise and sport science (143). Wearable technology is a huge industry in which large investments are made to develop and market products (143). Further, a plethora of smartphone fitness and exercise apps are used alone or paired with wearable technology to monitor training (143).

Akenhead and Nassis (3) investigated the practices and perceptions of practitioners working with football players (soccer in the United States). The survey was completed by practitioners at 41 high-level clubs throughout Europe, Australia, and the United States. Almost all reported using GPS and heart rate measures during training sessions. No universal approach to the use of this data

emerged, and a wide range of variables were used for analysis. In addition, 28 of the clubs used rating of perceived exertion (RPE) measures (3). In terms of support staff, all the clubs employed a fitness coach or sport scientist, but only 17 (21%) employed someone whose specific job was to analyze monitoring data. Anecdotally, it would seem that this would be the job of sport scientists or fitness coaches. More than 50% of the practitioners reported using wellness questionnaires daily for monitoring (3). Smartphones and tablets were commonly used to collect this information.

McCall and colleagues (94) reported on the most popular monitoring practices used by international Premier League football teams, specifically in relation to the prevention of noncontact injuries. The most common screening tests used were the functional movement screen, questionnaires, isokinetic dynamometry, physical tests, and flexibility assessments (94). Interestingly, in a follow-up study they evaluated the evidence for the most popular screening tests (93). Overall, they found limited evidence of successful screening for noncontact injuries for the functional movement screen, most questionnaires, and **isokinetics** (specialized assessment at constant speed) (93). This suggests that the efficacy of these monitoring tools is questionable.

Different approaches to assess the movements and techniques of athletes appear to be used for monitoring purposes (62, 94). The methods range from video analysis to simple movement screens. McCall and colleagues (94) found the functional movement screen to be the most popular tool used by football clubs (66%) for monitoring for noncontact injury risk. An additional

16% of the clubs were using some type of modified screening tool. Clearly, movement screening is widely used for monitoring athletes. What is less clear is how effective these screens are for informing decisions about programming and injury prevention. Practitioners appear to be using adaptations of screening tools, which has not helped to establish evidence for the efficacy of these methods.

Blood sampling does not appear to be widely implemented for monitoring purposes (3, 141). It seems to be used more as a clinical tool to investigate suspicious complaints in athletes (100). As discussed in chapter 5, repeated monitoring of blood markers requires that practitioners take into account within-athlete variability. Practitioners in high-performance sport also report the use of salivary analysis (3). Despite many research studies of hormone monitoring in athletes (32, 138, 151, 154), this practice is not widespread in high-performance sport.

Many simple practices for measuring both external and internal load are available for practitioners (see chapter 4). In baseball it is common practice to measure pitch counts across the course of a season (26, 131). In cricket, measures of the number of deliveries bowled can be useful for practitioners who want to manage injury risk (113, 114). External load measures, which include throw counts, can be routinely monitored in athletes involved in throwing sports and do not involve sophisticated measurement tools. Practitioners also routinely monitor other external load measures such as the number of jumps, sprints, loads, sets, and repetitions (62).

More data continue to be published on the training programs of elite athletes (104, 146, 147). These studies provide rich insights into the training practices of athletes but also the methods that can be used for monitoring. Questionnaires and training diaries are commonly used by practitioners and athletes for keeping training records (62, 127, 145). Digital data capture, which is also increasingly used (127), affords several advantages. Practitioners can perform more in-depth analyses of electronic training data to observe patterns and trends and organize training data in multiple ways to make reporting more efficient.

Although practitioners are using monitoring technology and tools in greater numbers, clarity about how to analyze the data is lacking (141). Practitioners report several approaches to data analysis, but a universal approach does not seem to exist. Some practitioners have reported using percentage change in measures, meaningful change, and z-scores, but these practices do not appear to be widespread (3, 141). Most of these methods seem to rely on visually identifying trends in the monitoring data from day to day or week to week (141). For example, a common approach is to use a series of flags or traffic lights, but without any clear consensus of what determines a red, yellow, or green light (141). Although there has been increasing support for the use of practical statistical approaches to analyzing monitoring data, how widely these approaches are used is unclear (3). Table 6.1 shows common monitoring practices reported by practitioners and their levels of use, levels of supporting evidence from the research literature, and practical value.

TABLE 6.1   Common Athlete Monitoring Practices

Monitoring variable	Level of use	Level of evidence	Practical value
GPS and accelerometry	High	Moderate	Moderate to high
RPE	High	High	High
Wellness questionnaires	High	High	High
Biochemical and hormonal markers	Low	Moderate	Low
Heart rate measures	High	Moderate to high	Moderate to high
Performance tests	Moderate	Moderate	Moderate
Movement screening	High	Low	Moderate
Neuromuscular assessments (e.g., jumps)	Moderate	Moderate	Moderate

Based on published reports from Akenhead and Nassis (3), McCall et al. (94), Saw et al. (127), and Taylor et al. (141).

Innovation and Athlete Monitoring

Innovation is an overused word in sport, and its meaning is often not clear. Many believe that technology is the focus of innovation and research. However, any approach that results in positive program changes can be considered innovative. One of the problems with technology is that early adopters may be left with obsolete equipment as the pace of change accelerates. Practical approaches that are as simple as recording data more systematically or using it in a different way can be very helpful.

Practitioners often cannot afford to wait for researchers to confirm the value of a particular monitoring system with a series of randomized controlled trials; thus, some degree of experimentation and use is required to gain a competitive advantage. A strategy proposed by Coutts (38) and based on the research of Kahnemann (77) is to use both fast and slow approaches to incorporating new developments in the field of athlete monitoring. The fast approach involves quickly adopting (and adapting) new ideas and technologies to inform decision making. The slow approach involves exercising caution to avoid purchasing unnecessary technology.

Case studies can be very useful in this context (79). Practitioners using the fast approach need to objectively assess what has worked. A scattergun approach involving measuring many variables and using several interventions, for example, would be difficult to assess. Coutts (38) suggested that a research program work with a fast-acting practitioner to determine the reliability and validity of a monitoring system. In-house methods for conducting these types of research projects are discussed in chapter 7.

Developing new metrics from existing technologies is an ongoing process in athlete monitoring. Consider the indices of heart rate (see chapter 5) and heart rate variability, which are often used in athlete populations (62). Using different aspects of heart rate variability may provide more sensitive measures of fatigue in athletes (130). Other measures such as maximal heart rate increase during exercise are proposed as potential markers of overreaching (18). Further research is required to confirm the value of many metrics for athlete monitoring.

Modeling

Modeling, which is increasingly used in athlete monitoring (12, 31), refers to any technique that explores the relationships and patterns within a data set. Methods range from fairly complicated ones, such as training impulse (12), to simple ones, such as session RPE. Although modeling can require advanced statistical analysis, it can be an extremely useful technique for obtaining richer insights from data.

A variety of modeling approaches lend themselves well to use with athlete monitoring. They are beneficial because they allow for some degree of prediction. For example, modeling has been used to predict oxygen uptake and energy expenditure from heart rate data (103) and to investigate pacing and fatigue in elite aerobic endurance athletes (136). Modeling can assist practitioners who are using different measuring equipment or testing under different conditions (66). Corrections can be made when monitoring is done with different types of equipment (66), although this not optimal. Practitioners should always try to use the same testing conditions; however, in the real world, alterations are often necessary. In such situations, practitioners must decide whether monitoring is useful. Allometric scaling is a form of modeling used to control for differences in body size (39).

Researchers often use modeling to investigate adaptations to training using quantifications of training and performance (2, 12, 30). Agostinho and colleagues (2) modeled the training responses of judo athletes over a 2-year period using competition performance, session RPE, fitness tests, and a judo fitness test. They identified factors that were useful for monitoring, including session RPE. However, practitioners do not necessarily need to use advanced statistical methods to gain insights into training adaptation. Simplified approaches, including obtaining overall score for a range of monitoring scores, can involve calculating z-scores for each test (chapter 2) and taking the sum of those scores (149).

Researchers have investigated a variety of modeling techniques that can be applied to monitoring data to predict injury in athletes (54, 150). Practitioners are often in search of a holy grail that predicts when an athlete will become injured or get sick and have to miss training or competition. Modeling takes into account all the variables measured and provides an estimate of the effect. It is important to remember that it is an estimate; error is associated with any model. In a sport environment it is impossible to account for all the variables, but a good model takes the important ones onto account. Monitoring and modeling daily performance is one approach to tracking athletes. This requires monitoring tools that can be used on a regular basis.

The fluctuations in the monitoring variables of athletes follow a nonlinear pattern (107). Le Meur and colleagues showed that increases in training load and performance in triathletes are not linear (82). Not surprisingly, in team sports, individual athletes differ in their training responses. An advantage of an athlete monitoring system is that it allows the practitioner to track these individual responses. Practitioners need to remember, though, that error is associated with any modeling approach (see chapter 2).

Monitoring Technologies

The use of technology is not new in sport. In the early part of the 20th century, A.V. Hill (1886-1977) used a timing setup to measure the speed of athletes in the field (70). Sprinters wore coils of wire and magnets in a design that would be recognized now as timing gates. The magnetic bands they wore around their chests could be considered one of the early examples of wearable technology. August Krogh (1874-1949) designed a cycle ergometer to measure exercise intensity and conducted studies with it (80, 81). Franklin Henry (1904-1993) undertook research in many areas related to athlete monitoring, including the use of a timing light set up over 50 yd, similar to that used by Hill (69). Henry also conducted research in the middle of the 20th century on the force–time characteristics of sprint starts by using pressure recording devices attached to the starting blocks (68). The last 50 years have seen many other examples of monitoring technology. $\dot{V}O_2$ testing has been used to monitor athletes by measuring the volume of oxygen consumed (121). Douglas bags have been popular portable approaches for measuring athletes' $\dot{V}O_2$ in the field (99). The bulk of the equipment limited its usefulness, however, resulting in the development of portable gas analysis systems (99).

Monitoring technologies for sport now have greater portability and utility, and many commercial companies now market equipment specifically for use in athlete monitoring. However, prac-titioners can benefit from learning how technology has developed historically and understanding the foundations of current technologies. The evolution of sprint monitoring is an interesting case study (65). Timing systems have progressed from handheld to fully automatic, and practitioners now use a variety of technologies to measure sprinting performance (65). Learning the history of monitoring technology and sport science can benefit practitioners by giving them a better understanding of the physiological and mechanical background of these monitoring approaches. Several excellent resources document the history of sport science (15, 91, 144).

Instrumented Sport Equipment

The integration of technology with sport equipment has provided practitioners with very interesting information (4, 59, 105). Morel and Hautier (105) used an instrumented scrum machine to measure neuromuscular fatigue in rugby union athletes. Attempts have been made to combine technology with sport equipment such as boats, oars, and paddles in rowing and kayaking (4, 59). Combat sport researchers have developed devices with **load cells**, which convert mechanical force into electrical signals, to assess striking and kicking forces (61, 137, 155) (see figure 6.1). In a case study, a professional boxer was monitored in the lead-up to a fight using a boxing-specific test that involved punching a custom-built apparatus mounted on a wall integrated with a load cell (61). The device's coefficient of variation for impact force and velocity was less than 1%, suggesting that it was very reliable. The monitoring tool, along with other performance tests, provided insight into

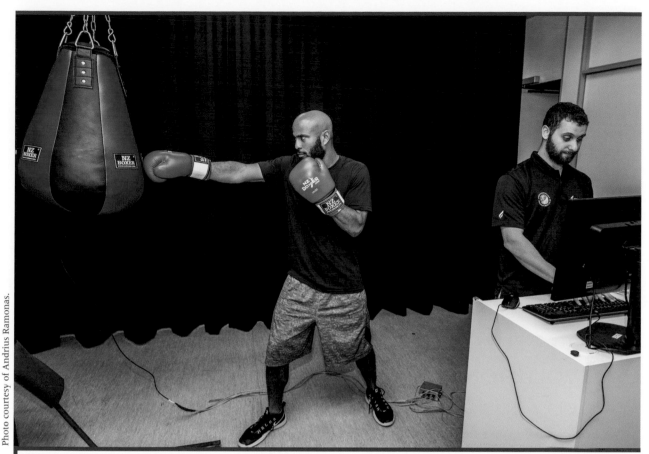

Photo courtesy of Andrius Ramonas.

Figure 6.1   Boxer punching an instrumented bag.

the athlete's peaking strategy. Such systems provide feedback on force profiles during training and competition. Practitioners can then use force–time profiles to calculate variables such as peak force, mean force, and time to peak force (35). Real-time feedback reveals athletes' movement techniques so that coaches can give them feedback during the training session to improve performance.

In the sport of skeleton, researchers have used instrumented sleds (55). In this event the practitioner can get feedback on the velocity of the sled during the push at the start of the race, which is particularly critical for performance (29).

An and colleagues (4) used strain gauge transducers in the foot stretch-ers of the rowers' boat. Peak force and average and peak loading rate were measured to quantify asymmetries (differences between limbs) and intralimb variability. The presence of asymmetries and the degree of performance variability during training sessions can show how the athlete produces force. This is an example of when practitioners need to be aware of overall changes in monitoring variables within a training session rather than a single measure such as peak power. Although such metrics are useful, a measure of variability (e.g., a standard deviation) in performance during the session or across the preceding week gives the practitioner a better indication of overarching factors such as pacing and fatigue (97) (see chapter 2).

In Paralympic sports, technology has played an important role in athlete monitoring. Researchers have investigated equipment instrumentation to quantify the demands of events (88). Activity sensors can be used to determine activity profiles in wheelchair court sports (e.g., rugby) (88). In one study, this technology was compared to an indoor tracking system (88). The devices accurately tracked variables such as distance covered and mean speed; however, they were less accurate in measuring the peak speeds produced by elite wheelchair athletes, which greatly limits the usefulness of the technology. Because different technologies can give different results for the same variable, practitioners should exercise caution when comparing them.

Load cell technology has been used to design novel equipment for athlete monitoring (112). Instrumentation of strength assessment equipment can provide important information about force production and imbalances (27, 112). Researchers have assessed the unilateral (single-leg) strength of the hamstrings in athlete populations using instrumented testing equipment (27, 112). Data on strength and potential imbalances may provide useful information for monitoring for fatigue and injury prevention.

EVOLUTION OF MONITORING TECHNOLOGY

Predicting how monitoring technology will develop and be used is somewhat futile because the rate of change is exponential. However, one thing is clear: If recent trends continue, monitoring will increasingly become a part of sport. The question is how this technology can be effectively integrated into overall sport programs. Transfers of laboratory-based technology to the field are likely. The value of laboratory-based research is that it is well controlled, although it may not have direct application to the practical sport setting. Smart watches, smart glasses, and smart fabrics will all continue to develop and have greater application in athlete monitoring. Wearable sensors that can measure biochemical markers will also continue to be developed and validated.

Rather than continually chase the most recent technological gadget, practitioners should keep in mind the most important people in sport: the athletes. Although wearable technology and the "quantified self" movement have created an awareness of monitoring data, the focus has been only on generating and collecting data. Less attention has been paid to how the data can be used to improve athletes' performance.

Practitioners would do well to ask themselves these questions:

- What types of technology do we currently use, and what will we be using in the future?
- What information produced by the technology is worthwhile reporting to the athlete?
- How can the information obtained from the monitoring technology be used to improve athlete performance?

Ultimately, the technology needs to help improve an athlete's performance. If it does not, it is not worth the investment.

Wearable Sensors

Wearable sensor technology is becoming increasingly prevalent in sport (143). A sensor is any device that transforms information into an analytically useful signal (10). This area has been researched extensively in a range of team and individual sports (33, 41). One of the advantages of wearable sensors is the ability to collect physiological and mechanical data such as heart rate, blood pressure, temperature, steps, distance covered, speed, and aspects of wellness such as sleep. These data, when processed by custom software, can then be summarized for the practitioner and athlete.

Wearable sensors have received a great deal of attention from researchers (10, 33, 42, 132). For example, sensors have been developed to use electromyography to measure the degree of muscular activity (108, 109, 140). This has led to developments in the area of smart clothing. Sensors have also been developed to measure impact forces (155) (see figure 6.2). Sensors that can be placed on the skin, such as patches, have significant applications for sport monitoring (9, 10, 56). One example is wearable devices that measure substrates, including lactate and hormones (23, 56). Feedback via these devices would be extremely useful for real-time monitoring of hormones, metabolites, and other markers to obtain a picture of athletes' physiological responses during training sessions (141). Research has shown that this technology can take valid measures of lactate, glucose, and electrolytes in addition to skin temperature and hydration status (10, 56).

A variety of wearable devices have been developed to analyze physiological factors such as temperature and sweat content (89). Sweat is an excellent candidate for analysis via sensors because it

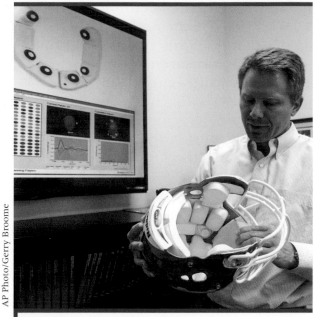

Figure 6.2   Wearable sensor.

AP Photo/Gerry Broome

contains many metabolites. To function well, sweat sensors require a good contact surface between the skin and the sensor surface. Measurement of sweat content could provide information on thermoregulation and hydration status, which is important for performance (19).

Wearable sensors can also be used to quantify movements in winter sports such as skiing (85, 86). In one study, skiers wore accelerometers; the differences in their characteristics were investigated with different techniques and validated against video analysis methods (86). The kinematic measures obtained via accelerometry were similar to those obtained with high-speed filming. The sensors provided information on technique selection and the rates and lengths of several kinematic variables (86).

Types of Sensors

Sensors for analyzing sweat consist of two major types: fabric and plastic devices and epidermal-based sensors (10).

Limitations of the technology include a lack of resiliency and stability in the devices and a limit to the metabolites that can be measured.

Gao and colleagues (56) used plastic-based sensors that interface with human skin. They performed real-time monitoring during cycling and rowing exercises and developed an app to use with the device (56). Researchers have developed temporary tattoos that may be able to directly detect chemicals on the skin (10) to monitor metabolites such as glucose (9) and lactate (72). Jia and colleagues collected sweat samples from a person during cycling exercise via a tattoo sensor, which revealed increases in lactate concentration with increased exercise intensity (72). Bandodkar and colleagues (9) showed that this technology could be used to detect glucose levels; they recorded increased levels after a meal. Further research is needed to validate these measures against levels in the blood and skeletal muscle, but the technology appears promising. Removing the need for invasive blood samples and complicated, expensive analyses would permit real-time assessments of athletes' physiological status. Currently, hormonal and biochemical monitoring appears to be minimal in high-performance sport because of these inherent limitations (3). However, it is not difficult to imagine increased adoption of this type of monitoring if cost-effective and accurate measures can be developed.

Saliva-based sensors offer another method for analyzing markers that may be of interest in athlete monitoring (10). Kim and colleagues (78) investigated the measurement of lactate in saliva using a mouthguard. Further work is needed to validate these approaches. Markers that are currently limited to saliva collection and then require subsequent analysis in the laboratory with complicated assays could be measured via this analysis (10).

Tears are another medium that can be analyzed to determine metabolite concentrations (64, 90). A contact lens sensor is one way to monitor glucose concentration (160). This technology could be incorporated into smart glasses for real-time monitoring. An obvious application would be to monitor glucose in people with diabetes, but athlete monitoring would be another application if additional metabolites could be measured in real time. Researchers have used a similar approach with lactate, which has even greater application to athlete monitoring (142).

Issues with sensors include resilience, power sources, and battery life (10). These are particularly important when this technology is used for real-time monitoring during long training sessions or competitions. As the technology develops, these limitations are less likely to be factors. Although several mediums can be used for measurement, and their noninvasive nature is appealing to practitioners, further validation of wearable sensors is required.

Placement of Sensors

The placement of sensors is an important consideration and has received attention from researchers (14, 133). As discussed in chapter 4, researchers have compared the position of GPS devices and accelerometry units (14, 133). The upper back and scapula region is a common site for wearing harnesses. Research suggests that location affects the data collected; thus, it needs to be consistent (14). Simons and Bradshaw (133) compared the reliability of impact loads during jumping and landing with an accelerometer placed on either the upper or lower back. They found the peak acceleration measurements to have moderate to good reliability for the tasks. The reliability was higher with the accelerometers on the lower back (133). Accelerometry technology can be useful for sports that involve a lot of landings such as gymnastics, figure skating, and dance. Monitoring the loads associated with these activities could have implications for injury prevention in these sports (133).

Researchers have investigated the use of inertial sensors for providing kinematic feedback during landings (46). A small-scale study suggested that after one session the feedback resulted in performers making alterations to their landing mechanics. Interestingly, only three parameters were used for feedback because the researchers found that this was the maximal number of parameters that could be modified during a single training session. This suggests that practitioners need to be careful not to overwhelm athletes with too much information from monitoring data (see chapter 7).

Athletes seem to prefer devices on the wrist, given their popularity (143). Some equipment is placed on equipment and clothing (e.g., on the cycle, in or on footwear, or embedded in clothing). Integrating technology with equipment the athlete uses regularly is logical. Earphones could be a good site given the common practice of listening to music during individual training sessions. Wearable technology that athletes don't notice is ideal.

Apps and Watches

Given that smartphones include GPS capability and often accelerometers, most practitioners and coaches have a readily available monitoring device in their pockets. Athlete monitoring apps track the metrics of an athlete over time and provide real-time feedback. A variety have been developed and validated for athlete monitoring (7, 8, 52). Even more advanced markers such as heart rate variability now have apps (51, 52). However, the validity and reliability of many apps have not been established. Practitioners should assess the accuracy of any app before using it. As research continues, the body of evidence on the validity and reliability of apps will be more complete so that practitioners can make more informed decisions about them.

Smart watches could be a good way to integrate monitoring data. Practitioners often want to monitor athletes during training sessions and competition, but monitoring at other times can also be helpful. Clearly, having an athlete wear a GPS device on the back or torso 24 hr a day is not feasible, but a smart watch could be a way to obtain regular monitoring data. Setting aside the ethics of constant surveillance of athletes, monitoring outside of training and competition appears to be increasing (127).

Force Plates

As discussed in chapter 5, force plates, position transducers, accelerometers, optical motion sensors, jump and reach devices, and jump mats can be used to assess neuromuscular fatigue during performance tests such as jump tests (17, 98). Measuring ground reaction forces using force plates has become more common in monitoring as technology has developed and become less expensive. Force plates measure triaxial forces, and force transducers convert mechanical information into an electrical signal. For example, a jump on a force plate results in a distortion to the load cells within the plate and causes a change in voltage that can be measured as a signal. Uni-axial plates measure the force output in one direction; triaxial plates measure all three planes of motion. Uniaxial plates are less expensive than triaxial plates, but they measure only vertical force, which can be a limitation (17). None-theless, they can still provide valuable information.

Dual force plates can be used for both bilateral and unilateral assessment (75) (see figure 6.3). They allow practitioners to monitor asymmetries, which can help them with program design (6, 95). Dual force plates are expensive, however, which has led to the development of more cost effective and portable options. Practitioners can use jump and reach devices for both bilateral and unilateral assessments, although they measure

only jump height. Jump height can be revealing, but greater insight can be obtained by tracking the underlying aspects of performance (111).

Calibration, which is important for determining the ground reaction forces measured from the voltage output, should be done over a range of loads and conditions (17)—for example, from the unloaded condition to the highest load athletes will use. This ensures that prac-titioners fully capture the highest forces athletes could produce. The calibration range will be somewhat different for a group of university-level gymnasts than it would be for an American football team because of the disparity in body mass. Ensuring appropriate calibration will help to reduce the errors associated with the measure.

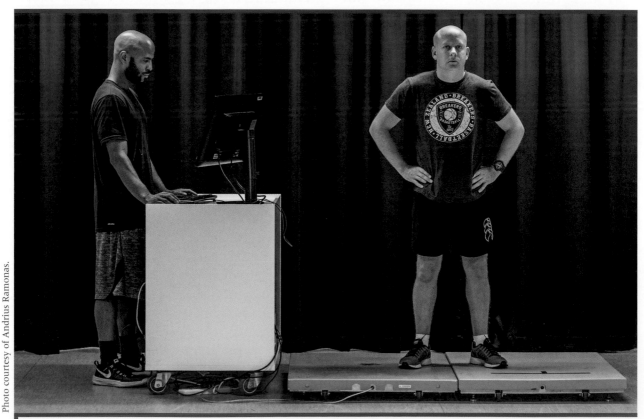

Photo courtesy of Andrius Ramonas.

Figure 6.3   Dual force plates for athlete monitoring.

Timing Systems

Infrared timing systems and contact mats can be used to measure flight time. Apps have been developed to estimate flight time, although more research is needed to determine their validity. When accurate measures of flight time are available, jump height can be calculated using the following formula (25):

$$\text{Jump height} = (9.81 \text{ m/s}^2 \times \text{flight time}^2) \div 8$$

If a flight time of 0.565 s is obtained, the jump height can be calculated as follows:

$$\text{Jump height} = (9.81 \text{ m/s}^2 \times 0.565^2) \div 8 = 0.39 \text{ m}$$

It is possible to estimate power from measures of flight time and jump height using equations (48, 129). Practitioners should use these equations with caution and be aware that they are simply an estimation of power output (49).

Data From Monitoring Technology

Focusing solely on the numbers produced by monitoring technologies can be tempting. However, an understanding of the technology and how it produces the information will help practitioners make sound decisions. Many systems use approaches that are not clear in terms of how the information is obtained and processed. This needs to be taken into account when interpreting the results of the monitoring. For example, when purchasing equipment it is useful for the practitioner to know how the data are being generated by the technology.

Sensing, Processing, and Visualizing

Sensing, processing, and visualizing data obtained from technology are important considerations. Sensing refers to the physical components such as a GPS device or a vest worn by the athlete. Processing occurs as the data are captured. Understanding these stages helps the practitioner determine whether the data are valid. An important part of this is having a fundamental understanding of the kinds of numbers to expect. The visualizing aspect refers to how the data appear to the end user. For example, is a single number produced, or do the data appear on a graph? A peak power result from a vertical countermovement jump of 20,000 watts should raise a red flag for the practitioner because normal results are below 10,000 watts. A limitation of approaches that produce a metric such as training load or stress is that there may be no way to determine how the measure was calculated and what a typical range should be for the results. The visualization aspect is important because it determines how the data are presented to the practitioner (see chapter 2).

Sampling Frequency

Monitoring any variable with technology requires collecting samples at regular intervals, which is also known as **sampling frequency**. The sampling frequency is how often the signal is recorded each second. A sampling rate of 50 Hz would mean that the signal is measured, or sampled, 50 times per second. Most human movement occurs at a range of 5 to 30 Hz (63). Research has been conducted to examine the effect of sampling frequency across a range of technologies in sport science (71, 74, 98). Differences in sampling frequency can affect the results of the monitoring (71).

The data obtained with monitoring technologies can be processed in several ways. Data collected are often filtered, smoothed, differentiated, and integrated to calculate and predict variables. Custom software can be used to perform signal processing and remove noise associated with the data signal. A wide range of sampling frequencies are used to collect and record monitoring data (120). The Nyquist-Shannon sampling theorem states that the critical sampling frequency should be at least two times the highest frequency of the signal being collected to obtain accurate information from the original signal (63). Fundamentally, what that means is that the required sampling frequency increases with increasing movement velocity. This accounts for why GPS devices are less accurate and less reliable with high-speed movements and accelerations and decelerations (153).

Recommendations can be made for sampling frequency ranges for several measures used in athlete monitoring (98). For example, the recommended sampling frequency range for vertical jumps is 350 to 700 Hz (98). To capture position changes of 5 mm (about 3/16 in.) for movements with velocities between 1.0 and 3.0 m/s, the monitoring device must sample at rates between 20 and 60 Hz (98). Using force plate testing, ground reaction force is recorded only at the time points determined by the sampling frequency. At a frequency of 500 Hz, this would be occurring every 0.002 s. Problems occur when the technology samples at rates below the critical frequency because it could distort the original signal and result in the loss of vital pieces of data. A rapid change in force could be missed at a given sampling frequency if the time from one sample to the next is too long. It is therefore recommended that the sampling frequency be at least five times higher than the frequency of the signal for athlete movements to ensure that peak values for aspects such as takeoff and landing forces are not missed (43). When measuring rate-dependent variables such as rate of force development, these ranges should be even higher (98).

Data Processing Methods

Built-in software systems can convert signals from analog to digital and then smooth and filter the digital data, which are adjusted to reduce the noise and distortion of the signal. Smoothing techniques include polynomial (e.g., Butterworth filters), splines (e.g., cubic splines), Fourier transform, moving averages, and digital filters. Filtered and smoothed data are then differentiated or integrated depending on the measurement system used to calculate the variables. Practitioners should keep in mind that as the number of calculations increases, so does the error. Although most practitioners do not need in-depth knowledge of these methods, a basic understanding of the key principles may be useful. More detailed information on these methods of data analysis can be found in other sources (43, 63, 120, 159).

Storing Data

Practitioners need to consider how they are going to store athlete monitoring data and records, especially given that many forms of technology generate a significant amount of data. Whether systems that track and store athlete monitoring information are being implemented effectively in sport is unclear. Injury surveillance systems have been found lacking as a result of inadequately stored data (50).

A variety of database solutions and products are used to store monitoring data and records (44). Commercial storage systems are available, and some organizations develop their own in-house systems. Adequate record keeping helps to build historical databases, which allow for even more sophisticated, as well as retrospective, analyses.

Because of the potential for high staff turnover, high-performance sport organizations should have systems in place to ensure that data are not lost when staff members move on. Systems should involve maintaining consistent record keeping, having policies governing the storage and backup of data (e.g., maintaining it in several locations), and using the approach consistently. Problems can occur when systems and technology change, so practitioners would be wise to use a system consistently for a period of time before changing to another.

Some monitoring systems require that a body of information be collected before informed decisions can be made about how to use it. Collecting information over a long period allows for data mining and more sophisticated analyses. Of course, this needs to be weighed against the program's short-term requirements. However, long-term strategic thinking can maximize the benefits of an athlete monitoring program.

Applications of Monitoring Technology

When implementing a monitoring system, some practitioners begin by purchasing equipment and technology. However, practitioners also need to consider how they will use the information gleaned from the technology to make decisions regarding athlete fatigue and training load. This section outlines several ways technology is used in athlete monitoring.

Technology to Analyze Skeletal Muscle

Characteristics of skeletal muscle can be of great interest to practitioners and researchers because of the critical role skeletal muscle plays in exercise. Traditionally in exercise science, muscle biopsies are used to measure aspects such as muscle fiber type and enzyme content (36, 53, 148). Skeletal muscle consists of a range of fiber types; the major ones are Type I, Type IIa, and Type IIx. Enzymes such as lactate dehydrogenase are important for speeding up chemical reactions in the body. Measures such as the content of myosin heavy chains (148) and titin (92) can provide insights into the structure and function of muscle. The expression of myosin heavy chains, which make up the thick filaments of skeletal muscle, can indicate responses to training (116). Titin is a structural protein found in skeletal muscle that is believed to have important roles in muscle elasticity (92). Obviously, the regular use of muscle biopsies is not a viable option for sport monitoring, so researchers have attempted to develop methods to assess skeletal muscle in athletes noninvasively (5, 67).

Connective tissues such as tendons and ligaments can be monitored using methods such as ultrasound (22), an imaging technique that uses high-frequency sound waves to visualize structures within the body. Magnetic resonance imaging (MRI) uses a magnetic field and radio frequency pulses to provide even more detailed images of internal body structures. Ultrasound and MRI can measure aspects of muscle and tendon architecture such as pennation angle, fascicle length, and muscle thickness, as well as tendon properties (110). Several of these measures change acutely in response to training sessions as well as over the long term. Ultrasound and MRI are noninvasive and can provide valuable information on how athletes are adapting to training. However, they are expensive (22), and trained personnel are needed to operate the equipment.

Measures of muscle carnosine determined from magnetic resonance spectroscopy may predict muscle fiber type (5). Using this noninvasive approach, Bex and colleagues (20) found differences in muscle carnosine content between athletes in different sports. Performance tests have also been used to estimate muscle fiber type and characteristics, which are of great interest to practitioners and researchers (24). It has been proposed that cycle tests and optimal cadence can be used as indirect estimators of muscle fiber type (67). Ultimately, tools that can be used regularly and are noninvasive to athletes are best for athlete monitoring.

Technology in the Weight Room

The increased use of technology has led to the development of equipment for monitoring strength and conditioning factors such as bar velocity. Attempts have been made to integrate this information with video analysis to monitor technique (126). Practitioners should pay attention to output from athlete monitoring (e.g., measures of force and velocity), but also to how the athlete is performing the movement. Being able to integrate this information and provide

real-time feedback would be extremely valuable. Variables such as strength, sets, and repetitions are relatively simple to monitor. However, technology is needed to monitor velocity, impulse, and power. A gradual transition has been made to using more practical and smaller devices to monitor athletes in these environments (98, 125). Devices require validation before they can be used confidently by practitioners, however. Rather than relying on a single study to confirm the validity of a device, practitioners would be better served by a process for replicating findings and building up a body of evidence.

Strength and conditioning practitioners have always been interested in exercise characteristics such as velocity (34, 123). Microsensors can be worn by the athlete or placed on the bar to measure these variables (8, 76) (see figure 6.4); for example, accelerometry can be used to measure weightlifting performance (125). However, practitioners must consider both reliability and validity before implementing any new technology into their monitoring systems.

Monitoring Running With Technology

Speed has always been of great interest to practitioners because of its fundamental importance in sport. A stopwatch is a simple but highly effective tool, but more sophisticated timing devices such as timing gates more accurately measure speed and acceleration (65) (figure 6.5).

Another metric to explore is the underlying force–time characteristics of running. Nonmotorized and torque treadmills have been used for this purpose in athlete monitoring (13, 84, 134, 135). Measures of force can be performed using specialized sprint treadmill ergometers

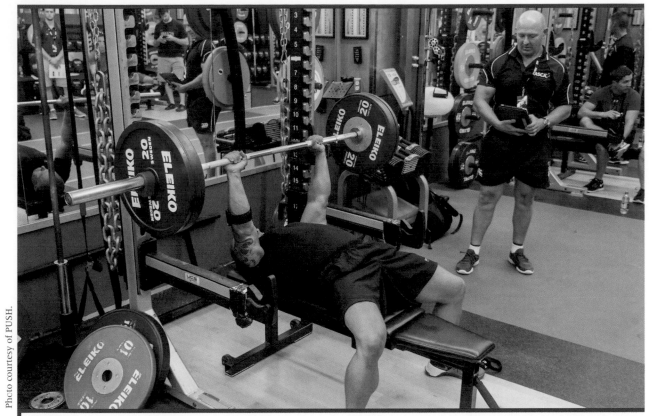

Figure 6.4 An athlete performing a bench press while a wearable device collects velocity data.

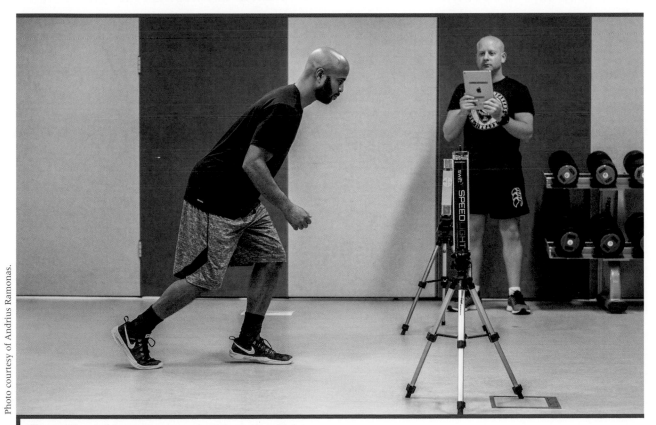

Figure 6.5 Athlete monitored with timing lights.

that allow athletes to drive the treadmill belt under them while remaining tethered in place. Technology can also be used to measure variables such as force as they are instrumented with load cells. Forces can be measured using either a tether-mounted strain gauge or force plates below the treadmill frame.

Given the importance of both horizontal and vertical force during sprinting, sprint treadmill ergometers can provide important information for athlete monitoring (106). Mangine and colleagues (84) used a 30-s sprint protocol on a nonmotorized treadmill and found good relationships with 30-m sprint time. Disadvantages of these systems include their high cost, an increased risk of injury (due to using maximal sprinting as a monitoring tool), and the difficulty of monitoring a large number of athletes unless several treadmills are available. Also, some have expressed concern about the change in running gait kinematics that can occur when running on different types of treadmills (96). All of these factors should be considered when making decisions regarding the implementation of this technology.

Recently validated field methods provide accurate and repeatable data on sprinting variables (106, 122). These methods estimate horizontal force and the associated force–velocity relationships via simple velocity–time data obtained from the movement of an athlete's center of mass (122). This means that common field testing equipment such as a **radar devices** can be used to calculate force–velocity profiles during sprinting as long as the sampling frequency is sufficient. Radar devices work by emitting radio waves and detecting changes in frequency as the waves bounce off the athlete.

Another way to assess running is with laser technology (134), which works by emitting a beam of infrared light that reflects off the athlete. Research has employed methods of quantifying force–velocity relationships and mechanical variables to delineate between injured and noninjured players (101, 102) and between positions in similar sports (e.g., rugby union and rugby league) (40). What makes methods such as this particularly useful is the ability to conduct testing in the field without the need for large amounts of equipment.

Researchers have looked at the use of GPS devices and accelerometry to assess stride variables and vertical stiffness during running in team sport athletes (28). As discussed in chapter 4, commercial GPS devices include accelerometers, gyroscopes, and magnetometers. Accelerometers and gyroscopes detect accelerations and angular velocities; magnetometers sense the strongest magnetic field. Buchheit and colleagues (28) compared data obtained from a GPS-embedded **triaxial** accelerometer with the vertical ground reaction force obtained from an instrumented force plate. *Triaxial* refers to three axes of rotation: vertical (x-axis), anteroposterior (y-axis), and mediolateral (z-axis). Algorithms were determined to calculate specific aspects of an athlete's stride (e.g., foot strike) from the accelerometry data. The results indicated that variables such as contact time, flight time, and vertical stiffness could be measured accurately (28). Obtaining these measures with lightweight GPS devices permits practitioners to test athletes in the field rather than relying on specialized and expensive equipment.

Running can be analyzed with accelerometry, and several studies have investigated the validity of some devices (83, 156). One study looked at the validity of an accelerometer compared with optical motion capture (83). The study showed the accelerometer to be a valid and reliable measure of running accelerations. Another study validated an accelerometer worn on the torso while athletes ran on an instrumented treadmill (156). The device provided valid measures of ground contact time, suggesting its potential as a field-based tool for athlete monitoring.

Researchers have investigated the use of inertial devices to measure fatigue in runners (139). In one study, runners ran on a treadmill and on an indoor track, and the two conditions were compared (139). Interestingly, differences in technique changes with fatigue were noted between the conditions. This highlights the importance of being specific when monitoring (139).

Using an accelerometer on the leg is another approach that can be used in the field and relies on laboratory validation. Giandolini and colleagues (57) investigated gait characteristics in a world-class trail runner using accelerometers on the runner's shoe and leg. They were able to track some interesting information on foot strikes and tibial acceleration throughout the 45-km (28 mile) race. Devices such as these are potential game changers for practitioners and athletes because they allow for the assessment of mechanical loading and impact during training and competition (58), which have been shown to be important in injury prevention (152). Simple monitoring of runners is informative, but when environmental factors such as terrain are taken into account, the picture of the external load on the athlete is far more complete. If this technology can be incorporated into runners' footwear, detailed measures of gait previously attainable only in controlled laboratory settings could be available in the field (58).

Insoles can be used to measure force characteristics such as plantar pressure distribution during running and jumping (87, 108). Martinez-Marti and colleagues (87) investigated the use of instrumented insoles to measure flight time during various types of vertical jumps; the results showed the potential of this technology for athlete monitoring. However, a great deal more research is required to validate these technologies and demonstrate their efficacy for athlete monitoring.

Monitoring Cycling With Technology

As discussed in chapter 4, cycling has been at the forefront of monitoring technology; measuring devices allow for continuous monitoring of power output. In cycling, the assessment of variables such as optimal power and cadence is most valuable when applied to training and competition (73). For example, a cycle-based assessment of power can replicate a competition scenario. Once determined, optimal conditions can be replicated to directly influence race performance. The targeted manipulation of factors such as crank length and gear ratios can enable the athlete to perform a cycle sprint in practically optimal conditions for power production (73).

Direct power measurement tools in the field are valuable for practitioners and used extensively in sports such as cycling (136). The timing and duration of force application can be particularly informative with this type of force and power profiling. Optimal cadence for road cyclists can be determined from training power output, heart rate, and cadence (119). Recently developed power profile monitoring tests may be able to predict performance (117, 118). As with other types of technology, practitioners need to exercise caution when comparing results between equipment (1). Abbiss and colleagues (1) compared a cycle ergometer and power meter and found different power measures. The magnitude of the difference was affected by the test type.

Researchers and practitioners use cycle ergometers to monitor athletes (45, 47, 157). Technology permits them to investigate asymmetries using instrumented pedals and cranks (21). Researchers have also developed multisensor cycle ergometers for monitoring. These systems allow for the integration of multiple sensors (e.g., instrumented cranks) and real-time monitoring. Technology for athlete monitoring should be adaptable and easy to set up and use.

Clinical Applications of Technology

Technology used in other fields is often developed or modified for athlete monitoring (11, 60). An example is **transcranial electrical stimulation**, which has been used with stroke patients and involves applying a weak electrical current (16). It may provide insights into the central nervous system adaptations that occur in response to training (60).

Wearable technology has been developed to provide direct feedback during activities (132). Haptic (touch), audio, and visual feedback have been investigated for providing feedback during gait (132). This information could be used to facilitate changes in gait and therefore be a useful tool for both athlete monitoring and training. In one study wearable sensors provided feedback to alter knee loading patterns during walking (158).

Having this type of real-time feedback has important applications to rehabilitation (132).

Clinical applications of wearable technology have scope in athlete monitoring for simplifying more complicated assessments. An example is smartphone apps that generate electrocardiograms that can be viewed remotely by cardiologists (115). Such technology can facilitate communication between athletic trainers and medical staff, helping them to monitor athletes during training and identify those who are at risk.

Activity monitors have been investigated for monitoring sleep in athletes (124). Sargent and colleagues (124) compared wrist activity monitors to **polysomnography**, which is considered the gold standard for sleep monitoring and is also used in sleep studies. It records a range of measures such as brain wave activity, oxygen level, heart rate, and respiration rate to determine the sleep quality. Activity monitors were shown to be a valid alternative for measuring the sleep of athletes, although selecting the correct sleep–wake threshold was important given the variations in sleep and wake durations (124). This highlights the importance of being cautious when comparing monitoring technologies. Practitioners needs to determine whether the technology provides more information than simply asking the athlete the simple question "How well did you sleep?" If the evidence suggests that a subjective tool can provide essentially the same information, practitioners need to question the value of additional technology (127).

FACTORS TO CONSIDER WHEN CHOOSING MONITORING TECHNOLOGY

With the wide variety of technology available for monitoring, practitioners should consider the following factors:

- Reliability, validity, and sensitivity of the technology
- Research evidence for its use
- Cost
- Ease of use
- Range of measures that can be obtained (functionality)
- Availability of a nontechnological alternative
- Extent of invasiveness
- Degree that the technology will interfere with training and competition
- Type of feedback provided to the practitioner (ideally, real-time)
- Quality and quantity of information about training load and fatigue (to help the practitioner make decisions regarding the athlete's training session and program)
- How the measures relate to performance
- Amount of athlete buy-in (acceptance)
- Durability
- Associated custom software for analysis and reporting
- Method of data collection (e.g., via smartphone or tablet)
- Battery life

A simple cost-benefit analysis is useful before making a final decision about the value of technology. A good strategy is to talk with other practitioners who have used the technology to get feedback on advantages and disadvantages. By weighing these factors, practitioners can make informed decisions about technology and its benefits for athlete monitoring.

Conclusion

Practitioners use a range of practices and technologies for athlete monitoring. How to use the monitoring data is a fundamental consideration. New technologies are being developed all the time, which presents challenges in terms of implementation. Wearable sensors are being used increasingly with athletes. Ideally, they should be small, lightweight, and inexpensive. Being able to collect the information via smartphone or tablet increases the utility of these systems for monitoring purposes. One of the major challenges for practitioners is the time required to learn how to use each new technology as well as to follow up with upgrades, maintenance, and the latest developments in the field of technology. All this is time away from other aspects of the practitioner's role. Although athlete monitoring is widely used in sport, large amounts of staff resources do not appear to be directed to this area (3). In most cases the additional work is incorporated into the practitioner's role. Therefore, practitioners are advised to keep things simple (37).

7

Integrating Monitoring With Coaching

A major purpose of athlete monitoring is to obtain both objective and subjective information to help coaches plan their athletes' training. Many monitoring programs focus on technology, but other approaches can contribute as well. Consider sitting in the cockpit of an airplane. It can be tempting to focus solely on all the numbers and flashing lights on the dashboard. However, sometimes just looking out the window (i.e., focusing on the most valuable monitoring tools and data) can provide all the needed information.

Other important issues in monitoring are communicating data to athletes, monitoring during training sessions, and conducting in-house research projects. All of these are addressed in this chapter, which focuses on integrating monitoring into the coaching process. In addition, the key aspects of a monitoring system are outlined.

Art and Science of Monitoring

Practitioners often refer to the *art of coaching*. Although this phrase is not always clear, it generally implies the use of experience and instincts to inform decisions. Ideally, this personal expertise should be combined with solid scientific evidence. However, practitioners sometimes have several options to choose from without any clear evidence to distinguish them. Such cases require the application of both the art and the science of monitoring—recognizing that there isn't necessarily a single correct solution. Effective coaching requires the practitioner to consider both approaches to guide an athlete's training.

The art of coaching can be useful when there is limited evidence for best practices. When there is an abundance of information, however, practitioners should be wary about using objective monitoring data to confirm findings based on intuition, or a gut feeling. This practice creates a **confirmation bias** when new information is used to confirm preexisting ideas or theories (51).

Practitioners should also guard against **cherry picking**—that is, accepting findings that agree with what they want to see and ignoring evidence that does not agree. This can occur when practitioners use **data dredging** (also called **data fishing**), especially when large amounts of data are available. Data dredging involves continuing to look for relationships and patterns in the monitoring information until they fit the picture the practitioner wants to create. One of the dangers of having a high volume of data is that false patterns can emerge and spurious (false) correlations can be created. Results that are interpreted without proper context can cause problems for practitioners.

Unfortunately, many aspects of athlete monitoring have not been researched extensively; as a result, an overwhelming body of evidence does not exist to support the implementation of some monitoring methods. This does not necessarily mean that these aspects are not important or useful. Practitioners can use **heuristics**, or rules of thumb, to help them integrate the art and science of monitoring (e.g., provide only three pieces of monitoring feedback to an athlete during the session). One of the research gaps relates to using monitoring data to inform decision making. To date, a great deal of focus has been on collecting data, and less has been on analyzing data. Many research studies have tracked athletes over the course of a season or, in some cases, multiple years (12, 26, 52, 56). Longitudinal data provide useful insights into monitoring measures and how they fluctuate over the course of the training cycle. However, these types of studies are only observational. Intervention studies can be more difficult to conduct (particularly in elite sports), and much of the information remains unpublished and outside of the public domain. To combat this, chapters 8 and 9 present case studies showing how monitoring data can be collected and used in a variety of sports.

A vital component of athlete monitoring is accurate data, which is why monitoring tools must be reliable, valid, and sensitive to change. It is important to use available evidence and not just rely on gut feel. On the other hand, it can be dangerous to rely solely on data, given that the human element remains a fundamental aspect of sport. The *coach's eye* is a term used to describe subjective monitoring approaches. Practitioners need to realize that they may not be able to accurately measure all important factors and that data sometimes provide insights but not answers.

late training performance scores. Agostinho and colleagues (2) developed a global training performance metric for judo athletes that took into account the intensity of key exercises and throws.

- *Appropriate analysis methods.* The smallest meaningful change in monitoring variables can be calculated for each athlete using appropriate baseline data; the process requires only a calculator.

Although commercial software platforms are available for athlete monitoring, practitioners can use simple tools such as Microsoft Excel or Google Docs to develop their own monitoring templates. Google Docs allows practitioners to develop their own training diaries and questionnaires that athletes can access on devices or smartphones. Moreover, questions can be presented in a variety of formats and layouts. An advantage of using simple tools such as this is that data reporting is relatively straightforward. Practitioners requiring more advanced analyses can convert the data to a .csv format. Although these systems require an initial time investment on the part of the practitioner, they can be very beneficial. As with any monitoring approach, it is advisable to begin with a simple set of questions and build on and refine them as needed.

In summary, using simple tools, practitioners can set up relatively sophisticated monitoring systems. The value of monitoring data is determined by how they are analyzed, interpreted, and implemented. Ultimately, a successful system is one that informs practitioner decision making and improves athlete performance.

Monitoring With Training Diaries

Data obtained from training diaries can be informative for practitioners, and the process is simple (16). An analysis of the training diaries of Olympic track and field athletes provided insights into the volumes of strength and power training across the year (5). The analyses showed that 50% to 60% of combined strength-based (high load) and power-based training volume undertaken in the preseason was enough to maintain strength and power throughout the 3-month season. Assigning training loads during the season is a critical consideration for practitioners. Retrospective analyses of training diaries can guide training program design. Fundamentally, at issue is not just the total training load but how the athlete gets there and how to vary the load across the season. Obtaining this information from simple training diaries can have implications for both performance enhancement and injury prevention.

Research studies that involve training diaries typically span periods of less than 1 year (39), although case studies have been published on single elite athletes for longer periods of time (26, 38). Keeping training diaries for several years or longer could provide rich details about athletes' evolution and reveal pictures of their training practices at various levels. Youth athletes, for example, could examine the training that elite athletes go through to see the intensities and loads they built up over time to arrive at the elite level. Further, athletes could compare training using different modes of exercise. A training diary can reveal the differences in the volume and intensity between aerobic endurance training and resistance training. Aerobic training volume (e.g., the total distance covered during a week) at a certain intensity (e.g., a percentage of $\dot{V}O_2max$) can be contrasted with the volume and loading of resistance training. Such analyses can help practitioners formulate training models for athletes.

Another way athletes keep track of their training is to record the intensity of their workouts based on zones (see chapter 4). Ideally, these zones are based on physiological measures such as heart rate. Tjelta (38) outlined five zones when documenting the training practices of elite distance runners. The zones were 1 = easy and continuous running (62% to 82% maximal heart rate), 2 = threshold training (82% to 92% maximal heart rate), 3 = intensive anaerobic intervals (92% to 97% maximal heart rate), 4 = anaerobic training (≥97% maximal heart rate), and 5 = sprinting. Using this approach, the practitioner can obtain a clear picture of the type and intensity of sessions simply by looking at the athlete's zone number in the training diary. As long as the practitioner or the athlete documents the intensity in some manner (e.g., RPE), a measure of internal load is available. The other factors that require consideration are the athlete's level of experience and his or her individual characteristics.

Tran and colleagues (43) analyzed the training practices of elite Australian rowers leading up to the 2012 Olympic Games. They documented external load by measuring training frequency, duration, and total distance rowed on the water and by using ergometers. Other forms of training, including resistance training and cycling, were also documented. Internal load was measured using an adaptation of the training impulse method (see pages 88-90 in chapter 4) (41, 42). Published research can give practitioners insights into the training practices of elite-level athletes (3, 39, 40, 43). Importantly, published studies providing data on both external load (training dosage) and internal load (training responses) can be particularly informative (43).

Applying Monitoring in Individual Sports

Although the general principles of athlete monitoring can be applied across a range of sports, specific nuances can be important to consider depending on the sport. The following sections outline how athlete monitoring is applied to some individual sports.

Weightlifting

Because no single measure is completely effective for monitoring athletes, practitioners should use a mixed-methods approach. They also need to strike a balance between the number of aspects measured and the practical value of their monitoring tools. An Olympic weightlifter might use a training diary to record essential information on exercises, sets, repetitions, and load. Session RPE measures can be obtained 10 to 30 min after each session and used to calculate training load, monotony, and strain. Neuromuscular fatigue can be tracked daily with a vertical countermovement jump test (35). In addition, a wellness questionnaire (e.g., addressing sleep, muscle soreness, fatigue, and stress) can be completed by the athlete three times per week.

For within-session monitoring, the practitioner can measure barbell velocity on one key set during each session using a linear position transducer (see figure 8.1). The exercise and the loading used for monitoring must be consistent. The practitioner might decide to use the snatch pull (Monday), clean pull (Wednesday), and jerk (Friday), all performed at 80% of 1RM over a 4-week microcycle.

Most important is that practitioners obtain direct measures of sport performance whenever possible. This is relatively straightforward in weightlifting because a 1RM snatch and clean and jerk can be measured directly on a regular basis or estimated using prediction equations from training (e.g.,

a 3RM). Measures of salivary testosterone and cortisol and blood creatine kinase can be considered, but cost and impracticality may be limitations. Table 8.1 outlines the frequency, purpose, analysis method, and practical interpretation of the monitoring variables for weightlifters.

Throwing Sports

In sports with high volumes of throwing (e.g., shot put, javelin), monitoring the training load can be vital for reducing injury risk and ensuring continued adaptation (31). It is possible to measure overall training load, but for throwing-based sports practitioners might also be interested in more specific aspects (e.g., the total number of throws) to calculate training load, monotony, and strain for that part of the athlete's training program (11) (see chapter 2).

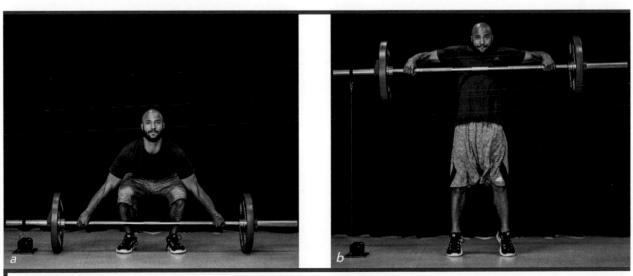

Photos courtesy of Andrius Ramonas.

Figure 8.1 Weightlifter training with a linear position transducer.

TABLE 8.1 Monitoring System for a Weightlifter

Variable	Assessment frequency	Purpose	Analysis method	Practical interpretation
1RM snatch and clean and jerk	Weekly or estimated from training	Measure of performance	Absolute change relative to reliability value and smallest meaningful change (determined from coefficient of variation of performance)	Smallest meaningful change (e.g., 1.5 kg [3.3 lb] for the snatch and 2 kg [4.4 lb] for the clean and jerk)
Volume load	Every session	Measure of external load	• Week-to-week change • Rolling 3-week average • Acute-to-chronic ratio (see chapter 9)	• Avoid >10% increase in volume load each week • Acute-to-chronic ratio <1.5 (see chapter 9)
Session RPE	Every session	Measure of perceived exertion of session	Z-score relative to baseline measure	Z-score ≤−1.5
Training load	Weekly	Measure of internal load	Z-score relative to baseline measure	Z-score ≤−1.5
Monotony	Weekly	Measure of sameness and variation of training	Z-score relative to baseline measure	Z-score ≤−1.5
Strain	Weekly	Overall product of training load and monotony	Z-score relative to baseline measure	Z-score ≤−1.5
Wellness (questionnaire)	Three times per week	Measure of overall wellness and quality of sleep, muscle soreness, fatigue, and stress	Z-score relative to baseline measure	Z-score ≤−1.5
Vertical countermovement jump (jump height)	Daily	Measure of neuromuscular fatigue	• Z-score relative to baseline measure • Smallest meaningful change relative to reliability	Z-score ≤−1.5
Training distress (scale)	Weekly	Measure of training-related distress and performance readiness	• Z-score relative to baseline measure • Week-to-week and chronic variability	Z-score ≤−1.5
Barbell velocity	Every session (one exercise)	Measure of velocity-based training to ensure quality of repetitions across the set	• Smallest meaningful change relative to reliability • Week-to-week variation • Percentage of decrement across sets	• Smallest meaningful change (e.g., 0.2 m/s) • Terminate set if greater than 20% loss in velocity

Table 8.2 shows a record of a shot put athlete's total number of throws of any type—throws with shots, medicine balls, or any projectile. By calculating the monotony, the practitioner was able to determine the variation of the load over the week.

In this example, the low monotony of 1.04 indicates a large degree of variation across the week. A good rule of thumb (heuristic) is to keep the monotony under 2.0, although this may differ across sports and individual athletes. Practitioners should also look at monotony over several weeks to get a full picture of how the training load is tracking. Research suggests the importance of avoiding large spikes in training loads (>10% per week), but also of avoiding too many periods of unloading, in which training load is dramatically reduced (12).

TABLE 8.2 Throw Monitoring for a Shot Put Athlete

Day	Training load (number of throws)
Monday	35
Tuesday	0
Wednesday	40
Thursday	0
Friday	45
Saturday	55
Sunday	0
Total weekly load	175.0
Daily mean load	24.1
Daily standard deviation	25.0
Monotony	1.04

Individual Aerobic Endurance Sports

Considering the difference between reality and an ideal scenario is important for practitioners. It is imperative to take into account the athlete's real-world situation when choosing which aspects of the monitoring system to implement. For example, research has shown that heart rate variability (HRV) should be monitored individually to see how each athlete is responding to training (27). Working with individual athletes makes this somewhat easier, although some practitioners are dealing with several individual athletes.

The method of data collection also needs to be considered. Obtaining resting HRV measures in both supine and standing positions, as recommended by some researchers, may be unrealistic because the process may take more than 15 min (8). Simpler methods in which data collection is faster may be preferable, as long as they are valid and reliable.

Establishing a baseline is an important part of any monitoring. One approach when measuring aspects such as HRV is to use the start of the training week (e.g., Monday morning) as a baseline. Another option is to establish a baseline period (e.g., over several sessions in the preseason). Having a defined baseline is important for making valid comparisons and detecting performance changes.

Combat Sports

Working with individual sport athletes competing in weight classes, such as in combat sports, often requires dealing with the issue of making weight. Body composition is important in many sports, but the additional layer of complexity provided by these weight sports can pose challenges for practitioners. Therefore, aspects of body composition must be monitored closely. Body weight should be measured on a regular basis (daily) leading up to weigh-in. Other metrics such as skinfold measurements can be obtained, but the tester must be trained in the technique and the protocols must be reliable and valid. Monitoring nutrition and hydration is also important, but the focus should be on performance and balanced with the athlete's health and well-being (36). Recommendations for working with athletes in sports with weight classes and strategies for making weight safely are available for practitioners (20, 36).

Regular monitoring of physical characteristics can identify specific responses to combat sport training programs. Ratamess and colleagues (30) tracked performance and physiological changes in university wrestlers over a training year. Maximal grip strength, Wingate peak power, and vertical countermovement jump force and power decreased over the course of the competitive season (30). Total testosterone, body fat, and body mass also declined as the season progressed. Interestingly, the periodized training program was designed to increase strength and power in the preseason period with a change to a circuit training program aimed to improve muscular endurance during the season. A monitoring program would have enabled the practitioner to assess the efficacy of the training program more regularly. In this instance, changing the in-season program to focus on maintaining strength and power would likely have been more appropriate.

Halperin and colleagues (15) documented a case study of a professional boxer preparing for a title fight in Australia. The boxer was monitored over 9 weeks leading up to the fight and then 8 days after the fight. Boxing-specific tests were completed using load cell technology to measure punching forces along with a variety of other performance tests. Body composition measures were also made on a regular basis (body weight, sum of skinfolds, and dual X-ray absorptiometry). Performance tests can be useful for tracking sport-specific changes in conjunction with body composition changes. In this example, the athlete was fighting at the 76.2-kg (168 lb) class and began the monitoring period at 80.8 kg (178 lb). The researchers were able to monitor the changes in body composition and relate them to the changes in performance. Decreases were seen in punching impact forces, maximal strength, and vertical countermovement jump height. Also interesting was that 8 days following the bout, the boxer had improved aerobic power and punching forces, possibly as a result of supercompensation and overcoming the accumulated fatigue of the lead-up to the fight. This type of monitoring information would enable practitioners to fine-tune tapering strategies for pinnacle events by taking into account individual differences.

Racket Sports

Tournament play can provide interesting scenarios for practitioners working with individual sport athletes. For example, in sports such as tennis, planning can be difficult because of many unknown factors such as when an athlete will exit the tournament and match duration and timing. Monitoring can allow the practitioner to gauge the athlete's fatigue and recovery, but it must present a minimal burden for the athlete, especially during a tournament. Short-form questionnaires such as the eight-item Short Recovery and Stress Scale can measure the degree of stress and recovery (44). Another option is a visual analog scale to measure the degree of delayed-onset muscle soreness (DOMS). Alternatively, practitioners can use their own custom wellness questionnaires (see table 4.1 for an example).

The choice of monitoring tools to use during a tournament should be driven by how the information can be used. Consider a practitioner who has a tennis player perform the vertical countermovement jump test each morning of a multiday tournament. A baseline score is determined at the beginning of a tournament (39 cm, or 15.4 in.), and the smallest meaningful change was previously calculated as 1.5 cm (0.6 in.). The athlete has the following scores over 6 days of tournament play:

Day 1 = 39 cm (baseline)
Day 2 = 39 cm (stable)
Day 3 = 38 cm (−1 cm)
Day 4 = 37 cm (−2 cm)
Day 5 = 37 cm (−2 cm)
Day 6 = 36 cm (−3 cm)

The results show that the smallest meaningful change was exceeded on day 4. However, the practitioner could have decided on day 3 that the 1-cm decrease warranted some type of intervention such as an increased focus on recovery strategies or a reduced training session on the morning of day 4. Ultimately, performance tests must be used for a purpose and not just for the sake of monitoring. Why use these monitoring tools if they do not improve the athlete's chance of success in tournament play? In this scenario, having a simple set of questions and one performance test would likely not be too onerous.

Motorsports

Monitoring motorsport athletes can present unique challenges for practitioners (28, 29). Determining the thermoregulation and the physiological stresses drivers are under during races has been of particular interest to researchers (6, 33). In motorsports, a great deal of attention has been given to the technology drivers use, but less to the drivers themselves. Monitoring methods that measure internal load, including heart rate and body temperature, would be useful for practitioners working in this sport (6, 33). In addition, simple wellness questionnaires to gain insights into athletes' fatigue as well as thermal discomfort could be informative (13).

Extreme Sports

The increasing popularity of extreme sports (e.g., skateboarding, surfing) and events such as the X Games has resulted in more focus on the training demands of these athletes (7, 14, 22, 34). Monitoring athletes in snowboarding (14) and surfing (10, 22) has received increased attention from researchers. Fatigue monitoring appears to have some value in these sports because of the high physical demands of training and competition (14). Although implementing a direct measure of performance on a regular basis may prove challenging, using a vertical countermovement jump to monitor fatigue has shown promise in these populations (14).

As discussed in chapter 3, fatigue is a complex topic, and designing appropriate monitoring tests to assess it can be challenging (9). Some experts believe that

PRACTICAL USE OF WELLNESS QUESTIONNAIRES

As discussed in chapter 4, practitioners often develop their own wellness questionnaires for athlete monitoring. Ideally, a wellness questionnaire is completed daily; however, doing so may burden the athlete. Therefore, the practitioner may consider a less-frequent approach with an individual sport athlete—say, three times per week. This schedule is frequent enough to obtain useful information but not so frequent that it results in questionnaire fatigue on the part of the athlete.

A practitioner may decide to use a wellness questionnaire (table 4.1) with an individual sport athlete for measures of sleep quality, muscle soreness, stress levels, and fatigue levels using a 1-5 scale. Initially, the practitioner has the athlete complete the questionnaire directly on a tablet or record responses on paper prior to a training session to ensure that he understands the purpose of the questionnaire; the athlete also has an opportunity to ask questions. Once satisfied that the athlete is familiar with the questionnaire, the practitioner sends a text to him on Monday, Thursday, and Saturday (at the same time each day) that asks him to text back the responses. The practitioner then calculates the z-score to determine the degree of day-to-day changes in his ratings.

The athlete rated the sleep, muscle soreness, stress, and fatigue questions as 1, 2, 3, and 2 (respectively) to give a sum of 8. The baseline mean and standard deviation (determined from a sum of scores taken over several occasions during the preseason) were 14 and 2.9, respectively. Therefore, the z-score is

(Current rating – baseline rating) ÷ standard deviation = (8 – 14) ÷ 2.9 = –2.1

Based on the recommendation to consider ≤1.5 a red flag (see chapter 4), the practitioner may consider an intervention (e.g., a decrease in training load for the day or some other recovery strategy).

Measures obtained are 14 on Thursday (z-score = 0.0) and 16 on Saturday (z-score = 0.69), which indicates that the athlete can train at full capacity.

Figure 8.2 shows the daily training load and z-score for wellness measures over a 3-week period. This provides a visual representation of the load fluctuation and its relationship to the athlete's perceived wellness.

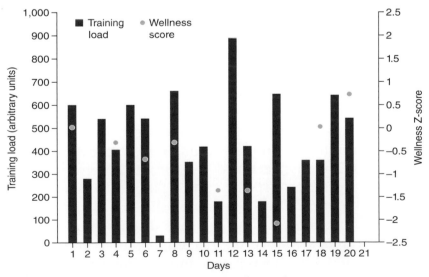

Figure 8.2 Training load and wellness scores over a training cycle.

training sessions designed for practicing technical aspects of sport performance should be undertaken in a nonfatigued state because the risk of injury may be greater when the athlete is fatigued (21). However, in extreme sports, athletes are required to perform technically under conditions of fatigue during competition. Because the goal of training is to prepare athletes to perform at their best during competition, training while fatigued would sometimes be necessary. Monitoring can help the practitioner first identify what fatigued conditions during competition look like.

It is unrealistic to expect a monitoring tool to assess fatigue in all circumstances, but a simple question of how fatigued the athlete feels is a good starting point. For example, a vertical countermovement jump with measures such as jump height and peak power may not be sensitive to fatigue in athletes (14), especially if the test is not performed using a force plate. Simple wellness measures have been shown to provide a good indicator of athlete fatigue (32).

Monitoring can be particularly useful when athletes undertake higher-than-normal training loads (tournaments in many individual sports include back-to-back performances over several days). Practitioners need to introduce training periods that simulate the demands of these periods. For athletes unaccustomed to this type of loading, back-to-back performances can pose an increased risk of injury; careful monitoring during these times may alleviate this risk.

Reporting One Week of Monitoring for an Athlete

Figure 8.3 shows a report provided to an athlete and other practitioners. Although electronic and paper formats are popular, practitioners should not be afraid to try alternative approaches to get their messages across. A short video or audio clip delivered to the athlete's mobile device may be a good way to relay information and highlight key aspects of the data. Being mindful of the athlete's preferences for how to receive the information is important. A good starting point would be a discussion with the athlete!

MONITORING AND REMOTE COACHING

Practitioners working with athletes in individual sports may sometimes work remotely (e.g., when traveling with athletes to competitions and training camps is not feasible). A monitoring system can keep the practitioner updated on the athlete's progress and may also facilitate communication. Although the efficacy of remote monitoring has not been established, some interesting case studies have been published. Adams and colleagues (1) presented a case study of a powerlifter who received virtual coaching following coronary artery bypass grafting. The athlete returned successfully to competition following a monitoring period in which he received a wrist blood pressure cuff for self-monitoring and regular advice on appropriate exercises and progressions. The effectiveness of remote coaching has been studied in rehabilitation, but less so in sport and with athlete populations (4, 18, 37).

Figure 8.3   Weekly monitoring report for a powerlifter.

Athlete: Kathryn Strong   **Training phase: Strength**
Sport: Powerlifting

	Result	Medal
Squat*	135 kg (298 lb)	Silver
Bench press*	70 kg (154 lb)	Silver
Deadlift*	145 kg (320 lb)	Gold
Training performance**	350 kg (772 lb)	Silver
Overall wellness score	6/10	Silver
Fatigue	7/10	Silver
Stress	7/10	Gold
Soreness	6/10	Silver
Sleep	4/10	Bronze
Training load	3,270 AU	Silver
Monotony	1.3	Gold
Strain	4,325 AU	Silver

*Estimated 1RMs based on training data
**Total of estimated 1RMs
AU = arbitrary units
Gold = exceeded expectations; silver = met the required standard; bronze = requires attention
Note: The overall wellness scores were converted to a score on a 1-10 scale to make it easier for the athlete to interpret.

Recommendations:
- Sleep needs attention this week.
- Focus for the week is triples for the main exercises and performing all exercises with technical perfection.

A weekly summary should contain all critical information, use an appropriate analysis method, be simple to interpret, and visually capture the key aspects of the monitoring data. Ultimately, the practitioner's goal should be to provide information that will make an impact and guide the programming and planning for the subsequent week.

Practitioners need to be careful not to go overboard with forms for reporting; they should use a format that will actually be used. Reports that are not used but are filed away and never looked at again are pointless. The report should include several important measures that are easily understood along with a brief explanation if needed.

Monitoring reports should provide usable information for the coming week. However, reporting is only one piece of the monitoring puzzle. The process should continue throughout the week to give the practitioner and athlete ongoing feedback so they can make training adjustments and note areas that need attention outside of training.

The results of the week could be presented using a medal system that denotes whether the result exceeded expectations (gold medal), met the required standard (silver medal), or requires attention (bronze medal). Figure 8.3 shows this system for a female powerlifter. Her performance is indicated by estimated 1RMs for the competition exercises (squat, bench press, and deadlift) based on training data; her overall training performance score is the estimated competition total.

Based on the wellness questionnaire, scores are given for the key areas, and a composite score is provided. In addition, training load, monotony, and strain are calculated as a weekly average but also measured relative to a 4-week rolling average. The practitioner could also include a figure that shows the major aspects of the report and the training for the year or training cycle so far. The benchmarking of the ratings (medals or flags or traffic signs) would be up to the practitioner to decide. Performance measures in sports such as powerlifting and weightlifting can simply be benchmarked against performance standards required for competition. Practitioners also need to consider the method of presentation (see chapter 2). Because many athletes may prefer electronic reports, practitioners would need to consider formatting to ensure that their reports appear correctly on mobile devices.

Modifying Training Based on Monitoring

One of the fundamental uses of athlete monitoring in individual sports is to inform adjustments to training prescription (23). Regular monitoring of an athlete's capacities may help optimize adaptations based on force–velocity (strength-speed or power) profiling (24).

Consider a practitioner who decides to use a vertical countermovement and static jump performed on a dual force plate at the start of each week for monitoring two heptathletes. If the practitioner does not have access to a force plate, more cost-effective technologies could be used (e.g., measuring jump height or distance). Monitoring shows that the eccentric utilization ratio (vertical countermovement jump to squat jump ratio) is 1.07 for athlete 1 and 0.93 for athlete 2. This suggests that the training of athlete 2 should include more exercises involving the stretch–shortening cycle (e.g., plyometrics) to improve the athlete's ability to utilize the stretch–shortening cycle. The training could incorporate exercises that focus on increasing the rate of force development using ballistic movements (e.g., jump squats). Depending on the training phase and periodization, the major focus for training should be those qualities requiring improvement. This is where regular monitoring data are particularly valuable. For example, if athlete 2 had low maximal strength in addition to the lower eccentric utilization ratio, the main training focus would be on maximal strength. Based on the monitoring data, athlete 1 might be considered to have an optimal eccentric utilization ratio. However, if these absolute numbers are below the benchmark required for that sport, then the training emphasis should be on improving these even though the ratio seems optimal.

Practitioners need to be wary of simply chasing numbers with training. Instead, they should always consider athlete monitoring data in the overall context of optimizing athlete performance.

Consider an athlete who is monitored over a 4-week period. The practitioner records the following results:

Week 1

- Countermovement jump = 55 watts/kg
- Static jump = 55 watts/kg
- Eccentric utilization ratio = countermovement jump ÷ static jump = 55 ÷ 55 = 1.00

The practitioner decides to incorporate more stretch–shortening cycle training that week. Because the relative results are also below the benchmark for that athlete (60 watts/kg), overall capacity still needs to be improved as well.

Week 2

- Countermovement jump = 56 watts/kg
- Static jump = 55 watts/kg
- Eccentric utilization ratio = 1.02

Week 3

- Countermovement jump = 57.5 watts/kg
- Static jump = 56 watts/kg
- Eccentric utilization ratio = 1.03

Week 4

- Countermovement jump = 58.5 watts/kg
- Static jump = 56.5 watts/kg
- Eccentric utilization ratio = 1.04

Each week adjustments are made to the training for that week to ensure continued adaptation. The results show a gradual improvement in both the capacities and the eccentric utilization ratio. However, practitioners should not become overly focused on a particular metric such as the eccentric utilization ratio. They need to also consider the actual numbers and how they fit with the other areas of athletic development.

With regard to unilateral versus bilateral monitoring, dual force plates can reveal any imbalances (see chapter 5); this can be applied across a range of individual sports. Ultimately, the practitioners must decide which variable to measure, such as displacement (jump height), impulse, power, or velocity. If a force plate is not available, the practitioner could use a tape measure or measuring stick to analyze single-leg vertical jumps. Broad or horizontal jump tests are also useful and do not require technology.

For example, a practitioner conducts a monitoring test to measure an athlete's single-leg broad jumps and records the following right leg to left leg ratios:

Week 1: 1.06

Week 2: 1.06

Week 3: 1.08

Week 4: 1.09

Having a perfect (1.0) right leg to left leg ratio is not a requirement, but a general guideline is that a difference greater than 15% is a red flag for the practitioner (17). Because the ratios in the example are within the 10% cutoff from one week to the next, the practitioner decides not to make any adjustments to the training program. If the ratio changes more than 15%, the practitioner could introduce more single-leg training for the weaker leg. Deciding which ratios are optimal is a challenge because many factors contribute to an imbalance, including sport requirements, limb dominance, and injury history.

However, a comparison should also be made between unilateral and bilateral performance (23). This can indicate a need for more emphasis on single-leg training. Comparing the sum of the right and left legs (e.g., adding the individual impulse scores for each leg in a long jumper) to the scores for bilateral vertical countermovement jump can identify differences in the bilateral deficit (see chapter 5). If one athlete produced 20% more impulse (noted in the sum of the unilateral jumps) and another athlete produced only 5% more, what could this mean to the practitioner? Depending on the sport, this could indicate that the first athlete should focus more on bilateral work in the next week, whereas the second athlete could be doing more unilateral exercises.

Practitioners working with individual sport athletes can often use more sophisticated strength and power monitoring tests than can practitioners dealing with larger numbers of athletes in team sports. For example, load profiling or measuring reactive strength capacity via drop jumps (25) over a range of heights is more challenging with a large squad of team sport athletes than with an individual athlete. Using these monitoring tests across a range of drop jump heights and comparing the results to vertical countermovement jump results can provide useful insights into the athlete's tolerance of stretch load. For example, a practitioner may decide to have an athlete complete a drop jump test using 30 cm (11.8 in.), 45 cm (17.7 in.), and 60 cm (23.6 in.) in addition to the vertical countermovement jump test. Performing these tests will reveal whether the athlete can tolerate the drop jump heights relative to vertical countermovement jump performance. If the athlete produces less jump height with increasing drop height, this suggests a lower tolerance to stretch load. This monitoring data would again need to be put into the context of other monitoring results to help understand the cause of this. It could be a lack of eccentric strength, which may be helped by including more maximal strength training. The lack of reactive strength could also be addressed by incorporating more reactive strength exercises in the next block of training.

Considerations for Monitoring Athletes in Individual Sports

Some practitioners deal with athletes from a variety of sports. For example, universities can have a range of sports, from swimming to wrestling to gymnastics to golf. Obviously, the physical demands of these sports are very different. Practitioners should take the time to understand the demands and culture of the sport they are working with by talking with other practitioners and athletes and observing the athletes in training and competition.

The best advice for monitoring athletes in individual sports is to keep things simple, at least in the beginning. At a minimum, having an athlete keep a training diary will provide indications of training load. With simple measures of session duration and RPE, other metrics can then be calculated.

An advantage of starting monitoring with a smaller number of tools is that it can create athlete buy-in and avoid both practitioners and athletes overrelying on the monitoring information. A good maxim for practitioners deciding whether to use a monitoring tool is "If in doubt, throw it out."

After completing the monitoring, one of the main considerations is the changes that need to be made to the training program, if any. Following are some fundamental questions to ask:

- How does the information guide the training for this session? For the week? For the training phase?

- Is it more important to focus on the identified weaknesses or continue to develop the athlete's strengths?

- Should the training program combine both aspects?

The underlying philosophy is to individualize training programs for athletes in individual sports. Practitioners need to take into account the athlete's years of training, the level of competition, the phase of the season, the impact of training individual capacities (e.g., muscular strength) on other physical capacities, and the athlete's needs based on performance priorities. Monitoring, if done well, provides the practitioner with regular feedback on the effects of the training program as well as insight into specific interventions needed.

Conclusion

Monitoring can provide important insights into the fatigue, fitness, and training readiness of athletes training for and competing in individual sports. A critical quality of a monitoring program is that it informs decisions about training. Ultimately, monitoring that can be incorporated into training sessions and competitions without creating extra work for the athlete and the practitioner is ideal. The monitoring tools should be reliable and valid and take into account the requirements of the athlete as well as be able to accurately discern a meaningful change in performance. Results of the monitoring tests need to be reported in a clear, meaningful, and timely manner to have maximal impact on the athlete's training. The practitioner can use this evidence-based information in conjunction with the art of coaching to maximize training program effectiveness for athletes in individual sports.

Athlete Monitoring Guidelines for Team Sports

This chapter focuses on athlete monitoring guidelines, approaches, challenges, and solutions in team sports. The general principles discussed in chapter 8 with respect to individual sport athletes can be applied in team sport environments, although often the circumstances are quite different.

Team Sport Athletes

For the purposes of this chapter, football, baseball, American football, rugby union, rugby league, basketball, volleyball, netball, handball, Australian rules football, ice hockey, field hockey, softball, and cricket are considered team sports. Typically, the greatest challenge facing practitioners working in team sports is the number of athletes they have to deal with. In individual sports, practitioners may be dealing with only several athletes, but team sport scenarios can involve playing groups with upwards of 30 athletes. In American football, more than 50 players may be training or practicing at the same time. Because large-scale monitoring systems can be difficult in such situations, practitioners often default to simple, but still effective, methods.

A crucial guideline in team sports is not to rely on a one-size-fits-all monitoring model. Ideally, the goal is to monitor team athletes individually and create individual training programs. Practitioners working with elite rugby union athletes identified the need for greater individualization (33), although this must be balanced with the realities of monitoring large numbers of athletes. Like practitioners working in individual sports, those working with teams need a good understanding of the demands of the sport and an appreciation of its culture.

Monitoring in Team Sports on a Budget

A large budget is not required to monitor athletes in team sports. With a few simple resources, a practitioner can implement a monitoring system that provides useful information. For example, the cost of obtaining measures of wellness and subjective internal training load is only the practitioner's time. With research supporting the value of subjective meas-

urements, practitioners can be confident that they provide valuable information on team sport athletes' responses to training load (23, 47, 50). Practitioners can also develop their own athlete monitoring databases using online tools (see chapter 8). Although dealing with data is not everyone's forte, doing so provides insight into how the information is generated and what it means so that practitioners do not have to simply accept the numbers.

Practitioners on a budget can develop a monitoring system gradually, adding aspects over time that they believe have value. The length of each phase is determined by the practitioner and the characteristics of the group of athletes. Ideally, each phase would last long enough (typically several weeks) to accustom the athletes to the monitoring tools. A practitioner working with a high school rugby union team, for example, might take the following approach:

- Phase 1: A simple training classification scale is assigned to the athletes at each session (e.g., A = full training, B = modified training, C = in rehabilitation, D = absent). The duration of each session is also recorded.

- Phase 2: A training diary that includes a place to record each session's duration and rating of perceived exertion (RPE) is introduced to the players.

- Phase 3: The training diary is expanded to include more detailed information about the content of each session such as the mode of training, exercises, sets, and repetitions. A wellness questionnaire is distributed and collected at the start of each week.

- Phase 4: The athletes continue filling out their training diaries, but now the wellness questionnaires are completed three times each week. For one training session, a smartphone app is used to monitor velocity in one upper-body exercise (e.g., speed bench press) and one lower-body exercise (e.g., vertical countermovement jump).

- Phase 5: Phase 4 continues with the addition of a 4-min submaximal running test (51), in which postexercise heart rate and RPE are measured. The test is performed as part of the athletes' warm-up for one training session every other week. A vertical countermovement jump test is also used to monitor fatigue and serve as a monitoring tool for one power training session.

- Future phases: Athletes can complete a more extensive wellness questionnaire (e.g., Recovery-Stress Questionnaire for Athletes) every 2 or 3 weeks.

Practitioners with more extensive budgets can start with a wider range of monitoring tools from which they can determine the ones that are particularly effective. In the majority of settings, however, a phased approach is more sensible.

Applying Monitoring in Team Sports

The general principles of athlete monitoring can be applied across a range of team sports. The following sections outline how athlete monitoring can be applied to some common team sports.

Jumping Sports

Practitioners are often interested in measuring jumping and landing volumes in sports such as basketball, volleyball, and netball to monitor training load. Inertial sensor technology can be used to count jumps during practices and matches (22). An alternative is to keep track of jumps performed during practice sessions by hand, but that may be too labor intensive with a large group of athletes. A more practical approach is to record jumps outside of team practice sessions, such as during conditioning workouts or specific jump training sessions. However, this assumes that the athletes are performing a standard number of jumps during practice sessions, which is unlikely. Doing some pilot work in which practice sessions are recorded (via video or direct observation) followed by a time–motion analysis of the number of jumps may prove informative. Another strategy is to classify session intensity in a general way (i.e., hard, moderate, or easy). However, the most accurate method is to obtain the number of jumps performed and calculate metrics such as load, monotony, and strain.

Table 9.1 shows an example of a week of jump monitoring for a volleyball player. The practitioner could conclude from this analysis that the volume and monotony of the week were too high. Targets could be set for the following week based on the data and published research (if available) on comparable athletes. For example, the practitioner may choose the following targets: total volume ≤3,600 jumps; monotony ≤1.50.

TABLE 9.1 Jump Monitoring for a Volleyball Athlete

Day	Training load (number of jumps)
Monday	600
Tuesday	935
Wednesday	805
Thursday	225
Friday	875
Saturday	400
Sunday	0
Total weekly load	3,840.0
Daily mean load	548.6
Daily standard deviation	354.0
Monotony	1.55

Unfortunately, for most measures, specific guidelines are not available. Practitioners can develop their own general guidelines from research on athletes in similar sports and adjust them as they collect more information over time.

Travel

One of the realities of sport is traveling to competitions, which places extra demands on athletes. Research has demonstrated that travel can have negative effects on athlete performance if not managed correctly (17-20); long-haul flights, in particular, can be very taxing. Athlete monitoring—especially of sleep quantity and quality (43)—can shed light on the effects of travel on team sport athletes (46). One of the advantages of monitoring while traveling is that it can make the athlete more mindful of good practice. For example, asking athletes to keep a record of their sleep, hydration, and activity (walking and stretching) during a long flight may help with adherence to guidelines.

Factors that need to be considered when traveling with a squad of athletes for competition or training camps include the number of time zones crossed, the availability of training facilities, the portability of monitoring equipment, the number of athletes, and athlete responses. At a minimum, monitoring player wellness reveals how athletes are coping with the demands of travel. Having performance plans based on monitoring information is also a good practice when traveling. An example is deciding to arrive earlier prior to competition to optimize acclimatization to the new time zone.

Injury Prevention

Athlete monitoring has tremendous potential for injury prevention. In team sports, the best athletes need to be available for the majority of the season (25, 53). A monitoring program that allows a practitioner to make sound decisions about return to performance, manage player workload, and avoid training errors can go a long way in achieving overall team health and athlete availability. Williams and colleagues (53) demonstrated a relationship between injury rates and team success in professional rugby union over a 7-year period. Having a reduced burden of injury (lost playing time due to injury) of 42 days per 1,000 playing hours resulted in a smallest meaningful change in the team's position in the competition. The relationship was also demonstrated over an 11-year period in professional European football (25). The teams with the lowest injury burdens performed better in both domestic leagues and international

European competitions (25). Windt and colleagues (54) showed that elite rugby league players who completed a greater number of sessions during the preseason had a reduced injury rate during the competitive season. This research shows that completing the preseason without interruption increases team sport athletes' availability for critical parts of the season.

The ratio of acute training load to chronic training load is emerging as an important measure and may help with injury prevention (6, 31). Avoiding large increases in workload is important for avoiding injury (30, 45). Drew and Finch suggested that increases in training load should not exceed 10% over the training load of the previous week (15). One of the issues with looking at training load in isolation (e.g., daily or weekly) is that practitioners are not able to determine how athletes are tolerating the overall workload. One way to remedy this is to examine the longitudinal patterns of the monitoring data such as comparing weekly training loads to a rolling average of training load over several weeks (31). Hulin and colleagues (31) demonstrated

that team sport athletes (rugby league) could tolerate high chronic loads as long as the acute-to-chronic training load ratio was maintained between 0.85 and 1.35. However, there is still no widely accepted range for all sports. The period of time used to calculate the chronic measure depends on the sport, but 3 weeks seems to provide an accurate picture for most (21). Measures of both internal and external load can be analyzed using this method.

Figure 9.1 shows 6 weeks of monitoring strain for a team sport athlete. Strain (training load × monotony) has been calculated for each week. A rolling 3-week average (also called a time series analysis; see page 32 in chapter 2) is calculated as a measure of the chronic strain on the athlete. In week 5 the acute-to-chronic training load ratio is greater than 1.5, which is a red flag for the practitioner (31). The picture may look quite different depending on the monitoring metric used in the calculation. This highlights the importance of not relying on a single measure for athlete monitoring. The use of ratios and metrics can be appealing, but they should not be used in isolation. Absolute

Figure 9.1   Acute and chronic monitoring of strain for a team sport athlete.

	WEEK					
	1	2	3	4	5	6
Weekly strain	4,132	6,669	3,512	6,737	11,066	9,273
Chronic strain (rolling 3-week average)	4,132	5,401	4,771	5,639	7,105	9,025
Acute-to-chronic training load ratio	1.00	1.23	0.74	1.19	1.56	1.03

values and athlete capacity are also important to consider when monitoring these aspects.

Managing the Workload of Starters and Nonstarters

The issue of starters and nonstarters is interesting to practitioners working in team sports. Research performed on football players revealed differences in training and match (game) load between starters and nonstarters (1). Over the course of the National Basketball Association (United States) season, differential responses in physical capacities (lower-body power, repeat jump ability, and reaction time) occur between starters and nonstarters (24). Athletes who sit on the bench during games may need additional training (sometimes called top-up sessions) outside of games to make up for this loss in training stress.

Some practitioners have nonstarters perform a conditioning session at the end of the game or as an additional session the following day. This requires an accurate gauge of the load experienced by the starters during the game. A simple monitoring tool is to track the number of minutes starting athletes play and obtain a measure of their internal load (e.g., RPE). The prescription for the extra conditioning session for nonstarters can be based on the load (number of minutes and RPE) handled by the starters during game time. Athletes who did not play at all would have different additional training prescriptions than those who did not start but played a significant amount of time later in the game.

Consider a practitioner who determines the number of minutes played by a squad of rugby league players. It may not be possible to fully replicate the demands of the match (although small-sided games and drills are good options), but using the minutes played as a starting point, the practitioner designs a session that takes into account differences in athletes' playing time. In this example, three athletes played the following number of minutes (note that the total match duration is 80 min):

$$\text{Athlete 1} = 80 \text{ min}$$

$$\text{Athlete 2} = 47 \text{ min}$$

$$\text{Athlete 3} = 15 \text{ min}$$

Looking at the number of minutes of playing time is helpful but not without limitations. Incorporating a measure of internal load such as RPE would more accurately calculate match load. Other factors that can be factored into the calculation (but are not included in this example) are the quality of the opposition and the intensity of the match (34).

Athletes 1, 2, and 3 had RPEs of 9, 10, and 7, respectively. Match load is calculated as follows:

$$\text{Athlete 1} = 80 \text{ min} \times 9 = 720 \text{ arbitrary units}$$

$$\text{Athlete 2} = 47 \text{ min} \times 10 = 470 \text{ arbitrary units}$$

$$\text{Athlete 3} = 15 \text{ min} \times 7 = 105 \text{ arbitrary units}$$

The calculations reveal that the top-up sessions for athletes 2 and 3 should be quite different; athlete 3 will need approximately 4.5 times more work than athlete 2.

Training Camps

Athletes are often required to handle high training volumes. Completing several shorter sessions is one way to disperse the volume. Monitoring can provide insight into the effect of performing multiple sessions in one day (32), particularly in situations such as training camps. In fact, athletes typically take on greater training loads in these situations than they do in the competitive season (12). Several research studies have investigated approaches for monitoring team sport athletes during training camps (8, 26, 44). These researchers state that no single measure can give a complete picture of the athlete's response to training; a one-size-fits-all training prescription in these environments is not considered best practice. Instead, monitoring across the squad of athletes can reveal how the athletes are coping with training and give the practitioner information to inform training and recovery decisions.

Competition and In-Season Periods

Practitioners sometimes face unique scenarios during competition and in-season periods. For example, the impact of different turnaround times between matches or games must be considered within the context of a team's training program (39). Although practitioners are often used to a standard 1-week turnaround between competitive events, the reality is quite different in many team sports.

Murray and colleagues (39) investigated the effects of different turnaround times between professional rugby league matches on match activity profiles using global positioning systems and injury rates. They discovered that athletes in some positions had higher injury rates with longer turnaround times, whereas those in other positions had higher rates with shorter turnaround times. Practitioners need to take these positional differences into account, and monitoring can help.

In sports such as football, basketball, ice hockey, softball, and cricket, teams may play more than two matches in a week (10). Research suggests that rates of injury increase with more congested match scheduling (5, 13). Although research shows that physical performance and technical ability are not affected, evidence points toward a greater risk of injury (9, 13). It may be possible to manage this increased risk, however, with appropriate attention to player rotation and postmatch recovery strategies (9). It is also important to consider the cumulative effect of these congested periods over the course of the season to manage fatigue and prevent injuries.

At the end of the regular season, teams may enter a tournament period in which they are playing matches with only 24 hr between them. In some sports, international championships have a very different schedule from that of the regular season; teams are expected to play several high-intensity games in a compressed time period. These scenarios present significant challenges for team sport practitioners. Sudden spikes in match load can increase the risk of injury and result in fatigue that contributes to decreased chances of team success. Athlete monitoring systems give practitioners a clearer understanding of the demands of match scheduling variations so they can make the necessary changes to the athletes' training programs.

Another common issue with team sport athletes during the competition season is the potential for decreases in physical fitness (37). Research has shown that physical qualities such as upper-body power and total-body mass can decrease across the competitive season in team sport athletes, indicating that match load stimulus is not sufficient to maintain physical fitness (28, 35). Athlete monitoring can provide more regular data on how athletes are tracking during the season to allow for more effective training management. Only by having up-to-date knowledge of their athletes' physical capacities can practitioners make the necessary week-to-week changes to ensure that they maintain fitness. A common misconception is that qualities such as aerobic endurance and maximal strength are difficult to maintain during the competition season. Researchers have demonstrated that with the necessary adjustments to programming, team sport athletes can maintain and even improve these qualities during the regular season (2, 4, 16, 24, 28, 29, 40).

Tactical Athletes and Workers

Although the focus of this book is on sport, the principles of monitoring can also be applied to other populations. Increasing focus on the physical preparation of tactical athletes (i.e., those in the military, law enforcement, and emergency services) reveals that more systematic approaches to monitoring (48) decrease injury rates and optimize performance (42). Several investigators have studied monitoring tools for tactical populations (41, 52). A mixed-methods approach appears to be optimal, but there are no clear guidelines for implementing or applying the methods in the field.

Monitoring approaches can also be applied in the workplace as employers increasingly appreciate the value of healthy workers. Therefore, methods for encouraging physical activity and improving lifestyle factors (e.g., getting more sleep) are gaining more attention.

When financial benefits are shown, employers have the incentive to increase efforts in these areas (14).

Monitoring System for Team Sports

Table 9.2 outlines the frequency, purpose, analysis methods, and practical interpretations of the monitoring variables for a squad of 25 football players. Training load was measured using session RPE and duration to allow for the calculation of monotony and strain. The practitioner decided to obtain wellness measures only twice a week because of the high number of players. A drop jump test was performed three times each week prior to the start of the training session to measure reactive strength. A submaximal running test, performed every second week, measured heart rate and RPE (51). This is based on the Yo-Yo intermittent recovery test, which the practitioner has been using as the aerobic endurance test. The test is performed for 4 min but using 18.5-m shuttles instead of 20-m shuttles.

Reporting One Week of Monitoring for a Team Sport

Figure 9.2 (page 198) shows a weekly monitoring report for a team athlete; the coach and practitioner summary report is shown in figure 9.3 (page 199). To avoid overwhelming the athlete with too much information, the summary is brief enough to appear on the athlete's device as a single screen capture. The coach and

TABLE 9.2 **Monitoring System for Football**

Variable	Assessment frequency	Purpose	Analysis method	Practical interpretation
Session RPE	Every session	Measure of perceived exertion of training session	Z-score relative to baseline measure	Z-score ≤–1.5
Training load	Weekly	Measure of internal load	• Z-score relative to baseline measure • Acute-to-chronic ratio	• Z-score ≤–1.5 • Acute-to-chronic ratio ≥1.5 is a yellow flag; ≥2.0 is a red flag
Monotony	Weekly	Measure of sameness and variation of training	Z-score relative to baseline measure	Z-score ≤–1.5
Strain	Weekly	Measure of overall product of training load and monotony	• Z-score relative to baseline measure • Acute-to-chronic ratio	• Z-score ≤–1.5 • Acute-to-chronic ratio ≥1.5 is a yellow flag; ≥2.0 is a red flag
Wellness (questionnaire)	Twice per week	Measure of overall wellness and quality of sleep, muscle soreness, fatigue, and stress	• Z-score relative to baseline measure • Change in raw score for individual items	Z-score ≤–1.5 ± 2 on individual item = positive or negative change
Vertical drop jump (jump height and contact time)*	Daily	Measure of neuromuscular fatigue	• Z-score relative to baseline measure • Smallest meaningful change relative to reliability	• Z-score ≤–1.5 • If contact time or jump height decreases greater than smallest meaningful change, investigation is needed.
Submaximal running test (average heart rate and RPE)	Every 2 weeks	Measure of running performance and fatigue	• For heart rate: z-score relative to baseline measure • For RPE: change in raw score	Z-score ≤–1.5 ± 2 on RPE scale = positive or negative change

*If a contact mat or similar technology is not available, the drop jump could be replaced with a vertical countermovement jump.

practitioner's report commonly includes more details about athletes in addition to the overall means and standard deviations. A traffic light system that incorporates the analysis measures discussed earlier can be used to point out flags for the coach and practitioner. The result is an easily digestible report that can be quickly scanned. A more detailed plot of the athlete's weekly monitoring z-scores and some key recommendations can also be provided (see figure 9.4, page 199).

Although the athlete's wellness score improved (see figure 9.2), the detailed report indicates that training loads, monotony, and strain were high (see figure 9.3). This highlights the problem of taking a snapshot of a single week (or day). It is not until the practitioner has detailed data or several weeks of monitoring information (or both) that patterns begin to emerge.

Modifying Training Based on Monitoring

With individual athletes it may be feasible to complete force–velocity (strength-speed or power) profiling using a range of loads; this is more challenging in the team sport environment (38). Simple approaches can be performed on a sem-iregular basis—for example, a high-force, low-velocity test (e.g., isometric mid-thigh pull); a moderate-force, moderate-velocity test (e.g., loaded vertical squat jump); or a high-force, high-velocity test (e.g., vertical squat jump). The data would provide a good overview of the athlete's force and velocity capabilities (3). Rather than relying on a single monitoring test to determine force–velocity capabilities, the practitioner could use two or three tests (36). A squad of players could be rotated through these exercises, or the exercises could be incorporated into a training session.

Figure 9.2   Weekly report for a soccer player.

Athlete: Nicky Speed (NS)   **Sport: Soccer**

	Result	Compared to previous week
Submaximal running test (% maximal heart rate)	<83%	↑↑
Submaximal running test (RPE)	6	→→
Training load	6,390 AU	↓↓
Monotony	2.10 AU	↓↓
Strain	13,421 AU	↓↓
Overall wellness score	7.5/10	↑↑
Fatigue	8/10	↑↑
Stress	6/10	↑↑
Soreness	8/10	↑↑
Sleep	8/10	↑↑

Key: ↑↑ = improved; →→ = maintained; ↓↓ = worsened

Note: The overall wellness scores were converted to a score on a 1-10 scale to make it easier for the athlete to interpret.

Observations and Recommendations
- The athlete coped well with the high training loads this week.
- Next week will have a more technical tactical focus; thus, overall training load will be lighter.

Figure 9.3 Weekly monitoring report for team coach and practitioner.

Sport: Soccer

Athlete	Submaximal running test (% maximal heart rate)	Submaximal running test (RPE)	Training load (arbitrary units)	Monotony (arbitrary units)	Strain (arbitrary units)	Overall wellness score*	Fatigue *	Stress *	Soreness *	Sleep *
NS	83	6	**6,390**	**2.10**	**13,421**	7.5	8	6	8	8
TP	81	3	5,565	1.94	10,814	**6**	6	6	6	6
MN	**89**	**7**	5,470	**2.22**	**12,135**	5	4	6	6	**4**
SC	77	5	3,880	1.89	7,316	8.5	8	10	8	8
JP	80	4	5,415	1.87	10,131	7.5	8	8	6	8
MR	81	4	5,910	1.62	9,576	8	8	8	8	8
AB	86	4	5,355	**2.22**	**11,877**	6	6	6	6	6
FT	84	3	4,675	**2.14**	9,993	**4.5**	**4**	6	**4**	**4**
JH	87	**7**	**6,080**	**2.09**	**12,724**	6	6	6	6	6
CJ	82	4	6,640	1.88	**12,499**	7	8	6	8	6
SM	DNC	DNC	1,500	1.81	2,716	**4.5**	6	4	4	4
Mean	83	4.7	4,740	1.98	9,434	6.41	6.55	6.55	6.36	6.18
Standard deviation	3.59	1.49	2,238	0.19	4,164	1.39	1.57	1.57	1.50	1.66

*Rating number is on a 1-10 scale.

DNC = did not complete

Summary: Red flags (results in bold) are identified for individual athletes and specific tests. Monotony and strain were high for the week, and overall sleep quality was lower than in previous weeks. In an actual report, practitioners would click on an athlete's initials for a graph of individual results.

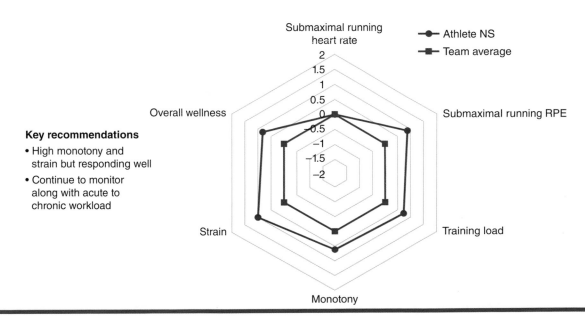

Key recommendations
- High monotony and strain but responding well
- Continue to monitor along with acute to chronic workload

Figure 9.4   Weekly monitoring z-scores for athlete NS.

Consider a practitioner working with a women's rugby sevens squad of 15 athletes who uses a monitoring battery in a training session every 2 weeks. The tests include the vertical squat jump performed with body weight and with a 20-kg (44 lb) load to determine the athletes' ability to tolerate external load.

Following testing, two athletes obtain the following ratios using jump height (although other variables could be used) calculated as loaded vertical squat jump divided by body weight vertical squat jump:

$$\text{Athlete 1} = 38 \text{ cm (15 in.)} \div 40 \text{ cm (15.7 in.)} = 0.95$$

$$\text{Athlete 2} = 40 \text{ cm (15.7 in.)} \div 51 \text{ cm (20.1 in.)} = 0.78$$

Athlete 1 tolerated the external load well, as shown in the similarity of the results on both tests. Athlete 2 had a decrease in performance with the addition of an external load. Based on this information, the practitioner decides to incorporate more exercises (e.g., loaded jump squats) into athlete 2's program to improve this capacity.

The practitioner decided to use an absolute load of 20 kg (44 lb) for the loaded vertical squat jump test. Although basing the external load on an athlete's strength (% of 1RM) or a percentage of body weight are options, these adjustments are time consuming for practitioners and athletes. What is required is a load high enough to discriminate the ability of the athletes in that sport (and playing position) to tolerate load. With athletes in sports that require the handling of high external loads, a heavier external load could be used. In American football a load of 60 kg (132 lb) might be used for the jump test.

Considerations for Monitoring Athletes in Team Sports

Because determining whether an athlete is struggling is more challenging in team sport environments than in individual sports, practitioners should use a mixed-methods approach when monitoring team sport athletes. No single measure can provide a complete picture of how a team is coping with the demands of training and competition. Practitioners need a range of monitoring methods, and they need to introduce athletes to them gradually to ensure adequate familiarization. This helps with compliance and athlete buy-in and improves the quality of the monitoring data.

A good example of a simple and inexpensive tool for monitoring stress is a questionnaire. Because the team sport environment involves working with large numbers of athletes, short-form questionnaires such as the four-item Perceived Stress Scale (11) are ideal because they are easy to complete and analyze.

Whenever possible, individual approaches should be used in team sport environments. This can occur only if athlete monitoring provides quantifiable data. Something as simple as monitoring sleep and providing strategies to improve sleep quality can be very valuable in helping athletes improve their performance (49).

With the emergence of more research on elite-level team sport athletes, especially women (27), practitioners now have a wealth of information at their disposal (7, 8). Having more data from a range of sports will help them understand how to monitor their athletes effectively.

Conclusion

Monitoring team sport athletes provides some interesting challenges for practitioners. Ideally, monitoring is done on an individual basis, but the logistics of the environment will dictate to what degree this can occur. Because no single monitoring tool can provide a complete picture of a team sport athlete, practitioners need to develop a toolbox of monitoring methods. The fundamental consideration is how the monitoring data can be used to inform decision making. Developing simple and effective monitoring systems can help practitioners manage the training load, reduce the injury rates, and optimize the performance of their team sport athletes.

REFERENCES

Chapter 1

1. Baker, D.G. 2013. 10-year changes in upper body strength and power in elite professional rugby league players—the effect of training age, stage, and content. *J Strength Cond Res* 27:285-92.

2. Baker, D.G., and R.U. Newton. 2006. Adaptations in upper-body maximal strength and power output resulting from long-term resistance training in experienced strength-power athletes. *J Strength Cond Res* 20:541-6.

3. Bamman, M.M., J.K. Petrella, J.S. Kim, D.L. Mayhew, and J.M. Cross. 2007. Cluster analysis tests the importance of myogenic gene expression during myofiber hypertrophy in humans. *J Appl Physiol* 102:2232-9.

4. Bourne, N.D. 2008. Fast science: A history of training theory and methods for elite runners through 1975. Doctor of Philosophy PhD thesis, University of Texas at Austin.

5. Box, G.E.P., and N.R. Draper. 1987. *Empirical model-building and response surfaces*, 424. New York: Wiley Series in Probability and Statistics.

6. Bradley, W.J., B.P. Cavanagh, W. Douglas, T.F. Donovan, J.P. Morton, and G.L. Close. 2015. Quantification of training load, energy intake, and physiological adaptations during a rugby preseason: A case study from an elite European rugby union squad. *J Strength Cond Res* 29:534-44.

7. Brink, M.S., W.G. Frencken, G. Jordet, and K.A. Lemmink. 2014. Coaches' and players' perceptions of training dose: Not a perfect match. *Int J Sports Physiol Perform* 9:497-502.

8. Buchheit, M., and P.B. Laursen. 2013. High-intensity interval training, solutions to the programming puzzle: Part I: Cardiopulmonary emphasis. *Sports Med* 43:313-38.

9. Buchheit, M., S. Racinais, J.C. Bilsborough, P.C. Bourdon, S.C. Voss, J. Hocking, J. Cordy, A. Mendez-Villanueva, and A.J. Coutts. 2013. Monitoring fitness, fatigue and running performance during a pre-season training camp in elite football players. *J Sci Med Sport* 16:550-5.

10. Buford, T.W., M.D. Roberts, and T.S. Church. 2013. Toward exercise as personalized medicine. *Sports Med* 43:157-65.

11. Carling, C., A. McCall, F. Le Gall, and G. Dupont. 2015. What is the extent of exposure to periods of match congestion in professional soccer players? *J Sports Sci* 20:2116-24.

12. Colby, M.J., B. Dawson, J. Heasman, B. Rogalski, and T.J. Gabbett. 2014. Accelerometer and GPS-derived running loads and injury risk in elite Australian footballers. *J Strength Cond Res* 28:2244-52.

13. Coutts, A.J. 2014. In the age of technology, Occam's razor still applies. *Int J Sports Physiol Perform* 9:741.

14. Coutts, A.J., and S. Cormack. 2014. Monitoring the training response. In *High-performance training for sports*, edited by D. Joyce and D. Lewindon, 85-96. Champaign, IL: Human Kinetics.

15. Cross, M.J., S. Williams, G. Trewartha, S.P. Kemp, and K.A. Stokes. 2016. The influence of in-season training loads on injury risk in professional rugby union. *Int J Sports Physiol Perform* 11:350-55.

16. Cunniffe, B., H. Griffiths, W. Proctor, B. Davies, J.S. Baker, and K.P. Jones. 2011. Mucosal immunity and illness incidence in elite rugby union players across a season. *Med Sci Sports Exerc* 43:388-97.

17. Dupont, G., M. Nedelec, A. McCall, D. McCormack, S. Berthoin, and U. Wisloff. 2010. Effect of 2 soccer matches in a week on physical performance and injury rate. *Am J Sports Med* 38:1752-8.

18. Erskine, R.M., D.A. Jones, A.G. Williams, C.E. Stewart, and H. Degens. 2010. Inter-individual variability in the adaptation of human muscle specific tension to progressive resistance training. *Eur J Appl Physiol* 110:1117-25.

19. Flatt, A.A., and M.R. Esco. 2015. Smartphone-derived heart rate variability and training load in a female soccer team. *Int J Sports Physiol Perform* 10:994-1000.

20. Foster, C., K.M. Heimann, P.L. Esten, G. Brice, and J.P. Porcari. 2001. Differences in perceptions of training by coaches and athletes. *S Afr J Sports Med* 8:3-7.

21. Gabbett, T.J. 2004. Reductions in pre-season training loads reduce training injury rates in rugby league players. *Br J Sports Med* 38:743-9.

22. Gabbett, T.J. 2010. The development and application of an injury prediction model for noncontact, soft-tissue injuries in elite collision sport athletes. *J Strength Cond Res* 24:2593-603.

23. Gabbett, T.J., and N. Domrow. 2007. Relationships between training load, injury, and fitness in sub-elite collision sport athletes. *J Sports Sci* 25:1507-19.

24. Gabbett, T.J., and D.G. Jenkins. 2011. Relationship between training load and injury in professional rugby league players. *J Sci Med Sport* 14:204-9.

25. Gabbett, T.J., and S. Ullah. 2012. Relationship between running loads and soft-tissue injury in elite team sport athletes. *J Strength Cond Res* 26:953-60.

26. Gleeson, M., N. Bishop, M. Oliveira, T. McCauley, P. Tauler, and A.S. Muhamad. 2012. Respiratory infection risk in athletes: Association with antigen-stimulated IL-10 production and salivary IgA secretion. *Scand J Med Sci Sports* 22:410-7.

27. Gleeson, M., N. Bishop, M. Oliveira, and P. Tauler. 2013. Influence of training load on upper respiratory tract infection incidence and antigen-stimulated cytokine production. *Scand J Med Sci Sports* 23:451-7.

28. Gleeson, M., and N.C. Bishop. 2013. URI in athletes: Are mucosal immunity and cytokine responses key risk factors? *Exerc Sport Sci Rev* 41:148-53.

29. Gomes, R.V., A. Moreira, L. Lodo, K. Nosaka, A.J. Coutts, and M.S. Aoki. 2013. Monitoring training loads, stress, immune-endocrine responses and performance in tennis players. *Biol Sport* 30:173-80.

30. Halson, S.L. 2014. Monitoring training load to understand fatigue in athletes. *Sports Med* 44 Suppl 2:S139-47.

31. Halson, S.L., and A.E. Jeukendrup. 2004. Does overtraining exist? An analysis of overreaching and overtraining research. *Sports Med* 34:967-81.

32. Hopkins, W.G. 1991. Quantification of training in competitive sports. Methods and applications. *Sports Med* 12:161-83.

33. Hubal, M.J., H. Gordish-Dressman, P.D. Thompson, T.B. Price, E.P. Hoffman, T.J. Angelopoulos, P.M. Gordon, N.M. Moyna, L.S. Pescatello, P.S. Visich, R.F. Zoeller, R.L. Seip, and P.M. Clarkson. 2005. Variability in muscle size and strength gain after unilateral resistance training. *Med Sci Sports Exerc* 37:964-72.

34. Kellmann, M. 2010. Preventing overtraining in athletes in high-intensity sports and stress/recovery monitoring. *Scand J Med Sci Sports* 20 Suppl 2:95-102.

35. Killen, N.M., T.J. Gabbett, and D.G. Jenkins. 2010. Training loads and incidence of injury during the preseason in professional rugby league players. *J Strength Cond Res* 24:2079-84.

36. Lombard, W.P. 1892. Some of the influences which affect the power of voluntary muscular contractions. *J Physiol* 13:1-58 8.

37. Mann, J.B., K. Bryant, B. Johnstone, P. Ivey, and S.P. Sayers. 2016. The effect of physical and academic stress on illness and injury in Division 1 college football players. *J Strength Cond Res* 30:20-25.

38. McGuigan, M.R., S. Cormack, and N.D. Gill. 2013. Strength and power profiling of athletes. *Strength Cond J* 35:7-14.

39. McLean, B.D., A.J. Coutts, V. Kelly, M.R. McGuigan, and S.J. Cormack. 2010. Neuromuscular, endocrine, and perceptual fatigue responses during different length between-match microcycles in professional rugby league players. *Int J Sports Physiol Perform* 5:367-83.

40. Meeusen, R., M. Duclos, C. Foster, A. Fry, M. Gleeson, D. Nieman, J. Raglin, G. Rietjens, J. Steinacker, A. Urhausen, S. European College of Sport Science, and American College of Sports Medicine. 2013. Prevention, diagnosis, and treatment of the overtraining syndrome: Joint consensus statement of the European College of Sport Science and the American College of Sports Medicine. *Med Sci Sports Exerc* 45:186-205.

41. Moreira, A., J.C. Bilsborough, C.J. Sullivan, M. Ciancosi, M.S. Aoki, and A.J. Coutts. 2015. Training periodization of professional Australian football players during an entire Australian Football League season. *Int J Sports Physiol Perform* 10:566-71.

42. Murphy, A.P., R. Duffield, A. Kellett, and M. Reid. 2014. Comparison of athlete-coach perceptions of internal and external load markers for elite junior tennis training. *Int J Sports Physiol Perform* 9:751-6.

43. Murray, A., and M. Cardinale. 2015. Cold applications for recovery in adolescent athletes: A systematic review and meta analysis. *Extrem Physiol Med* 4:17.

44. Neville, V., M. Gleeson, and J.P. Folland. 2008. Salivary IgA as a risk factor for upper respiratory infections in elite professional athletes. *Med Sci Sports Exerc* 40:1228-36.

45. Newton, R.U., and E. Dugan. 2002. Application of strength diagnosis. *Strength Cond J* 24:50-59.

46. Plews, D.J., P.B. Laursen, Y. Le Meur, C. Hausswirth, A.E. Kilding, and M. Buchheit. 2014. Monitoring training with heart rate-variability: How much compliance is needed for valid assessment? *Int J Sports Physiol Perform* 9:783-90.

47. Plews, D.J., P.B. Laursen, J. Stanley, A.E. Kilding, and M. Buchheit. 2013. Training adaptation and heart rate variability in elite endurance athletes: Opening the door to effective monitoring. *Sports Med* 43:773-81.

48. Roberts, L.A., T. Raastad, J.F. Markworth, V.C. Figueiredo, I.M. Egner, A. Shield, D. Cameron-Smith, J.S. Coombes, and J.M. Peake. 2015. Post-exercise cold water immersion attenuates acute anabolic signalling and long-term adaptations in muscle to strength training. *J Physiol* 593:4285-301.

49. Rogalski, B., B. Dawson, J. Heasman, and T.J. Gabbett. 2013. Training and game loads and injury risk in elite Australian footballers. *J Sci Med Sport* 16:499-503.

50. Saw, A.E., L.C. Main, and P.B. Gastin. 2016. Monitoring the athlete training response: Subjective self-reported measures trump commonly used objective measures: A systematic review. *Br J Sports Med* 50:281-91.

51. Selye, H. 1956. *The stress of life*. London: Longmans Green.

52. Suchomel, T.J., and C.A. Bailey. 2014. Monitoring and managing fatigue in baseball players. *Strength Cond J* 36:39-45.

53. Svendsen, I.S., M. Gleeson, T.A. Haugen, and E. Tonnessen. 2015. Effect of an intense period of competition on race performance and self-reported illness in elite cross-country skiers. *Scand J Med Sci Sports* 25:846-53.

54. Tonnessen, E., I.S. Svendsen, B.R. Ronnestad, J. Hisdal, T.A. Haugen, and S. Seiler. 2015. The annual training periodization of 8 world champions in orienteering. *Int J Sports Physiol Perform* 10:29-38.

55. Tonnessen, E., O. Sylta, T.A. Haugen, E. Hem, I.S. Svendsen, and S. Seiler. 2014. The road to gold: Training and peaking characteristics in the year prior to a gold medal endurance performance. *PLoS One* 9:e101796.

56. Veugelers, K.R., W.B. Young, B. Fahrner, and J.T. Harvey. 2015. Different methods of training load quantification and their relationship to injury and illness in elite Australian football. *J Sci Med Sport*.

57. West, D.J., C.V. Finn, D.J. Cunningham, D.A. Shearer, M.R. Jones, B.J. Harrington, B.T. Crewther, C.J. Cook, and L.P. Kilduff. 2014. Neuromuscular function, hormonal, and mood responses to a professional rugby union match. *J Strength Cond Res* 28:194-200.

Chapter 2

1. Atkinson, G., and A.M. Nevill. 1998. Statistical methods for assessing measurement error (reliability) in variables relevant to sports medicine. *Sports Med* 26:217-38.

2. Batterham, A.M., and W.G. Hopkins. 2006. Making meaningful inferences about magnitudes. *Int J Sports Physiol Perform* 1:50-57.

3. Baumgartner, T.A., and A.S. Jackson. 2016. *Measurement for evaluation in physical education and exercise science*. 9th ed. Madison, WI: Brown & Benchmark.

4. Blanch, P., and T.J. Gabbett. 2016. Has the athlete trained enough to return to play safely? The acute:chronic workload ratio permits clinicians to quantify a player's risk of subsequent injury. *Br J Sports Med* 50:471-75.

5. Box, G.E.P., and G.M. Jenkins. 1976. *Time series analysis: Forecasting and control*. San Francisco: Holden-Day.

6. Chandler, T.J., and L.E. Brown. 2013. *Conditioning for strength and human performance*. 2nd ed. Philadelphia: Lippincott Williams and Wilkins.

7. Chiu, L.Z., and G.J. Salem. 2010. Time series analysis: Evaluating performance trends within resistance exercise sessions. *J Strength Cond Res* 24:230-4.

8. Church, J.B. 2008. Basic statistics for the strength and conditioning professional. *Strength Cond J* 30:51-53.

9. Cohen, J.A. 1988. *Statistical power analysis for the behavioural sciences*. 2nd ed. Hillsdale, NJ: Lawrence Erlbaum Associates.

10. Coutts, A.J., and S. Cormack. 2014. Monitoring the training response. In *High-performance training for sports*, edited by D. Joyce and D. Lewindon, 85-96. Champaign, IL: Human Kinetics.

11. Flanagan, E. 2013. The effect size statistic—applications for the strength and conditioning coach. *Strength Cond J* 35:37-40.

12. Haddad, M., A. Chaouachi, C. Castagna, P. Wong del, D.G. Behm, and K. Chamari. 2011. The construct validity of session RPE during an intensive camp in young male taekwondo athletes. *Int J Sports Physiol Perform* 6:252-63.

13. Halperin, I., D.B. Pyne, and D.T. Martin. 2015. Threats to internal validity in exercise science: A review of overlooked confounding variables. *Int J Sports Physiol Perform* 10:823-9.

14. Handcock, P., and T. Cassidy. 2014. Reflective practice for rugby union strength and conditioning coaches. *Strength Cond J* 36:41-45.

15. Hopkins, W. 2004. How to interpret changes in an athletic performance test. *Sportscience* 8:1-7.

16. Hopkins, W. 2012. http://sportsci.org/resource/stats/xrely.xls.

17. Hopkins, W. 2015. Confidence limits and clinical chances. http://sportsci.org/resource/stats/xcl.xls.

18. Hopkins, W., J. Hawley, and L. Burke. 1999. Design and analysis of research on sport performance enhancement. *Med Sci Sports Exerc* 31:472-85.

19. Hopkins, W., S. Marshall, A. Batterham, and J. Hanin. 2009. Progressive statistics for studies in sports medicine and exercise science. *Med Sci Sports Exerc* 41:3-13.

20. Hopkins, W.G. 2015. Assessing an individual. http://sportsci.org/resource/stats/xprecisionsubject.xls.

21. Hopkins, W.G. 2015. A new view of statistics. http://sportsci.org/resource/stats/index.html.

22. Hulin, B.T., T.J. Gabbett, D.W. Lawson, P. Caputi, and J.A. Sampson. 2016. The acute:chronic workload ratio predicts injury: High chronic workload may decrease injury risk in elite rugby league players. *Br J Sports Med* 50:231-36.

23. Lakens, D. 2013. Calculating and reporting effect sizes to facilitate cumulative science: A practical primer for t-tests and anovas. *Front Psychol* 4:863.

24. Lythe, J. 2015. Excel tricks for sports. www.youtube.com/channel/UCagflprv_C-UPPdzSJ0bMCA.

25. Malcata, R.M., and W.G. Hopkins. 2014. Variability of competitive performance of elite athletes: A systematic review. *Sports Med* 44:1763-74.

26. Montgomery, D.C. 2012. *Introduction to statistical quality control*. 7th ed. Hoboken, NJ: Wiley.

27. Nibali, M.L., D.W. Chapman, R.A. Robergs, and E.J. Drinkwater. 2013. A rationale for assessing the lower-body power profile in team sport athletes. *J Strength Cond Res* 27:388-97.

28. Nibali, M.L., T. Tombleson, P.H. Brady, and P. Wagner. 2015. Influence of familiarization and competitive level on the reliability of countermovement vertical jump kinetic and kinematic variables. *J Strength Cond Res* 29:2827-35.

29. Nuzzo, J.L., J.H. Anning, and J.M. Scharfenberg. 2011. The reliability of three devices used for measuring vertical jump height. *J Strength Cond Res* 25:2580-90.

30. Patton, M.Q. 2015. *Qualitative research and evaluation methods*. 4th ed. Thousand Oaks, CA: Sage.

31. Pettitt, R.W. 2010. Evaluating strength and conditioning tests with z scores: Avoiding common pitfalls. *Strength Cond J* 32:100-03.

32. Pettitt, R.W. 2010. The standard difference score: A new statistic for evaluating strength

and conditioning programs. *J Strength Cond Res* 24:287-91.

33. Reaburn, P., B. Dascombe, R. Reed, A. Jones, and J. Weyers. 2011. *Practical skills in sport and exercise science.* Essex, UK: Pearson Education Limited.

34. Saw, A.E., L.C. Main, and P.B. Gastin. 2016. Monitoring the athlete training response: Subjective self-reported measures trump commonly used objective measures: A systematic review. *Br J Sports Med* 50:281-91.

35. Singh, F., C. Foster, D. Tod, and M.R. McGuigan. 2007. Monitoring different types of resistance training using session rating of perceived exertion. *Int J Sports Physiol Perform* 2:34-45.

36. Stone, M.H., M. Stone, and W.A. Sands. 2006. *Principles and practice of resistance training.* Champaign, IL: Human Kinetics.

37. Taylor, K.L., D.W. Chapman, J.B. Cronin, M.J. Newton, and N. Gill. 2012. Fatigue monitoring in high performance sport: A survey of current trends. *J Aust Strength Cond* 20:12-23.

38. Taylor, K.L., J. Cronin, N.D. Gill, D.W. Chapman, and J. Sheppard. 2010. Sources of variability in iso-inertial jump assessments. *Int J Sports Physiol Perform* 5:546-58.

39. Thomas, J.R., J.K. Nelson, and S.J. Silverman. 2015. *Research methods in physical activity.* 7th ed. Champaign, IL.: Human Kinetics.

40. Tod, D.A., K.A. Bond, and D. Lavallee. 2012. Professional development themes in strength and conditioning coaches. *J Strength Cond Res* 26:851-60.

41. Tufte, E. 2001. *The visual display of quantitative information.* 2nd ed. Cheshire, CT: Graphics Press.

42. Turner, A., J. Brazier, C. Bishop, S. Chavda, J. Cree, and P. Read. 2015. Data analysis for strength and conditioning coaches: Using excel to analyze reliability, differences and relationships. *Strength Cond J* 37:76-83.

43. Wallace, L.K., K.M. Slattery, F.M. Impellizzeri, and A.J. Coutts. 2014. Establishing the criterion validity and reliability of common methods for quantifying training load. *J Strength Cond Res* 28:2330-7.

44. Weissgerber, T.L., N.M. Milic, S.J. Winham, and V.D. Garovic. 2015. Beyond bar and line graphs: Time for a new data presentation paradigm. *PLoS Biol* 13:e1002128.

45. Yau, N. 2013. *Data points: Visualization that means something.* Indianapolis: Wiley.

Chapter 3

1. Andersen, J.L., and P. Aagaard. 2000. Myosin heavy chain IIX overshoot in human skeletal muscle. *Muscle Nerve* 23:1095-104.

2. Andersen, L.L., J.L. Andersen, S.P. Magnusson, C. Suetta, J.L. Madsen, L.R. Christensen, and P. Aagaard. 2005. Changes in the human muscle force-velocity relationship in response to resistance training and subsequent detraining. *J Appl Physiol* 99:87-94.

3. Aubry, A., C. Hausswirth, J. Louis, A.J. Coutts, and L.E.M. Y. 2014. Functional overreaching: The key to peak performance during the taper? *Med Sci Sports Exerc* 46:1769-77.

4. Banister, E.W., T.W. Calvert, M.V. Savage, and T. Bach. 1975. A system model of training for athletic performance. *Aust J Sports Med* 7:170-76.

5. Bartholomew, J.B., M.A. Stults-Kolehmainen, C.C. Elrod, and J.S. Todd. 2008. Strength gains after resistance training: The effect of stressful, negative life events. *J Strength Cond Res* 22:1215-21.

6. Bosquet, L., S. Merkari, D. Arvisais, and A.E. Aubert. 2008. Is heart rate a convenient tool to monitor overreaching? A systematic review of the literature. *Br J Sports Med* 42:709-14.

7. Bruin, G., H. Kuipers, H.A. Keizer, and G.J. Vander Vusse. 1994. Adaptation and overtraining in horses subjected to increasing training loads. *J Appl Physiol* 76:1908-13.

8. Buchheit, M., W. Morgan, J. Wallace, M. Bode, and N. Poulos. 2015. Physiological, psychometric, and performance effects of the Christmas break in Australian football. *Int J Sports Physiol Perform* 10:120-3.

9. Buchheit, M., S. Racinais, J.C. Bilsborough, P.C. Bourdon, S.C. Voss, J. Hocking, J. Cordy, A. Mendez-Villanueva, and A.J. Coutts. 2013. Monitoring fitness, fatigue and running performance during a pre-season training camp in elite football players. *J Sci Med Sport* 16:550-5.

10. Budgett, R., E. Newsholme, M. Lehmann, C. Sharp, D. Jones, T. Peto, D. Collins, R. Nerurkar, and P. White. 2000. Redefining the overtraining syndrome as the unexplained underperformance syndrome. *Br J Sports Med* 34:67-8.

11. Cairns, S.P. 2013. Holistic approaches to understanding mechanisms of fatigue in high-intensity sport. *Fatigue: Biomed Health Behav* 1:148-67.

12. Calvert, T.W., E.W. Banister, M.V. Savage, and T. Bach. 1976. A systems model of the effects of training on physical performance. *IEEE Trans Syst Man Cybern* 6:94-102.

13. Chiu, L.Z., and J.L. Barnes. 2003. The fitness-fatigue model revisited: Implications for planning short- and long-term training. *Strength Cond J* 25:42-51.

14. Chiu, L.Z., A.C. Fry, L.W. Weiss, B.K. Schilling, L.E. Brown, and S.L. Smith. 2003. Postactivation potentiation response in athletic and recreationally trained individuals. *J Strength Cond Res* 17:671-7.

15. Cormack, S.J., R.U. Newton, M.R. McGuigan, and P. Cormie. 2008. Neuromuscular and endocrine responses of elite players during an Australian rules football season. *Int J Sports Physiol Perform* 3:439-53.

16. Coutts, A.J., and S. Cormack. 2014. Monitoring the training response. In *High-performance training for sports*, edited by D. Joyce and D. Lewindon, 85-96. Champaign, IL: Human Kinetics.

17. Coutts, A.J., and R. Duffield. 2010. Validity and reliability of GPS devices for measuring movement demands of team sports. *J Sci Med Sport* 13:133-5.

18. Coutts, A.J., P. Reaburn, T.J. Piva, and G.J. Rowsell. 2007. Monitoring for overreaching in rugby league players. *Eur J Appl Physiol* 99:313-24.

19. Crewther, B., J. Keogh, J. Cronin, and C. Cook. 2006. Possible stimuli for strength and power adaptation: Acute hormonal responses. *Sports Med* 36:215-38.

20. Cross, M.J., S. Williams, G. Trewartha, S.P. Kemp, and K.A. Stokes. 2016. The influence of in-season training loads on injury risk in professional rugby union. *Int J Sports Physiol Perform* 11:350-55.

21. Elloumi, M., N. El Elj, M. Zaouali, F. Maso, E. Filaire, Z. Tabka, and G. Lac. 2005. IGFBP-3, a sensitive marker of physical training and overtraining. *Br J Sports Med* 39:604-10.

22. Enoka, R.M., and J. Duchateau. 2008. Muscle fatigue: What, why and how it influences muscle function. *J Physiol* 586:11-23.

23. Foster, C. 1998. Monitoring training in athletes with reference to overtraining syndrome. *Med Sci Sports Exerc* 30:1164-8.

24. Foster, C., E. Daines, L. Hector, A.C. Snyder, and R. Welsh. 1996. Athletic performance in relation to training load. *Wis Med J* 95:370-4.

25. Fowler, P., R. Duffield, K. Howle, A. Waterson, and J. Vaile. 2015. Effects of northbound long-haul international air travel on sleep quantity and subjective jet lag and wellness in professional Australian soccer players. *Int J Sports Physiol Perform* 10:648-54.

26. Fowler, P.M., R. Duffield, D. Lu, J.A. Hickmans, and T.J. Scott. 2016. Effects of long-haul transmeridian travel on subjective jet-lag and self-reported sleep and upper respiratory symptoms in professional rugby league players. *Int J Sports Physiol Perform*.

27. Frohlich, M., O. Faude, M. Klein, A. Pieter, E. Emrich, and T. Meyer. 2014. Strength training adaptations after cold-water immersion. *J Strength Cond Res* 28:2628-33.

28. Fry, A.C., and W.J. Kraemer. 1997. Resistance exercise overtraining and overreaching. Neuroendocrine responses. *Sports Med* 23:106-29.

29. Fry, A.C., W.J. Kraemer, and L.T. Ramsey. 1998. Pituitary-adrenal-gonadal responses to high-intensity resistance exercise overtraining. *J Appl Physiol* 85:2352-9.

30. Fry, A.C., W.J. Kraemer, M.H. Stone, B.J. Warren, S.J. Fleck, J.T. Kearney, and S.E. Gordon. 1994. Endocrine responses to overreaching before and after 1 year of weightlifting. *Can J Appl Physiol* 19:400-10.

31. Fry, A.C., W.J. Kraemer, F. van Borselen, J.M. Lynch, J.L. Marsit, E.P. Roy, N.T. Triplett, and H.G. Knuttgen. 1994. Performance decrements with high-intensity resistance exercise overtraining. *Med Sci Sports Exerc* 26:1165-73.

32. Fry, A.C., J.M. Webber, L.W. Weiss, M.D. Fry, and Y. Li. 2000. Impaired performances with excessive high-intensity free weight training. *J Strength Cond Res* 14:54-61.

33. Fullagar, H.H., S. Skorski, R. Duffield, D. Hammes, A.J. Coutts, and T. Meyer. 2015. Sleep and athletic performance: The effects of sleep loss on exercise performance, and physiological and cognitive responses to exercise. *Sports Med* 45:161-86.

34. Gandevia, S.C. 2001. Spinal and supraspinal factors in human muscle fatigue. *Physiol Rev* 81:1725-89.

35. Gleeson, M., and N.P. Walsh. 2012. The BASES expert statement on exercise, immunity, and infection. *J Sports Sci* 30:321-4.

36. Grandys, M., J. Majerczak, J. Kulpa, K. Duda, U. Rychlik, and J.A. Zoladz. 2016. The importance of the training-induced decrease in basal cortisol concentration in the improvement in muscular performance in humans. *Physiological Res* 65:109-20.

37. Haff, G.G. 2012. Training integration and periodization. In *NSCA's guide to program design*, edited by J.R. Hoffman, 213-49. Champaign, IL: Human Kinetics.

38. Halperin, I., D.W. Chapman, and D.G. Behm. 2015. Non-local muscle fatigue: Effects and possible mechanisms. *Eur J Appl Physiol* 115:2031-48.

39. Halson, S., D.T. Martin, A.S. Gardner, K. Fallon, and J. Gulbin. 2006. Persistent fatigue in a female sprint cyclist after a talent-transfer initiative. *Int J Sports Physiol Perform* 1:65-9.

40. Halson, S.L. 2014. Monitoring training load to understand fatigue in athletes. *Sports Med* 44 Suppl 2:S139-47.

41. Halson, S.L., and A.E. Jeukendrup. 2004. Does overtraining exist? An analysis of overreaching and overtraining research. *Sports Med* 34:967-81.

42. Halson, S.L., G.I. Lancaster, A.E. Jeukendrup, and M. Gleeson. 2003. Immunological responses to overreaching in cyclists. *Med Sci Sports Exerc* 35:854-61.

43. Harre, D. 1982. *Principles of sports training: Introduction to the theory and methods of training*. Berlin: Sportverlag.

44. Hartmann, U., and J. Mester. 2000. Training and overtraining markers in selected sport events. *Med Sci Sports Exerc* 32:209-15.

45. Hausswirth, C., J. Louis, A. Aubry, G. Bonnet, R. Duffield, and L.E.M. Y. 2014. Evidence of disturbed sleep and increased illness in overreached endurance athletes. *Med Sci Sports Exerc* 46:1036-45.

46. Henckens, M.J., F. Klumpers, D. Everaerd, S.C. Kooijman, G.A. van Wingen, and G. Fernandez. 2016. Inter-individual differences in stress sensitivity: Basal and stress-induced cortisol levels differentially predict neural vigilance processing under stress. *Soc Cogn Affect Neurosci* 11:663-73.

47. Hodgson, M., D. Docherty, and D. Robbins. 2005. Post-activation potentiation: Underlying physiology and implications for motor performance. *Sports Med* 35:585-95.

48. Hooper, S.L., L.T. Mackinnon, A. Howard, R.D. Gordon, and A.W. Bachmann. 1995. Markers for monitoring overtraining and recovery. *Med Sci Sports Exerc* 27:106-12.

49. Hough, J., R. Corney, A. Kouris, and M. Gleeson. 2013. Salivary cortisol and testosterone responses to high-intensity cycling before and after an 11-day intensified training period. *J Sports Sci* 31:1614-23.

50. Hough, J.P., E. Papacosta, E. Wraith, and M. Gleeson. 2011. Plasma and salivary steroid hormone responses of men to high-intensity cycling and resistance exercise. *J Strength Cond Res* 25:23-31.

51. Impellizzeri, F.M., E. Rampinini, A.J. Coutts, A. Sassi, and S.M. Marcora. 2004. Use of RPE-based training load in soccer. *Med Sci Sports Exerc* 36:1042-7.

52. Jones, D.A. 1996. High- and low-frequency fatigue revisited. *Acta Physiol Scand* 156:265-70.

53. Jurimae, J., J. Maestu, T. Jurimae, B. Mangus, and S.P. von Duvillard. 2011. Peripheral signals of energy homeostasis as possible markers of training stress in athletes: A review. *Metabolism* 60:335-50.

54. Kelly, V.G., and A.J. Coutts. 2007. Planning and monitoring training loads during the competition phase in team sports. *Strength Cond J* 29:32-37.

55. Kentta, G., and P. Hassmen. 1998. Overtraining and recovery: A conceptual model. *Sports Med* 26:1-16.

56. Killer, S.C., I.S. Svendsen, A.E. Jeukendrup, and M. Gleeson. 2015. Evidence of disturbed sleep and mood state in well-trained athletes during short-term intensified training with and without a high carbohydrate nutritional intervention. *J Sports Sci* 25:1-9.

57. Knicker, A.J., I. Renshaw, A.R. Oldham, and S.P. Cairns. 2011. Interactive processes link the multiple symptoms of fatigue in sport competition. *Sports Med* 41:307-28.

58. Koutedakis, Y., and N.C. Sharp. 1998. Seasonal variations of injury and overtraining in elite athletes. *Clin J Sport Med* 8:18-21.

59. Kraemer, W.J., L. Marchitelli, S.E. Gordon, E. Harman, J.E. Dziados, R. Mello, P. Frykman, D. McCurry, and S.J. Fleck. 1990. Hormonal and growth factor responses to heavy resistance exercise protocols. *J Appl Physiol* 69:1442-50.

60. Kraemer, W.J., and N.A. Ratamess. 2005. Hormonal responses and adaptations to resistance exercise and training. *Sports Med* 35:339-61.

61. Le Meur, Y., C. Hausswirth, F. Natta, A. Couturier, F. Bignet, and P.P. Vidal. 2013. A multidisciplinary approach to overreaching detection in endurance trained athletes. *J Appl Physiol* 114:411-20.

62. Le Meur, Y., A. Pichon, K. Schaal, L. Schmitt, J. Louis, J. Gueneron, P.P. Vidal, and C. Hausswirth. 2013. Evidence of parasympathetic hyperactivity in functionally overreached athletes. *Med Sci Sports Exerc* 45:2061-71.

63. Lewis, N.A., D. Collins, C.R. Pedlar, and J.P. Rogers. 2015. Can clinicians and scientists explain and prevent unexplained underperformance syndrome in elite athletes: An interdisciplinary perspective and 2016 update. *BMJ Open Sport & Exercise Medicine* 1:e000063.

64. Loturco, I., L.A. Pereira, R. Kobal, H. Martins, K. Kitamura, C.C. Cal Abad, and F.Y. Nakamura. 2015. Effects of detraining on neuromuscular performance in a selected group of elite women pole-vaulters: A case study. *J Sports Med Phys Fitness*.

65. Mahlfeld, K., J. Franke, and F. Awiszus. 2004. Postcontraction changes of muscle architecture in human quadriceps muscle. *Muscle Nerve* 29:597-600.

66. Mann, J.B., K. Bryant, B. Johnstone, P. Ivey, and S.P. Sayers. 2016. The effect of physical and academic stress on illness and injury in Division 1 college football players. *J Strength Cond Res* 30:20-25.

67. Marcora, S.M., W. Staiano, and V. Manning. 2009. Mental fatigue impairs physical performance in humans. *J Appl Physiol* 106:857-64.

68. Matos, N.F., R.J. Winsley, and C.A. Williams. 2011. Prevalence of nonfunctional overreaching/overtraining in young English athletes. *Med Sci Sports Exerc* 43:1287-94.

69. McKeown, I., D.W. Chapman, K. Taylor, and N. Ball. 2016. Time course of improvements in power characteristics in elite development netball players entering a full time training program. *J Strength Cond Res* 30:1308-15.

70. Meeusen, R., and K. De Pauw. 2013. Overtraining syndrome. In *Recovery for performance in sport*, edited by C. Hauusswirth and I. Mujika, 9-20. Champaign, IL: Human Kinetics.

71. Meeusen, R., M. Duclos, C. Foster, A. Fry, M. Gleeson, D. Nieman, J. Raglin, G. Rietjens, J. Steinacker, A. Urhausen, S. European College of Sport Science, and American College of Sports Medicine. 2013. Prevention, diagnosis, and treatment of the overtraining syndrome: Joint consensus statement of the European College of Sport Science and the American College of Sports Medicine. *Med Sci Sports Exerc* 45:186-205.

72. Meeusen, R., E. Nederhof, L. Buyse, B. Roelands, G. de Schutter, and M.F. Piacentini. 2010. Diagnosing overtraining in athletes using the two-bout exercise protocol. *Br J Sports Med* 44:642-8.

73. Meeusen, R., M.F. Piacentini, B. Busschaert, L. Buyse, G. De Schutter, and J. Stray-Gundersen. 2004. Hormonal responses in athletes: The use of a two bout exercise protocol to detect subtle differences in (over)training status. *Eur J Appl Physiol* 91:140-6.

74. Milanez, V.F., S.P. Ramos, N.M. Okuno, D.A. Boullosa, and F.Y. Nakamura. 2014.

Evidence of a non-linear dose-response relationship between training load and stress markers in elite female futsal players. *J Sports Sci Med* 13:22-29.

75. Milewski, M.D., D.L. Skaggs, G.A. Bishop, J.L. Pace, D.A. Ibrahim, T.A. Wren, and A. Barzdukas. 2014. Chronic lack of sleep is associated with increased sports injuries in adolescent athletes. *J Pediatr Orthop* 34:129-33.

76. Moore, C.A., and A.C. Fry. 2007. Nonfunctional overreaching during off-season training for skill position players in collegiate American football. *J Strength Cond Res* 21:793-800.

77. Morgan, W.P., D.L. Costill, M.G. Flynn, J.S. Raglin, and P.J. O'Connor. 1988. Mood disturbance following increased training in swimmers. *Med Sci Sports Exerc* 20:408-14.

78. Morgan, W.P., P.J. O'Connor, P.B. Sparling, and R.R. Pate. 1987. Psychological characterization of the elite female distance runner. *Int J Sports Med* 8 Suppl 2:124-31.

79. Mountjoy, M., J. Sundgot-Borgen, L. Burke, S. Carter, N. Constantini, C. Lebrun, N. Meyer, R. Sherman, K. Steffen, R. Budgett, and A. Ljungqvist. 2014. The IOC consensus statement: Beyond the female athlete triad—relative energy deficiency in sport (red-s). *Br J Sports Med* 48:491-7.

80. Mountjoy, M., J. Sundgot-Borgen, L. Burke, S. Carter, N. Constantini, C. Lebrun, N. Meyer, R. Sherman, K. Steffen, R. Budgett, and A. Ljungqvist. 2015. Authors' 2015 additions to the IOC consensus statement: Relative energy deficiency in sport (red-s). *Br J Sports Med* 49:417-20.

81. Mujika, I. 2010. Intense training: The key to optimal performance before and during the taper. *Scand J Med Sci Sports* 20 Suppl 2:24-31.

82. Nederhof, E., K.A. Lemmink, C. Visscher, R. Meeusen, and T. Mulder. 2006. Psychomotor speed: Possibly a new marker for overtraining syndrome. *Sports Med* 36:817-28.

83. Nederhof, E., J. Zwerver, M. Brink, R. Meeusen, and K. Lemmink. 2008. Different diagnostic tools in nonfunctional overreaching. *Int J Sports Med* 29:590-7.

84. Nimmerichter, A., R.G. Eston, N. Bachl, and C. Williams. 2011. Longitudinal monitoring of power output and heart rate profiles in elite cyclists. *J Sports Sci* 29:831-40.

85. Noakes, T.D. 2007. The central governor model of exercise regulation applied to the marathon. *Sports Med* 37:374-7.

86. Otter, R.T., M.S. Brink, R.L. Diercks, and K.A. Lemmink. 2016. A negative life event impairs psychosocial stress, recovery and running economy of runners. *Int J Sports Med* 37:224-29.

87. Perl, J. 2001. PerPot: A metamodel for simulation of load performance interaction. *Eur J Sport Sci* 1:1-13.

88. Pfeiffer, M. 2008. Modeling the relationship between training and performance—a comparison of two antagonistic concepts. *Int J Comp Sci in Sport* 7:13-32.

89. Piacentini, M.F., O.C. Witard, C. Tonoli, S.R. Jackman, J.E. Turner, A.K. Kies, A.E. Jeukendrup, K.D. Tipton, and R. Meeusen. 2016. Intensive training affects mood with no effect on brain-derived neurotrophic factor. *Int J Sports Physiol Perform* 11:824-30.

90. Plews, D.J., P.B. Laursen, J. Stanley, A.E. Kilding, and M. Buchheit. 2013. Training adaptation and heart rate variability in elite endurance athletes: Opening the door to effective monitoring. *Sports Med* 43:773-81.

91. Pyne, D.B., I. Mujika, and T. Reilly. 2009. Peaking for optimal performance: Research limitations and future directions. *J Sports Sci* 27:195-202.

92. Reid, V.L., M. Gleeson, N. Williams, and R.L. Clancy. 2004. Clinical investigation of athletes with persistent fatigue and/or recurrent infections. *Br J Sports Med* 38:42-5.

93. Robbins, D.W. 2005. Postactivation potentiation and its practical applicability: A brief review. *J Strength Cond Res* 19:453-8.

94. Roberts, L.A., T. Raastad, J.F. Markworth, V.C. Figueiredo, I.M. Egner, A. Shield, D. Cameron-Smith, J.S. Coombes, and J.M. Peake. 2015. Post-exercise cold water immersion attenuates acute anabolic signalling and long-term adaptations in muscle to strength training. *J Physiol* 593:4285-301.

95. Ruuska, P.S., A.J. Hautala, A.M. Kiviniemi, T.H. Makikallio, and M. Tulppo. 2012. Self-rated mental stress and exercise training response in healthy subjects. *Front Physiol* 3:1-7.

96. Saw, A.E., L.C. Main, and P.B. Gastin. 2016. Monitoring the athlete training response: Subjective self-reported measures trump commonly used objective measures: A systematic review. *Br J Sports Med* 50:281-91.

97. Schmikli, S.L., M.S. Brink, W.R. de Vries, and F.J. Backx. 2011. Can we detect non-functional overreaching in young elite soccer players and middle-long distance runners using field performance tests? *Br J Sports Med* 45:631-6.

98. Schmikli, S.L., W.R. de Vries, M.S. Brink, and F.J. Backx. 2012. Monitoring performance, pituitary-adrenal hormones and mood profiles: How to diagnose non-functional over-reaching in male elite junior soccer players. *Br J Sports Med* 46:1019-23.

99. Seitz, L.B., and G.G. Haff. 2016. Factors modulating post-activation potentiation of jump, sprint, throw, and upper-body ballistic performances: A systematic review with meta-analysis. *Sports Med* 46:231-40.

100. Selye, H. 1950. Stress and the general adaptation syndrome. *British Medical Journal* June 17:1383-92.

101. Selye, H. 1956. *The stress of life*. London: Longmans Green.

102. Smith, L.L. 2000. Cytokine hypothesis of overtraining: A physiological adaptation to excessive stress? *Med Sci Sports Exerc* 32:317-31.

103. Smith, L.L. 2004. Tissue trauma: The underlying cause of overtraining syndrome? *J Strength Cond Res* 18:185-93.

104. Smith, M.R., A.J. Coutts, M. Merlini, D. Deprez, M. Lenoir, and S.M. Marcora. 2016. Mental fatigue impairs soccer-specific physical and technical performance. *Med Sci Sports Exerc* 48:267-76.

105. Steinacker, J.M., W. Lormes, S. Reissnecker, and Y. Liu. 2004. New aspects of the hormone and cytokine response to training. *Eur J Appl Physiol* 91:382-91.

106. Stone, M.H., M. Stone, and W.A. Sands. 2006. *Principles and practice of resistance training*. Champaign, IL: Human Kinetics.

107. Stults-Kolehmainen, M.A., and J.B. Bartholomew. 2012. Psychological stress impairs short-term muscular recovery from resistance exercise. *Med Sci Sports Exerc* 44:2220-7.

108. Stults-Kolehmainen, M.A., J.B. Bartholomew, and R. Sinha. 2014. Chronic psychological stress impairs recovery of muscular function and somatic sensations over a 96-hour period. *J Strength Cond Res* 28:2007-17.

109. Thomas, K., A. Toward, D.J. West, G. Howatson, and S. Goodall. 2015. Heavy-resistance exercise-induced increases in jump performance are not explained by changes in neuromuscular function. *Scand J Med Sci Sports*.

110. Thornton, H.R., J.A. Delaney, G.M. Duthie, B.R. Scott, W.J. Chivers, C.E. Sanctuary, and B.J. Dascombe. 2016. Predicting self-reported illness for professional team-sport athletes. *Int J Sports Physiol Perform* 11:543-50.

111. Thorpe, R.T., A.J. Strudwick, M. Buchheit, G. Atkinson, B. Drust, and W. Gregson. 2015. Monitoring fatigue during the in-season competitive phase in elite soccer players. *Int J Sports Physiol Perform* 10:958-64.

112. Tillin, N.A., and D. Bishop. 2009. Factors modulating post-activation potentiation and its effect on performance of subsequent explosive activities. *Sports Med* 39:147-66.

113. Turner, A. 2011. The science and practice of periodization: A brief review. *Strength Cond J* 33:34-46.

114. Urhausen, A., and W. Kindermann. 2002. Diagnosis of overtraining: What tools do we have? *Sports Med* 32:95-102.

115. Walburn, J., K. Vedhara, M. Hankins, L. Rixon, and J. Weinman. 2009. Psychological stress and wound healing in humans: A systematic review and meta-analysis. *J Psychosom Res* 67:253-71.

116. Walsh, N.P., M. Gleeson, D.B. Pyne, D.C. Nieman, F.S. Dhabhar, R.J. Shephard, S.J. Oliver, S. Bermon, and A. Kajeniene. 2011. Position statement. Part two: Maintaining immune health. *Exerc Immunol Rev* 17:64-103.

117. Walsh, N.P., M. Gleeson, R.J. Shephard, M. Gleeson, J.A. Woods, N.C. Bishop, M. Fleshner, C. Green, B.K. Pedersen, L. Hoffman-Goetz, C.J. Rogers, H. Northoff, A. Abbasi, and P. Simon. 2011. Position statement. Part one: Immune function and exercise. *Exerc Immunol Rev* 17:6-63.

118. Zoladz, J.A., A.J. Sargeant, J. Emmerich, J. Stoklosa, and A. Zychowski. 1993. Changes in acid-base status of marathon runners during an incremental field test. Relationship to mean competitive marathon velocity. *Eur J Appl Physiol Occup Physiol* 67:71-6.

Chapter 4

1. Akenhead, R., and G.P. Nassis. 2016. Training load and player monitoring in high-level football: Current practice and perceptions. *Int J Sports Physiol Perform* 11:587-93.

2. Akubat, I., S. Barrett, and G. Abt. 2014. Integrating the internal and external training loads in soccer. *Int J Sports Physiol Perform* 9:457-62.

3. Alexiou, H., and A.J. Coutts. 2008. A comparison of methods used for quantifying internal training load in women soccer players. *Int J Sports Physiol Perform* 3:320-30.

4. Arcos, A.L., R. Martinez-Santos, J. Yanci, J. Mendiguchia, and A. Mendez-Villanueva. 2015. Negative associations between perceived training load, volume and changes in physical fitness in professional soccer players. *J Sports Sci Med* 14:394-401.

5. Arcos, A.L., J. Yanci, J. Mendiguchia, and E.M. Gorostiaga. 2014. Rating of muscular and respiratory perceived exertion in professional soccer players. *J Strength Cond Res* 28:3280-8.

6. Atlaoui, D., V. Pichot, L. Lacoste, F. Barale, J.R. Lacour, and J.C. Chatard. 2007. Heart rate variability, training variation and performance in elite swimmers. *Int J Sports Med* 28:394-400.

7. Aughey, R.J. 2011. Applications of GPS technologies to field sports. *Int J Sports Physiol Perform* 6:295-310.

8. Aughey, R.J., G.P. Elias, A. Esmaeili, B. Lazarus, and A.M. Stewart. 2015. Does the recent internal load and strain on players affect match outcome in elite Australian football? *J Sci Med Sport.*

9. Austin, D., T. Gabbett, and D. Jenkins. 2011. Repeated high-intensity exercise in professional rugby union. *J Sports Sci* 29:1105-12.

10. Banister, E.W., T.W. Calvert, M.V. Savage, and T. Bach. 1975. A system model of training for athletic performance. *Aust J Sports Med* 7:170-76.

11. Barrett, S., A. Midgley, and R. Lovell. 2014. Playerload: Reliability, convergent validity, and influence of unit position during treadmill running. *Int J Sports Physiol Perform* 9:945-52.

12. Barrett, S., A.W. Midgley, C. Towlson, A. Garrett, M. Portas, and R. Lovell. 2015. Within-match playerload patterns during a simulated soccer match (SAFT90): Potential implications for unit positioning and fatigue management. *Int J Sports Physiol Perform.*

13. Bautista, I.J., I.J. Chirosa, L.J. Chirosa, I. Martin, A. Gonzalez, and R.J. Robertson. 2014. Development and validity of a scale of perception of velocity in resistance exercise. *J Sports Sci Med* 13:542-9.

14. Bautista, I.J., I.J. Chirosa, J.E. Robinson, L.J. Chirosa, and I.M. Martin. 2016. Concurrent validity of a perception velocity scale to monitor squat exercise intensity in young skiers. *J Strength Cond Res* 30:421-9.

15. Blanch, P., and T.J. Gabbett. 2016. Has the athlete trained enough to return to play safely? The acute:chronic workload ratio permits clinicians to quantify a player's risk of subsequent injury. *Br J Sports Med* 50:471-75.

16. Borg, E., and G. Borg. 2002. A comparison of AME and CR100 for scaling perceived exertion. *Acta Psychol (Amst)* 109:157-75.

17. Borg, E., G. Borg, K. Larsson, M. Letzter, and B.M. Sundblad. 2010. An index for breathlessness and leg fatigue. *Scand J Med Sci Sports* 20:644-50.

18. Borg, E., and L. Kaijser. 2006. A comparison between three rating scales for perceived exertion and two different work tests. *Scand J Med Sci Sports* 16:57-69.

19. Borg, G. 1990. Psychophysical scaling with applications in physical work and the perception of exertion. *Scand J Work Environ Health* 16 Suppl 1:55-8.

20. Borg, G., P. Hassmen, and M. Lagerstrom. 1987. Perceived exertion related to heart rate and blood lactate during arm and leg exercise. *Eur J Appl Physiol Occup Physiol* 56:679-85.

21. Borg, G.A. 1982. Psychophysical bases of perceived exertion. *Med Sci Sports Exerc* 14:377-81.

22. Borg, G.A., and B.J. Noble. 1974. Perceived exertion. *Exerc Sport Sci Rev* 2:131-53.

23. Borges, N.R., and M.W. Driller. 2016. Wearable lactate threshold predicting device is valid and reliable in runners. *J Strength Cond Res* 30:2212-8.

24. Borresen, J., and M. Lambert. 2006. Validity of self-reported training duration. *Int J Sports Sci Coaching* 1:353-59.

25. Borresen, J., and M.I. Lambert. 2008. Quantifying training load: A comparison of subjective and objective methods. *Int J Sports Physiol Perform* 3:16-30.

26. Borresen, J., and M.I. Lambert. 2009. The quantification of training load, the training response and the effect on performance. *Sports Med* 39:779-95.

27. Boyd, L.J., K. Ball, and R.J. Aughey. 2011. The reliability of MinimaxX accelerometers for measuring physical activity in Australian football. *Int J Sports Physiol Perform* 6:311-21.

28. Brink, M.S., W.G. Frencken, G. Jordet, and K.A. Lemmink. 2014. Coaches' and players' perceptions of training dose: Not a perfect match. *Int J Sports Physiol Perform* 9:497-502.

29. Buchheit, M., A. Gray, and J.B. Morin. 2015. Assessing stride variables and vertical stiffness with GPS-embedded accelerometers: Preliminary insights for the monitoring of neuromuscular fatigue on the field. *J Sports Sci Med* 14:698-701.

30. Busso, T., K. Hakkinen, A. Pakarinen, C. Carasso, J.R. Lacour, P.V. Komi, and H. Kauhanen. 1990. A systems model of training responses and its relationship to hormonal responses in elite weight-lifters. *Eur J Appl Physiol Occup Physiol* 61:48-54.

31. Calvert, T.W., E.W. Banister, M.V. Savage, and T. Bach. 1976. A systems model of the effects of training on physical performance. *IEEE Trans Syst Man Cybern* 6:94-102.

32. Chatard, J.C., D. Atlaoui, V. Pichot, C. Gourne, M. Duclos, and Y.C. Guezennec. 2003. Training follow up by questionnaire fatigue, hormones and heart rate variability measurements. *Sci Sports* 18:302-04.

33. Chen, M.J., X. Fan, and S.T. Moe. 2002. Criterion-related validity of the Borg rat-

ings of perceived exertion scale in healthy individuals: A meta-analysis. *J Sports Sci* 20:873-99.

34. Clarke, A.C., J. Anson, and D. Pyne. 2015. Physiologically based GPS speed zones for evaluating running demands in women's rugby sevens. *J Sports Sci* 33:1101-8.

35. Clarke, A.C., J.M. Anson, and D.B. Pyne. 2015. Neuromuscular fatigue and muscle damage after a women's rugby sevens tournament. *Int J Sports Physiol Perform* 10:808-14.

36. Cleather, D.J., and S.R. Guthrie. 2007. Quantifying delayed-onset muscle soreness: A comparison of unidimensional and multidimensional instrumentation. *J Sports Sci* 25:845-50.

37. Cormack, S.J., R.L. Smith, M.M. Mooney, W.B. Young, and B.J. O'Brien. 2014. Accelerometer load as a measure of activity profile in different standards of netball match play. *Int J Sports Physiol Perform* 9:283-91.

38. Coutts, A.J., and S. Cormack. 2014. Monitoring the training response. In *High-performance training for sports*, edited by D. Joyce and D. Lewindon, 85-96. Champaign, IL: Human Kinetics.

39. Coutts, A.J., T. Kempton, C. Sullivan, J. Bilsborough, J. Cordy, and E. Rampinini. 2015. Metabolic power and energetic costs of professional Australian football match-play. *J Sci Med Sport* 18:219-24.

40. Cross, M.J., S. Williams, G. Trewartha, S.P. Kemp, and K.A. Stokes. 2016. The influence of in-season training loads on injury risk in professional rugby union. *Int J Sports Physiol Perform* 11:350-55.

41. Cummins, C., and R. Orr. 2015. Analysis of physical collisions in elite national rugby league match play. *Int J Sports Physiol Perform* 10:732-9.

42. Cummins, C., R. Orr, H. O'Connor, and C. West. 2013. Global positioning systems (GPS) and microtechnology sensors in team sports: A systematic review. *Sports Med* 43:1025-42.

43. Day, M.L., M.R. McGuigan, G. Brice, and C. Foster. 2004. Monitoring exercise intensity during resistance training using the session RPE scale. *J Strength Cond Res* 18:353-8.

44. de Jong, J., L. van der Meijden, S. Hamby, S. Suckow, C. Dodge, J.J. de Koning, and C. Foster. 2015. Pacing strategy in short cycling time trials. *Int J Sports Physiol Perform* 10:1015-22.

45. Driller, M.W., C.K. Argus, and C.M. Shing. 2013. The reliability of a 30-s sprint test on the Wattbike cycle ergometer. *Int J Sports Physiol Perform* 8:379-83.

46. Dwyer, D.B., and T.J. Gabbett. 2012. Global positioning system data analysis: Velocity ranges and a new definition of sprinting for field sport athletes. *J Strength Cond Res* 26:818-24.

47. Edwards, S. 1992. *The heart rate monitor book*. Sacramento, CA: Polar CIC.

48. Ekegren, C.L., A. Donaldson, B.J. Gabbe, and C.F. Finch. 2014. Implementing injury surveillance systems alongside injury prevention programs: Evaluation of an online surveillance system in a community setting. *Inj Epidemiol* 1:19.

49. Ekegren, C.L., B.J. Gabbe, and C.F. Finch. 2014. Injury reporting via SMS text messaging in community sport. *Inj Prev* 20:266-71.

50. Elloumi, M., N. El Elj, M. Zaouali, F. Maso, E. Filaire, Z. Tabka, and G. Lac. 2005. IGFBP-3, a sensitive marker of physical training and overtraining. *Br J Sports Med* 39:604-10.

51. Eston, R. 2012. Use of ratings of perceived exertion in sports. *Int J Sports Physiol Perform* 7:175-82.

52. Evenson, K.R., M.M. Goto, and R.D. Furberg. 2015. Systematic review of the validity and reliability of consumer-wearable activity trackers. *Int J Behav Nutr Phys Act* 12:159.

53. Fanchini, M., I. Ferraresi, R. Modena, F. Schena, A.J. Coutts, and F.M. Impellizzeri. 2016. Use of CR100 scale for session—RPE in soccer and interchangeability with CR10. *Int J Sports Physiol Perform* 11:388-92.

54. Foster, C. 1998. Monitoring training in athletes with reference to overtraining syndrome. *Med Sci Sports Exerc* 30:1164-8.

55. Foster, C., E. Daines, L. Hector, A.C. Snyder, and R. Welsh. 1996. Athletic performance in relation to training load. *Wis Med J* 95:370-4.

56. Foster, C., J.A. Florhaug, J. Franklin, L. Gottschall, L.A. Hrovatin, S. Parker, P. Doleshal, and C. Dodge. 2001. A new approach to monitoring exercise training. *J Strength Cond Res* 15:109-15.

57. Foster, C., L.L. Hector, R. Welsh, M. Schrager, M.A. Green, and A.C. Snyder. 1995. Effects of specific versus cross-training on running performance. *Eur J Appl Physiol Occup Physiol* 70:367-72.

58. Foster, C., K.M. Heimann, P.L. Esten, G. Brice, and J.P. Porcari. 2001. Differences in perceptions of training by coaches and athletes. *South Afr J Sports Med* 8:3-7.

59. Fry, R.W., J.R. Grove, A.R. Morton, P.M. Zeroni, S. Gaudieri, and D. Keast. 1994. Psychological and immunological correlates of acute overtraining. *Br J Sports Med* 28:241-6.

60. Gabbett, T.J. 2010. The development and application of an injury prediction model for noncontact, soft-tissue injuries in elite collision sport athletes. *J Strength Cond Res* 24:2593-603.

61. Gabbett, T.J. 2015. Relationship between accelerometer load, collisions, and repeated high-intensity effort activity in rugby league players. *J Strength Cond Res* 29:3424-31.

62. Gabbett, T.J., and N. Domrow. 2007. Relationships between training load, injury, and fitness in sub-elite collision sport athletes. *J Sports Sci* 25:1507-19.

63. Gabbett, T.J., and D.G. Jenkins. 2011. Relationship between training load and injury in professional rugby league players. *J Sci Med Sport* 14:204-9.

64. Gabbett, T.J., D.G. Jenkins, and B. Abernethy. 2012. Physical demands of professional rugby league training and competition using microtechnology. *J Sci Med Sport* 15:80-6.

65. Gabbett, T.J., and S. Ullah. 2012. Relationship between running loads and soft-tissue injury in elite team sport athletes. *J Strength Cond Res* 26:953-60.

66. Gallo, T., S. Cormack, T. Gabbett, M. Williams, and C. Lorenzen. 2015. Characteristics impacting on session rating of perceived exertion training load in Australian footballers. *J Sports Sci* 33:467-75.

67. Gastin, P.B., D. Meyer, and D. Robinson. 2013. Perceptions of wellness to monitor adaptive responses to training and competition in elite Australian football. *J Strength Cond Res* 27:2518-26.

68. Gaudino, P., F.M. Iaia, G. Alberti, A.J. Strudwick, G. Atkinson, and W. Gregson. 2013. Monitoring training in elite soccer players: Systematic bias between running speed and metabolic power data. *Int J Sports Med* 34:963-8.

69. Gaudino, P., F.M. Iaia, A.J. Strudwick, R.D. Hawkins, G. Alberti, G. Atkinson, and W. Gregson. 2015. Factors influencing perception of effort (session rating of perceived exertion) during elite soccer training. *Int J Sports Physiol Perform* 10:860-4.

70. Gil-Rey, E., A. Lezaun, and A. Los Arcos. 2015. Quantification of the perceived training load and its relationship with changes in physical fitness performance in junior soccer players. *J Sports Sci* 33:2125-32.

71. Gomes, R.V., A. Moreira, L. Lodo, K. Nosaka, A.J. Coutts, and M.S. Aoki. 2013. Monitoring training loads, stress, immune-endocrine responses and performance in tennis players. *Biol Sport* 30:173-80.

72. Grove, J.R., L.C. Main, K. Partridge, D.J. Bishop, S. Russell, A. Shepherdson, and L. Ferguson. 2014. Training distress and performance readiness: Laboratory and field validation of a brief self-report measure. *Scand J Med Sci Sports* 24:e483-e90.

73. Haddad, M., A. Chaouachi, C. Castagna, P. Wong del, D.G. Behm, and K. Chamari. 2011. The construct validity of session RPE during an intensive camp in young male taekwondo athletes. *Int J Sports Physiol Perform* 6:252-63.

74. Haff, G.G. 2010. Quantifying workloads in resistance training: A brief review. *UK Strength Cond Assoc J* 19:31-40.

75. Haile, L., F.L. Goss, R.J. Robertson, J.L. Andreacci, M. Gallagher, Jr., and E.F. Nagle. 2013. Session perceived exertion and affective responses to self-selected and imposed cycle exercise of the same intensity in young men. *Eur J Appl Physiol* 113:1755-65.

76. Halson, S.L. 2014. Monitoring training load to understand fatigue in athletes. *Sports Med* 44 Suppl 2:S139-47.

77. Halson, S.L., M.W. Bridge, R. Meeusen, B. Busschaert, M. Gleeson, D.A. Jones, and A.E. Jeukendrup. 2002. Time course of performance changes and fatigue markers during intensified training in trained cyclists. *J Appl Physiol* 93:947-56.

78. Hausler, J., M. Halaki, and R. Orr. 2016. Application of global positioning system and microsensor technology in competitive rugby league match-play: A systematic review and meta-analysis. *Sports Med* 46:559-88.

79. Hiscock, D.J., B. Dawson, C.J. Donnelly, and P. Peeling. 2015. Muscle activation, blood lactate, and perceived exertion responses to changing resistance training programming variables. *Eur J Sport Sci*:1-9.

80. Hiscock, D.J., B. Dawson, and P. Peeling. 2015. Perceived exertion responses to changing resistance training programming variables. *J Strength Cond Res* 29:1564-9.

81. Hooper, S.L., L.T. Mackinnon, A. Howard, R.D. Gordon, and A.W. Bachmann. 1995. Markers for monitoring overtraining and recovery. *Med Sci Sports Exerc* 27:106-12.

82. Hopkins, W.G. 1991. Quantification of training in competitive sports. Methods and applications. *Sports Med* 12:161-83.

83. Howatson, G., and K.A. van Someren. 2008. The prevention and treatment of exercise-induced muscle damage. *Sports Med* 38:483-503.

84. Hulin, B.T., T.J. Gabbett, P. Blanch, P. Chapman, D. Bailey, and J.W. Orchard. 2014. Spikes in acute workload are associated with increased injury risk in elite cricket fast bowlers. *Br J Sports Med* 48:708-12.

85. Hulin, B.T., T.J. Gabbett, S. Kearney, and A. Corvo. 2015. Physical demands of match play in successful and less-successful elite rugby league teams. *Int J Sports Physiol Perform* 10:703-10.

86. Impellizzeri, F.M., and N.A. Maffiuletti. 2007. Convergent evidence for construct validity of a 7-point Likert scale of lower limb muscle soreness. *Clin J Sport Med* 17:494-6.

87. Impellizzeri, F.M., E. Rampinini, A.J. Coutts, A. Sassi, and S.M. Marcora. 2004. Use of RPE-based training load in soccer. *Med Sci Sports Exerc* 36:1042-7.

88. Jennings, D., S. Cormack, A.J. Coutts, L. Boyd, and R.J. Aughey. 2010. The validity and reliability of GPS units for measuring distance in team sport specific running patterns. *Int J Sports Physiol Perform* 5:328-41.

89. Jennings, D., S. Cormack, A.J. Coutts, L.J. Boyd, and R.J. Aughey. 2010. Variability of GPS units for measuring distance in team sport movements. *Int J Sports Physiol Perform* 5:565-9.

90. Jennings, D., S.J. Cormack, A.J. Coutts, and R.J. Aughey. 2012. GPS analysis of an international field hockey tournament. *Int J Sports Physiol Perform* 7:224-31.

91. Jobson, S.A., L. Passfield, G. Atkinson, G. Barton, and P. Scarf. 2009. The analysis and utilization of cycling training data. *Sports Med* 39:833-44.

92. Johnston, R.J., M.L. Watsford, D. Austin, M.J. Pine, and R.W. Spurrs. 2015. Player acceleration and deceleration profiles in professional Australian football. *J Sports Med Phys Fitness* 55:931-9.

93. Johnston, R.J., M.L. Watsford, D.J. Austin, M.J. Pine, and R.W. Spurrs. 2015. An examination of the relationship between movement demands and rating of perceived exertion in Australian footballers. *J Strength Cond Res* 29:2026-33.

94. Johnston, R.J., M.L. Watsford, D.J. Austin, M.J. Pine, and R.W. Spurrs. 2015. Movement demands and metabolic power comparisons between elite and subelite Australian footballers. *J Strength Cond Res* 29:2738-44.

95. Johnston, R.J., M.L. Watsford, S.J. Kelly, M.J. Pine, and R.W. Spurrs. 2014. Validity and interunit reliability of 10 Hz and 15 Hz GPS units for assessing athlete movement demands. *J Strength Cond Res* 28:1649-55.

96. Kellmann, M., ed. 2002. *Enhancing recovery: Preventing underperformance in athletes.* Champaign, IL: Human Kinetics.

97. Kempton, T., A.C. Sirotic, E. Rampinini, and A.J. Coutts. 2015. Metabolic power demands of rugby league match play. *Int J Sports Physiol Perform* 10:23-8.

98. Kentta, G., and P. Hassmen. 1998. Overtraining and recovery: A conceptual model. *Sports Med* 26:1-16.

99. Kolling, S., B. Hitzschke, T. Holst, A. Ferrauti, T. Meyer, M. Pfeiffer, and M. Kellmann. 2015. Validity of the acute recovery and stress scale: Training monitoring of the German junior national field hockey team. *Int J Sports Sci Coaching* 10:529-42.

100. Kolling, S., J.M. Steinacker, S. Endler, A. Ferrauti, T. Meyer, and M. Kellmann. 2016. The longer the better: Sleep-wake patterns during preparation of the world rowing junior championships. *Chronobiol Int*:1-12.

101. Kraemer, W.J., S.J. Fleck, and M.R. Deschenes. 2012. *Exercise physiology: Integrating theory and application.* Baltimore, MD: Lippincott Williams & Wilkins.

102. Kraft, J.A., J.M. Green, and T.M. Gast. 2014. Work distribution influences session ratings of perceived exertion response during resistance exercise matched for total volume. *J Strength Cond Res* 28:2042-6.

103. Lambert, M., and J. Borresen. 2006. A theoretical basis of monitoring fatigue: A practical approach for coaches. *Int J Sports Sci Coaching* 1:371-88.

104. Lambert, M.I., P. Marcus, T. Burgess, and T.D. Noakes. 2002. Electro-membrane microcurrent therapy reduces signs and symptoms of muscle damage. *Med Sci Sports Exerc* 34:602-7.

105. Lan, M.F., A.M. Lane, J. Roy, and N.A. Hanin. 2012. Validity of the Brunel Mood Scale for use with Malaysian athletes. *J Sports Sci Med* 11:131-5.

106. Larsson, P. 2003. Global positioning system and sport-specific testing. *Sports Med* 33:1093-101.

107. Lau, W.Y., A.J. Blazevich, M.J. Newton, S.S. Wu, and K. Nosaka. 2015. Assessment of muscle pain induced by elbow-flexor eccentric exercise. *J Athl Train* 50:1140-8.

108. Laurent, C.M., J.M. Green, P.A. Bishop, J. Sjokvist, R.E. Schumacker, M.T. Richardson, and M. Curtner-Smith. 2011. A practical approach to monitoring recovery: Development of a perceived recovery status scale. *J Strength Cond Res* 25:620-8.

109. Lockie, R.G., A.J. Murphy, B.R. Scott, and X.A. Janse de Jonge. 2012. Quantifying session ratings of perceived exertion for field-based speed training methods in team sport athletes. *J Strength Cond Res* 26:2721-8.

110. Lovell, R., and G. Abt. 2013. Individualization of time-motion analysis: A case-cohort example. *Int J Sports Physiol Perform* 8:456-8.

111. Lovell, T.W., A.C. Sirotic, F.M. Impellizzeri, and A.J. Coutts. 2013. Factors affecting perception of effort (session rating of perceived exertion) during rugby league training. *Int J Sports Physiol Perform* 8:62-9.

112. Lucia, A., J. Hoyos, A. Santalla, C. Earnest, and J.L. Chicharro. 2003. Tour de France versus Vuelta a Espana: Which is harder? *Med Sci Sports Exerc* 35:872-8.

113. Manzi, V., A. Bovenzi, C. Castagna, P.S. Salimei, M. Volterrani, and F. Iellamo. 2015. Training-load distribution in endurance runners: Objective versus subjective assessment. *Int J Sports Physiol Perform* 10:1023-8.

114. Maso, F., G. Lac, E. Filaire, O. Michaux, and A. Robert. 2004. Salivary testosterone and cortisol in rugby players: Correlation with psychological overtraining items. *Br J Sports Med* 38:260-3.

115. McArdle, W.D., F.I. Katch, and V.L. Katch. 2014. *Exercise physiology: Energy, nutrition, and human performance*. 8th ed. Baltimore: Lippincott Williams & Wilkins.

116. McGuigan, M.R., A.D. Egan, and C. Foster. 2004. Salivary cortisol responses and perceived exertion during high intensity and low intensity bouts of resistance exercise. *J Sports Sci Med* 3:8-15.

117. McLaren, S.J., M. Weston, A. Smith, R. Cramb, and M.D. Portas. 2015. Variability of physical performance and player match loads in professional rugby union. *J Sci Med Sport*.

118. McLean, B.D., A.J. Coutts, V. Kelly, M.R. McGuigan, and S.J. Cormack. 2010. Neuromuscular, endocrine, and perceptual fatigue responses during different length between-match microcycles in professional rugby league players. *Int J Sports Physiol Perform* 5:367-83.

119. McNair, D.M., M. Lorr, and L.F. Droppleman. 1971. *Manual for the profile of mood states*. San Diego, CA: Educational and Industrial Testing Service.

120. McNamara, D.J., T.J. Gabbett, G. Naughton, P. Farhart, and P. Chapman. 2013. Training and competition workloads and fatigue responses of elite junior cricket players. *Int J Sports Physiol Perform* 8:517-26.

121. Meeusen, R., M. Duclos, C. Foster, A. Fry, M. Gleeson, D. Nieman, J. Raglin, G. Rietjens, J. Steinacker, A. Urhausen, S. European College of Sport Science, and American College of Sports Medicine. 2013. Prevention, diagnosis, and treatment of the overtraining syndrome: Joint consensus statement of the European college of sport science and the American College of Sports Medicine. *Med Sci Sports Exerc* 45:186-205.

122. Melzack, R. 1975. The McGill pain questionnaire: Major properties and scoring methods. *Pain* 1:277-99.

123. Milanez, V.F., S.P. Ramos, N.M. Okuno, D.A. Boullosa, and F.Y. Nakamura. 2014. Evidence of a non-linear dose-response relationship between training load and stress markers in elite female futsal players. *J Sports Sci Med* 13:22-29.

124. Minganti, C., L. Capranica, R. Meeusen, S. Amici, and M.F. Piacentini. 2010. The validity of session rating of perceived exertion method for quantifying training load in teamgym. *J Strength Cond Res* 24:3063-8.

125. Minganti, C., L. Capranica, R. Meeusen, and M.F. Piacentini. 2011. The use of session-RPE method for quantifying training load in diving. *Int J Sports Physiol Perform* 6:408-18.

126. Montgomery, P.G., and W.G. Hopkins. 2013. The effects of game and training loads on perceptual responses of muscle soreness in Australian football. *Int J Sports Physiol Perform* 8:312-8.

127. Mooney, M., S. Cormack, B. O'Brien, and A.J. Coutts. 2013. Do physical capacity and interchange rest periods influence match exercise-intensity profile in Australian football? *Int J Sports Physiol Perform* 8:165-72.

128. Mooney, M., B. O'Brien, S. Cormack, A. Coutts, J. Berry, and W. Young. 2011. The relationship between physical capacity and match performance in elite Australian football: A mediation approach. *J Sci Med Sport* 14:447-52.

129. Mooney, R., G. Corley, A. Godfrey, L.R. Quinlan, and O.L. G. 2015. Inertial sensor technology for elite swimming performance analysis: A systematic review. *Sensors (Basel)* 16.

130. Moreira, A., J.C. Bilsborough, C.J. Sullivan, M. Ciancosi, M.S. Aoki, and A.J. Coutts. 2015. Training periodization of professional Australian football players during an entire Australian football league season. *Int J Sports Physiol Perform* 10:566-71.

131. Moreira, A., N.R. de Moura, A. Coutts, E.C. Costa, T. Kempton, and M.S. Aoki. 2013.

Monitoring internal training load and mucosal immune responses in futsal athletes. *J Strength Cond Res* 27:1253-9.

132. Moreira, A., M.R. McGuigan, A.F. Arruda, C.G. Freitas, and M.S. Aoki. 2012. Monitoring internal load parameters during simulated and official basketball matches. *J Strength Cond Res* 26:861-6.

133. Morton, R.H., J.R. Fitz-Clarke, and E.W. Banister. 1990. Modeling human performance in running. *J Appl Physiol* 69:1171-77.

134. Murray, N.B., T.J. Gabbett, and K. Chamari. 2014. Effect of different between-match recovery times on the activity profiles and injury rates of national rugby league players. *J Strength Cond Res* 28:3476-83.

135. Neely, G., G. Ljunggren, C. Sylven, and G. Borg. 1992. Comparison between the visual analogue scale (VAS) and the category ratio scale (CR-10) for the evaluation of leg exertion. *Int J Sports Med* 13:133-6.

136. Nimmerichter, A., R.G. Eston, N. Bachl, and C. Williams. 2011. Longitudinal monitoring of power output and heart rate profiles in elite cyclists. *J Sports Sci* 29:831-40.

137. Nimmerichter, A., and C.A. Williams. 2015. Comparison of power output during ergometer and track cycling in adolescent cyclists. *J Strength Cond Res* 29:1049-56.

138. Noble, B.J., G.A. Borg, I. Jacobs, R. Ceci, and P. Kaiser. 1983. A category-ratio perceived exertion scale: Relationship to blood and muscle lactates and heart rate. *Med Sci Sports Exerc* 15:523-8.

139. Nosaka, K., M. Newton, and P. Sacco. 2002. Delayed-onset muscle soreness does not reflect the magnitude of eccentric exercise-induced muscle damage. *Scand J Med Sci Sports* 12:337-46.

140. Padulo, J., H. Chaabene, M. Tabben, M. Haddad, C. Gevat, S. Vando, L. Maurino, A. Chaouachi, and K. Chamari. 2014. The construct validity of session RPE during an intensive camp in young male karate athletes. *Muscles Ligaments Tendons J* 4:121-6.

141. Paulson, T.A., B. Mason, J. Rhodes, and V.L. Goosey-Tolfrey. 2015. Individualized internal and external training load relationships in elite wheelchair rugby players. *Front Physiol* 6:388.

142. Pinot, J., and F. Grappe. 2015. A six-year monitoring case study of a top-10 cycling Grand Tour finisher. *J Sports Sci* 33:907-14.

143. Polglaze, T., B. Dawson, and P. Peeling. 2016. Gold standard or fool's gold? The efficacy of displacement variables as indicators of energy expenditure in team sports. *Sports Med* 46:657-70.

144. Pritchett, R.C., J.M. Green, P.J. Wickwire, K.L. Pritchett, and M.S. Kovacs. 2009. Acute and session RPE responses during resistance training: Bouts to failure at 60% and 90% of 1RM. *South Afr J Sports Med* 21:23-26.

145. Putlur, P., C. Foster, J.A. Miskowski, M.K. Kane, S.E. Burton, T.P. Scheett, and M.R. McGuigan. 2004. Alteration of immune function in women collegiate soccer players and college students. *J Sports Sci Med* 3:234-43.

146. Rabelo, F.N., B.N. Pasquarelli, B. Goncalves, F. Matzenbacher, F.A. Campos, J. Sampaio, and F.Y. Nakamura. 2016. Monitoring the intended and perceived training load of a professional futsal team over 45 weeks: A case study. *J Strength Cond Res* 30:134-40.

147. Rampinini, E., G. Alberti, M. Fiorenza, M. Riggio, R. Sassi, T.O. Borges, and A.J. Coutts. 2015. Accuracy of GPS devices for measuring high-intensity running in field-based team sports. *Int J Sports Med* 36:49-53.

148. Rampinini, E., F.M. Impellizzeri, C. Castagna, A.J. Coutts, and U. Wisloff. 2009. Technical performance during soccer matches of the Italian Serie A league: Effect of fatigue and competitive level. *J Sci Med Sport* 12:227-33.

149. Rebelo, A., J. Brito, A. Seabra, J. Oliveira, B. Drust, and P. Krustrup. 2012. A new tool to measure training load in soccer training and match play. *Int J Sports Med* 33:297-304.

150. Rietjens, G.J., H. Kuipers, J.J. Adam, W.H. Saris, E. van Breda, D. van Hamont, and H.A. Keizer. 2005. Physiological, biochemical and psychological markers of strenuous training-induced fatigue. *Int J Sports Med* 26:16-26.

151. Robertson, R.J. 2004. *Perceived exertion for practitioners*. Champaign, IL: Human Kinetics.

152. Robertson, R.J., F.L. Goss, J. Dube, J. Rutkowski, M. Dupain, C. Brennan, and J. Andreacci. 2004. Validation of the adult OMNI scale of perceived exertion for cycle ergometer exercise. *Med Sci Sports Exerc* 36:102-8.

153. Robertson, R.J., F.L. Goss, J. Rutkowski, B. Lenz, C. Dixon, J. Timmer, K. Frazee, J. Dube, and J. Andreacci. 2003. Concurrent validation of the OMNI perceived exertion scale for resistance exercise. *Med Sci Sports Exerc* 35:333-41.

154. Rodriguez-Marroyo, J.A., G. Villa, J. Garcia-Lopez, and C. Foster. 2012. Comparison of heart rate and session rating of perceived exertion methods of defining exercise load in cyclists. *J Strength Cond Res* 26:2249-57.

155. Rogalski, B., B. Dawson, J. Heasman, and T.J. Gabbett. 2013. Training and game loads and injury risk in elite Australian footballers. *J Sci Med Sport* 16:499-503.

156. Rosenberger, M.E., M.P. Buman, W.L. Haskell, M.V. McConnell, and L.L. Carstensen. 2016. 24 hours of sleep, sedentary behavior, and physical activity with nine wearable devices. *Med Sci Sports Exerc* 48:547-65.

157. Ross, A., N. Gill, and J. Cronin. 2015. The match demands of international rugby sevens. *J Sports Sci* 33:1035-41.

158. Sato, K., W.A. Sands, and M.H. Stone. 2012. The reliability of accelerometry to measure weightlifting performance. *Sports Biomech* 11:524-31.

159. Saw, A.E., L.C. Main, and P.B. Gastin. 2015. Monitoring athletes through self-report: Factors influencing implementation. *J Sports Sci Med* 14:137-46.

160. Saw, A.E., L.C. Main, and P.B. Gastin. 2016. Monitoring the athlete training response: Subjective self-reported measures trump commonly used objective measures: A systematic review. *Br J Sports Med* 50:281-91.

161. Schwarz, N. 1999. Self reports: How questions shape the answers. *Am Psychol* 54:93-105.

162. Scott, M.T., T.J. Scott, and V.G. Kelly. 2016. The validity and reliability of global positioning systems in team sport: A brief review. *J Strength Cond Res* 30:1470-90.

163. Scott, T.J., C.R. Black, J. Quinn, and A.J. Coutts. 2013. Validity and reliability of the session-RPE method for quantifying training in Australian football: A comparison of the cr10 and CR100 scales. *J Strength Cond Res* 27:270-6.

164. Semark, A., T.D. Noakes, A. St Clair Gibson, and M.I. Lambert. 1999. The effect of a prophylactic dose of flurbiprofen on muscle soreness and sprinting performance in trained subjects. *J Sports Sci* 17:197-203.

165. Sikorski, E.M., J.M. Wilson, R.P. Lowery, J.M. Joy, C.M. Laurent, S.M. Wilson, D. Hesson, M.A. Naimo, B. Averbuch, and P. Gilchrist. 2013. Changes in perceived recovery status scale following high-volume muscle damaging resistance exercise. *J Strength Cond Res* 27:2079-85.

166. Singh, F., C. Foster, D. Tod, and M.R. McGuigan. 2007. Monitoring different types of resistance training using session rating of perceived exertion. *Int J Sports Physiol Perform* 2:34-45.

167. Stone, M.H., M. Stone, and W.A. Sands. 2006. *Principles and practice of resistance training.* Champaign, IL: Human Kinetics.

168. Sweet, T.W., C. Foster, M.R. McGuigan, and G. Brice. 2004. Quantitation of resistance training using the session rating of perceived exertion method. *J Strength Cond Res* 18:796-802.

169. Taylor, K.L., D.W. Chapman, J.B. Cronin, M.J. Newton, and N. Gill. 2012. Fatigue monitoring in high performance sport: A survey of current trends. *J Aust Strength Cond* 20:12-23.

170. Terbizan, D.J., B.A. Dolezal, and C. Albano. 2002. Validity of seven commercially available heart rate monitors. *Meas Phys Educ Exerc Sci* 6:243-47.

171. Terry, P.C., A.M. Lane, and G.J. Fogarty. 2003. Construct validity of the profile of mood states—adolescents for use with adults. *Psyc Sport Exerc* 4:125-39.

172. Terry, P.C., A.M. Lane, H.J. Lane, and L. Keohane. 1999. Development and validation of a mood measure for adolescents. *J Sports Sci* 17:861-72.

173. Thornton, H.R., J.A. Delaney, G.M. Duthie, B.R. Scott, W.J. Chivers, C.E. Sanctuary, and B.J. Dascombe. 2016. Predicting self-reported illness for professional team-sport athletes. *Int J Sports Physiol Perform* 11:543-50.

174. Twist, C., and J. Highton. 2013. Monitoring fatigue and recovery in rugby league players. *Int J Sports Physiol Perform* 8:467-74.

175. Uchida, M.C., L.F. Teixeira, V.J. Godoi, P.H. Marchetti, M. Conte, A.J. Coutts, and R.F. Bacurau. 2014. Does the timing of measurement alter session-RPE in boxers? *J Sports Sci Med* 13:59-65.

176. Utter, A.C., R.J. Robertson, J.M. Green, R.R. Suminski, S.R. McAnulty, and D.C. Nieman. 2004. Validation of the adult OMNI scale of perceived exertion for walking/running exercise. *Med Sci Sports Exerc* 36:1776-80.

177. Varley, M.C., T. Gabbett, and R.J. Aughey. 2014. Activity profiles of professional soccer, rugby league and Australian football match play. *J Sports Sci* 32:1858-66.

178. Vescovi, J.D., and T. Goodale. 2015. Physical demands of women's rugby sevens matches: Female Athletes in Motion (FAIM) study. *Int J Sports Med* 36:887-92.

179. Veugelers, K.R., W.B. Young, B. Fahrner, and J.T. Harvey. 2016. Different methods of training load quantification and their relationship to injury and illness in elite Australian football. *J Sci Med Sport* 19:24-8.

180. Wallace, L.K., K.M. Slattery, and A.J. Coutts. 2009. The ecological validity and application of the session-RPE method for quantifying training loads in swimming. *J Strength Cond Res* 23:33-8.

181. Wallace, L.K., K.M. Slattery, and A.J. Coutts. 2014. A comparison of methods for quantifying training load: Relationships between modelled and actual training responses. *Eur J Appl Physiol* 114:11-20.

182. Weaving, D., P. Marshall, K. Earle, A. Nevill, and G. Abt. 2014. Combining internal- and external-training-load measures in professional rugby league. *Int J Sports Physiol Perform* 9:905-12.

183. Wellman, A.D., S.C. Coad, G.C. Goulet, and C.P. McLellan. 2016. Quantification of competitive game demands of NCAA Division I college football players using global positioning systems. *J Strength Cond Res* 30:11-9.

184. Weston, M., J. Siegler, A. Bahnert, J. McBrien, and R. Lovell. 2015. The application of differential ratings of perceived exertion to Australian football league matches. *J Sci Med Sport* 18:704-8.

185. Wilkerson, G.B., A. Gupta, J.R. Allen, C.M. Keith, and M.A. Colston. 2016. Utilization of practice session average inertial load to quantify college football injury risk. *J Strength Cond Res* 30:2369-74.

186. Zourdos, M.C., A. Klemp, C. Dolan, J.M. Quiles, K.A. Schau, E. Jo, E. Helms, B. Esgro, S. Duncan, S. Garcia Merino, and R. Blanco. 2016. Novel resistance training-specific rating of perceived exertion scale measuring repetitions in reserve. *J Strength Cond Res* 30:267-75.

Chapter 5

1. Akenhead, R., and G.P. Nassis. 2016. Training load and player monitoring in high-level football: Current practice and perceptions. *Int J Sports Physiol Perform* 11:587-93.

2. Al Haddad, H., P.B. Laursen, D. Chollet, S. Ahmaidi, and M. Buchheit. 2011. Reliability of resting and postexercise heart rate measures. *Int J Sports Med* 32:598-605.

3. Bailey, C., K. Sato, R. Alexander, C. Chiang, and M.H. Stone. 2013. Isometric force production in symmetry and jump performance in collegiate athletes. *J Trainology* 2:1-5.

4. Baker, D.G., and R.U. Newton. 2007. Change in power output across a high-repetition set of bench throws and jump squats in highly trained athletes. *J Strength Cond Res* 21:1007-11.

5. Balsalobre-Fernandez, C., M. Glaister, and R.A. Lockey. 2015. The validity and reliability of an iPhone app for measuring vertical jump performance. *J Sports Sci* 33:1574-9.

6. Bautista, I.J., I.J. Chirosa, I.M. Tamayo, A. Gonzalez, J.E. Robinson, L.J. Chirosa, and R.J. Robertson. 2014. Predicting power output of upper body using the OMNI-RES scale. *J Hum Kinet* 44:161-9.

7. Bazyler, C.D., G.K. Beckham, and K. Sato. 2015. The use of the isometric squat as a measure of strength and explosiveness. *J Strength Cond Res* 29:1386-92.

8. Beaven, C.M., C.J. Cook, and N.D. Gill. 2008. Significant strength gains observed in rugby players after specific resistance exercise protocols based on individual salivary testosterone responses. *J Strength Cond Res* 22:419-25.

9. Beaven, C.M., N.D. Gill, and C.J. Cook. 2008. Salivary testosterone and cortisol responses in professional rugby players after four resistance exercise protocols. *J Strength Cond Res* 22:426-32.

10. Beckham, G., T. Suchomel, and S. Mizuguchi. 2014. Force plate use in performance monitoring and sport science testing. *New Stud Athlet* 29:25-37.

11. Bellenger, C.R., J.T. Fuller, R.L. Thomson, K. Davison, E.Y. Robertson, and J.D. Buckley. 2016. Monitoring athletic training status through autonomic heart rate regulation: A systematic review and meta-analysis. *Sports Med* 46:1461-86.

12. Borer, K. 2013. *Advanced exercise endocrinology*. 2nd ed. Champaign, IL: Human Kinetics.

13. Borresen, J., and M.I. Lambert. 2007. Changes in heart rate recovery in response to acute changes in training load. *Eur J Appl Physiol* 101:503-11.

14. Borresen, J., and M.I. Lambert. 2008. Autonomic control of heart rate during and after exercise: Measurements and implications for monitoring training status. *Sports Med* 38:633-46.

15. Bosco, C., A. Belli, M. Astrua, J. Tihanyi, R. Pozzo, S. Kellis, O. Tsarpela, C. Foti, R. Manno, and C. Tranquilli. 1995. A dynamometer for evaluation of dynamic muscle work. *Eur J Appl Physiol Occup Physiol* 70:379-86.

16. Brancaccio, P., G. Lippi, and N. Maffulli. 2010. Biochemical markers of muscular damage. *Clin Chem Lab Med* 48:757-67.

17. Brancaccio, P., N. Maffulli, and F.M. Limongelli. 2007. Creatine kinase monitoring in sport medicine. *Br Med Bull* 81-82:209-30.

18. Bressel, E., J.C. Yonker, J. Kras, and E.M. Heath. 2007. Comparison of static and dynamic balance in female collegiate soccer, basketball, and gymnastics athletes. *J Athl Train* 42:42-6.

19. Bruinvels, G., R. Burden, N. Brown, T. Richards, and C. Pedlar. 2016. The prevalence and impact of heavy menstrual bleeding (menorrhagia) in elite and non-elite athletes. *PLoS One* 11:e0149881.

20. Buchheit, M. 2014. Monitoring training status with HR measures: Do all roads lead to Rome? *Front Physiol* 5:73.

21. Buchheit, M. 2015. Sensitivity of monthly heart rate and psychometric measures for monitoring physical performance in highly trained young handball players. *Int J Sports Med* 36:351-6.

22. Buchheit, M., Y. Cholley, M. Nagel, and N. Poulos. 2016. The effect of body mass on eccentric knee flexor strength assessed with an instrumented Nordic hamstring device (Nordbord) in football players. *Int J Sports Physiol Perform* 11:721-6.

23. Buchheit, M., S. Racinais, J.C. Bilsborough, P.C. Bourdon, S.C. Voss, J. Hocking, J. Cordy, A. Mendez-Villanueva, and A.J. Coutts. 2013. Monitoring fitness, fatigue and running performance during a pre-season training camp in elite football players. *J Sci Med Sport* 16:550-5.

24. Buchheit, M., M.B. Simpson, H. Al Haddad, P.C. Bourdon, and A. Mendez-Villanueva. 2012. Monitoring changes in physical performance with heart rate measures in young soccer players. *Eur J Appl Physiol* 112:711-23.

25. Bush, J.A., W.J. Kraemer, A.M. Mastro, N.T. Triplett-McBride, J.S. Volek, M. Putukian, W.J. Sebastianelli, and H.G. Knuttgen. 1999. Exercise and recovery responses of adrenal medullary neurohormones to heavy resistance exercise. *Med Sci Sports Exerc* 31:554-9.

26. Butler, R.J., P.J. Plisky, C. Southers, C. Scoma, and K.B. Kiesel. 2010. Biomechanical analysis of the different classifications of the functional movement screen deep squat test. *Sports Biomech* 9:270-9.

27. Cairns, S.P. 2013. Holistic approaches to understanding mechanisms of fatigue in high-intensity sport. *Fatigue: Biomed Health Behav* 1:148-67.

28. Cardinale, M., and M.H. Stone. 2006. Is testosterone influencing explosive performance? *J Strength Cond Res* 20:103-7.

29. Clarke, A.C., J.M. Anson, and D.B. Pyne. 2015. Neuromuscular fatigue and muscle damage after a women's rugby sevens tournament. *Int J Sports Physiol Perform* 10:808-14.

30. Clarke, N., J.P. Farthing, J.L. Lanovaz, and J.R. Krentz. 2015. Direct and indirect measurement of neuromuscular fatigue in Canadian football players. *Appl Physiol Nutr Metab* 40:464-73.

31. Claudino, J.G., J.B. Cronin, B. Mezencio, J.P. Pinho, C. Pereira, L. Mochizuki, A.C. Amadio, and J.C. Serrao. 2016. Auto-regulating jump performance to induce functional overreaching. *J Strength Cond Res* 30:2242-9.

32. Claudino, J.G., B. Mezencio, R. Soncin, J.C. Ferreira, B.P. Couto, and L.A. Szmuchrowski. 2012. Pre vertical jump performance to regulate the training volume. *Int J Sports Med* 33:101-7.

33. Coad, S., B. Gray, and C. McLellan. 2016. Seasonal analysis of mucosal immunological function and physical demands in professional Australian rules footballers. *Int J Sports Physiol Perform* 11:574-80.

34. Coad, S., B. Gray, G. Wehbe, and C. McLellan. 2015. Physical demands and salivary immunoglobulin a responses of elite Australian rules football athletes to match play. *Int J Sports Physiol Perform* 10:613-7.

35. Conceicao, F., J. Fernandes, M. Lewis, J.J. Gonzalez-Badillo, and P. Jimenez-Reyes. 2015. Movement velocity as a measure of exercise intensity in three lower limb exercises. *J Sports Sci*:1-8.

36. Cook, C.J., and C.M. Beaven. 2013. Salivary testosterone is related to self-selected training load in elite female athletes. *Physiol Behav* 116-117:8-12.

37. Cook, C.J., B.T. Crewther, and A.A. Smith. 2012. Comparison of baseline free testosterone and cortisol concentrations between elite and non-elite female athletes. *Am J Hum Biol* 24:856-8.

38. Cormack, S.J., M.G. Mooney, W. Morgan, and M.R. McGuigan. 2013. Influence of neuromuscular fatigue on accelerometer load in elite Australian football players. *Int J Sports Physiol Perform* 8:373-8.

39. Cormack, S.J., R.U. Newton, and M.R. McGuigan. 2008. Neuromuscular and endocrine responses of elite players to an Australian rules football match. *Int J Sports Physiol Perform* 3:359-74.

40. Cormack, S.J., R.U. Newton, M.R. McGuigan, and P. Cormie. 2008. Neuromuscular and endocrine responses of elite players during an Australian rules football season. *Int J Sports Physiol Perform* 3:439-53.

41. Cormack, S.J., R.U. Newton, M.R. McGuigan, and T.L. Doyle. 2008. Reliability of measures obtained during single and repeated countermovement jumps. *Int J Sports Physiol Perform* 3:131-44.

42. Cormie, P., J.M. McBride, and G.O. McCaulley. 2008. Power-time, force-time, and velocity-time curve analysis during the jump squat: Impact of load. *J Appl Biomech* 24:112-20.

43. Cormie, P., M.R. McGuigan, and R.U. Newton. 2010. Changes in the eccentric phase contribute to improved stretch-shorten cycle performance after training. *Med Sci Sports Exerc* 42:1731-44.

44. Coughlan, G.F., E. Delahunt, B.M. Caulfield, C. Forde, and B.S. Green. 2014. Normative adductor squeeze test values in elite junior rugby union players. *Clin J Sport Med* 24:315-9.

45. Coutts, A.J., and S. Cormack. 2014. Monitoring the training response. In *High-performance training for sports*, edited by D. Joyce and D. Lewindon, 85-96. Champaign, IL: Human Kinetics.

46. Coutts, A.J., P. Reaburn, T.J. Piva, and G.J. Rowsell. 2007. Monitoring for overreaching in rugby league players. *Eur J Appl Physiol* 99:313-24.

47. Coutts, A.J., L.K. Wallace, and K.M. Slattery. 2007. Monitoring changes in performance, physiology, biochemistry, and psychology during overreaching and recovery in triathletes. *Int J Sports Med* 28:125-34.

48. Crewther, B., J. Keogh, J. Cronin, and C. Cook. 2006. Possible stimuli for strength and power adaptation: Acute hormonal responses. *Sports Med* 36:215-38.

49. Crewther, B.T., and C. Christian. 2010. Relationships between salivary testosterone and cortisol concentrations and training performance in Olympic weightlifters. *J Sports Med Phys Fitness* 50:371-5.

50. Crewther, B.T., and C. Cook. 2010. Measuring the salivary testosterone and cortisol concentrations of weightlifters using an enzyme-immunoassay kit. *Int J Sports Med* 31:486-9.

51. Crewther, B.T., D. Hamilton, K. Casto, L.P. Kilduff, and C.J. Cook. 2015. Effects of oral contraceptive use on the salivary testosterone and cortisol responses to training sessions and competitions in elite women athletes. *Physiol Behav* 147:84-90.

52. Crewther, B.T., L.P. Kilduff, and C.J. Cook. 2014. Trained and untrained males show reliable salivary testosterone responses to a physical stimulus, but not a psychological stimulus. *J Endocrinol Invest* 37:1065-72.

53. Crewther, B.T., M.R. McGuigan, and N.D. Gill. 2011. The ratio and allometric scaling of speed, power, and strength in elite male rugby union players. *J Strength Cond Res* 25:1968-75.

54. Crewther, B.T., C.E. Sanctuary, L.P. Kilduff, J.S. Carruthers, C.M. Gaviglio, and C.J. Cook. 2013. The workout responses of salivary-free testosterone and cortisol concentrations and their association with the subsequent competition outcomes in professional rugby league. *J Strength Cond Res* 27:471-6.

55. Cunniffe, B., H. Griffiths, W. Proctor, B. Davies, J.S. Baker, and K.P. Jones. 2011. Mucosal immunity and illness incidence in elite rugby union players across a season. *Med Sci Sports Exerc* 43:388-97.

56. Daanen, H.A., R.P. Lamberts, V.L. Kallen, A. Jin, and N.L. Van Meeteren. 2012. A systematic review on heart-rate recovery to monitor changes in training status in athletes. *Int J Sports Physiol Perform* 7:251-60.

57. Dalleau, G., A. Belli, F. Viale, J.R. Lacour, and M. Bourdin. 2004. A simple method for field measurements of leg stiffness in hopping. *Int J Sports Med* 25:170-6.

58. Delahunt, E., B.L. McEntee, C. Kennelly, B.S. Green, and G.F. Coughlan. 2011. Intrarater reliability of the adductor squeeze test in Gaelic Games athletes. *J Athl Train* 46:241-5.

59. Edwards, D.A., and K.V. Casto. 2013. Women's intercollegiate athletic competition: Cortisol, testosterone, and the dual-hormone hypothesis as it relates to status among teammates. *Horm Behav* 64:153-60.

60. Edwards, D.A., and K.V. Casto. 2015. Baseline cortisol moderates testosterone reactivity to women's intercollegiate athletic competition. *Physiol Behav* 142:48-51.

61. Edwards, D.A., and L.S. Kurlander. 2010. Women's intercollegiate volleyball and tennis: Effects of warm-up, competition, and practice on saliva levels of cortisol and testosterone. *Horm Behav* 58:606-13.

62. Edwards, D.A., K. Wetzel, and D.R. Wyner. 2006. Intercollegiate soccer: Saliva cortisol and testosterone are elevated during competition, and testosterone is related to status and social connectedness with team mates. *Physiol Behav* 87:135-43.

63. Elloumi, M., N. El Elj, M. Zaouali, F. Maso, E. Filaire, Z. Tabka, and G. Lac. 2005. IGFBP-3, a sensitive marker of physical training and overtraining. *Br J Sports Med* 39:604-10.

64. Esco, M.R., and A.A. Flatt. 2014. Ultra-short-term heart rate variability indexes at rest and post-exercise in athletes: Evaluating the agreement with accepted recommendations. *J Sports Sci Med* 13:535-41.

65. Filho, E., S. di Fronso, F. Forzini, M. Murgia, T. Agostini, L. Bortoli, C. Robazza, and M. Bertollo. 2015. Athletic performance and recovery-stress factors in cycling: An ever changing balance. *Eur J Sport Sci* 15:671-80.

66. Foster, C. 1998. Monitoring training in athletes with reference to overtraining syndrome. *Med Sci Sports Exerc* 30:1164-8.

67. Fowles, J.R. 2006. Technical issues in quantifying low-frequency fatigue in athletes. *Int J Sports Physiol Perform* 1:169-71.

68. French, D.N., A.L. Gomez, J.S. Volek, M.R. Rubin, N.A. Ratamess, M.J. Sharman, L.A. Gotshalk, W.J. Sebastianelli, M. Putukian, R.U. Newton, K. Hakkinen, S.J. Fleck, and W.J. Kraemer. 2004. Longitudinal tracking of muscular power changes of NCAA Division I collegiate women gymnasts. *J Strength Cond Res* 18:101-7.

69. French, D.N., W.J. Kraemer, J.S. Volek, B.A. Spiering, D.A. Judelson, J.R. Hoffman, and C.M. Maresh. 2007. Anticipatory responses of catecholamines on muscle force production. *J Appl Physiol* 102:94-102.

70. Frohm, A., A. Heijne, J. Kowalski, P. Svensson, and G. Myklebust. 2012. A nine-test screening battery for athletes: A reliability study. *Scand J Med Sci Sports* 22:306-15.

71. Fry, A.C., B.K. Schilling, S.J. Fleck, and W.J. Kraemer. 2011. Relationships between competitive wrestling success and neuroendocrine responses. *J Strength Cond Res* 25:40-5.

72. Gathercole, R., B. Sporer, and T. Stellingwerff. 2015. Countermovement jump performance with increased training loads in elite female rugby athletes. *Int J Sports Med* 36:722-8.

73. Gathercole, R., B. Sporer, T. Stellingwerff, and G. Sleivert. 2015. Alternative countermovement-jump analysis to quantify acute neuromuscular fatigue. *Int J Sports Physiol Perform* 10:84-92.

74. Gathercole, R.J., B.C. Sporer, T. Stellingwerff, and G.G. Sleivert. 2015. Comparison of the capacity of different jump and sprint field tests to detect neuromuscular fatigue. *J Strength Cond Res* 29:2522-31.

75. Gathercole, R.J., T. Stellingwerff, and B.C. Sporer. 2015. Effect of acute fatigue and training adaptation on countermovement jump performance in elite snowboard cross athletes. *J Strength Cond Res* 29:37-46.

76. Gaviglio, C.M., and C.J. Cook. 2014. Relationship between midweek training measures of testosterone and cortisol concentrations and game outcome in professional rugby union matches. *J Strength Cond Res* 28:3447-52.

77. Gaviglio, C.M., B.T. Crewther, L.P. Kilduff, K.A. Stokes, and C.J. Cook. 2014. Relationship between pregame concentrations of free testosterone and outcome in rugby union. *Int J Sports Physiol Perform* 9:324-31.

78. Gibson, N.E., A.J. Boyd, and A.M. Murray. 2016. Countermovement jump is not affected during final competition preparation periods in elite rugby sevens players. *J Strength Cond Res* 30:777-83.

79. Gleeson, M., and N.C. Bishop. 2013. URI in athletes: Are mucosal immunity and cytokine responses key risk factors? *Exerc Sport Sci Rev* 41:148-53.

80. Gleeson, M., N.P. and Walsh. 2012. The BASES expert statement on exercise, immunity, and infection. *J Sports Sci* 30:321-4.

81. Gonzalez-Badillo, J.J., and L. Sanchez-Medina. 2010. Movement velocity as a measure of loading intensity in resistance training. *Int J Sports Med* 31:347-52.

82. Gouarne, C., C. Groussard, A. Gratas-Delamarche, P. Delamarche, and M. Duclos. 2005. Overnight urinary cortisol and cortisone add new insights into adaptation to training. *Med Sci Sports Exerc* 37:1157-67.

83. Grandys, M., J. Majerczak, J. Kulpa, K. Duda, U. Rychlik, and J.A. Zoladz. 2015. The importance of the training-induced decrease in basal cortisol concentration in the improvement in muscular performance in humans. *Physiological Res*.

84. Gribble, P.A., J. Hertel, and P. Plisky. 2012. Using the star excursion balance test to assess dynamic postural-control deficits and outcomes in lower extremity injury: A literature and systematic review. *J Athl Train* 47:339-57.

85. Guilhem, G., C. Hanon, N. Gendreau, D. Bonneau, A. Guevel, and M. Chennaoui. 2015. Salivary hormones response to preparation and pre-competitive training of world-class level athletes. *Front Physiol* 6:333.

86. Haff, G.G., J.M. Carlock, M.J. Hartman, J.L. Kilgore, N. Kawamori, J.R. Jackson, R.T. Morris, W.A. Sands, and M.H. Stone. 2005. Force-time curve characteristics of dynamic and isometric muscle actions of elite women Olympic weightlifters. *J Strength Cond Res* 19:741-8.

87. Haff, G.G., R.P. Ruben, J. Lider, C. Twine, and P. Cormie. 2015. A comparison of methods for determining the rate of force development during isometric midthigh clean pulls. *J Strength Cond Res* 29:386-95.

88. Hakkinen, K. 1989. Neuromuscular and hormonal adaptations during strength and power training. A review. *J Sports Med Phys Fitness* 29:9-26.

89. Hakkinen, K., A. Pakarinen, M. Alen, H. Kauhanen, and P.V. Komi. 1988. Neuromuscular and hormonal adaptations in athletes to strength training in two years. *J Appl Physiol* 65:2406-12.

90. Halperin, I., K. Williams, D.T. Martin, and D.W. Chapman. 2016. The effects of attentional focusing instructions on force production during the isometric mid-thigh pull. *J Strength Cond Res* 30:919-23.

91. Halson, S.L. 2014. Monitoring training load to understand fatigue in athletes. *Sports Med* 44 Suppl 2:S139-47.

92. Halson, S.L., M.W. Bridge, R. Meeusen, B. Busschaert, M. Gleeson, D.A. Jones, and A.E. Jeukendrup. 2002. Time course of performance changes and fatigue markers during intensified training in trained cyclists. *J Appl Physiol* 93:947-56.

93. Halson, S.L., G.I. Lancaster, A.E. Jeukendrup, and M. Gleeson. 2003. Immunological responses to overreaching in cyclists. *Med Sci Sports Exerc* 35:854-61.

94. Hamilton, D. 2009. Drop jump as an indicator of neuromuscular fatigue and recovery in elite youth soccer athletes following tournament match play. *J Aust Strength Cond* 17:3-8.

95. Harris, N.K., J. Cronin, K. Taylor, J. Boris, and J. Sheppard. 2010. Understanding linear position transducer technology for strength and conditioning practitioners. *Strength Cond J* 32:66-79.

96. Haugen, T., and M. Buchheit. 2016. Sprint running performance monitoring: Methodological and practical considerations. *Sports Med* 46:641-56.

97. Hegedus, E.J., S. McDonough, C. Bleakley, G.D. Baxter, J.T. DePew, I. Bradbury, and C. Cook. 2016. Physical performance tests predict injury in national collegiate athletic association athletes: A three-season prospective cohort study. *Br J Sports Med*.

98. Hertel, J., R.A. Braham, S.A. Hale, and L.C. Olmsted-Kramer. 2006. Simplifying the star excursion balance test: Analyses of subjects with and without chronic ankle instability. *J Orthop Sports Phys Ther* 36:131-37.

99. Hoffman, J.R., C.M. Maresh, R.U. Newton, M.R. Rubin, D.N. French, J.S. Volek, J. Sutherland, M. Robertson, A.L. Gomez, N.A. Ratamess, J. Kang, and W.J. Kraemer. 2002. Performance, biochemical, and endocrine changes during a competitive football game. *Med Sci Sports Exerc* 34:1845-53.

100. Hogarth, L.W., B.J. Burkett, and M.R. McKean. 2015. Neuromuscular and perceptual fatigue responses to consecutive tag football matches. *Int J Sports Physiol Perform* 10:559-65.

101. Hooper, S.L., L.T. Mackinnon, A. Howard, R.D. Gordon, and A.W. Bachmann. 1995. Markers for monitoring overtraining and recovery. *Med Sci Sports Exerc* 27:106-12.

102. Jidovtseff, B., N.K. Harris, J.M. Crielaard, and J.B. Cronin. 2011. Using the load-velocity relationship for 1RM prediction. *J Strength Cond Res* 25:267-70.

103. Jimenez-Reyes, P., F. Pareja-Blanco, C. Balsalobre-Fernandez, V. Cuadrado-Penafiel, M.A. Ortega-Becerra, and J.J. Gonzalez-Badillo. 2015. Jump-squat performance and its relationship with relative training intensity in high-level athletes. *Int J Sports Physiol Perform* 10:1036-40.

104. Jones, D.A. 1996. High-and low-frequency fatigue revisited. *Acta Physiol Scand* 156:265-70.

105. Jordan, M.J., P. Aagaard, and W. Herzog. 2015. Lower limb asymmetry in mechanical muscle function: A comparison between ski racers with and without ACL reconstruction. *Scand J Med Sci Sports* 25:e301-9.

106. Jovanavic, M., and E. Flanagan. 2014. Researched applications of velocity based strength training *J Aust Strength Cond* 22:58-69.

107. Jurimae, J., J. Maestu, and T. Jurimae. 2003. Leptin as a marker of training stress in highly trained male rowers? *Eur J Appl Physiol* 90:533-8.

108. Jurimae, J., J. Maestu, T. Jurimae, B. Mangus, and S.P. von Duvillard. 2011. Peripheral signals of energy homeostasis as possible markers of training stress in athletes: A review. *Metabolism* 60:335-50.

109. Kargotich, S., D. Keast, C. Goodman, C.I. Bhagat, D.J. Joske, B. Dawson, and A.R. Morton. 2007. Monitoring 6 weeks of progressive endurance training with plasma glutamine. *Int J Sports Med* 28:211-6.

110. Kawamori, N., S.J. Rossi, B.D. Justice, E.E. Haff, E.E. Pistilli, H.S. O'Bryant, M.H. Stone, and G.G. Haff. 2006. Peak force and rate of force development during isometric and

dynamic mid-thigh clean pulls performed at various intensities. *J Strength Cond Res* 20:483-91.

111. Kiesel, K., P.J. Plisky, and M.L. Voight. 2007. Can serious injury in professional football be predicted by a preseason functional movement screen? *North American Journal of Sports Physical Therapy* 2:147-58.

112. Kipp, K., M.T. Kiely, and C.F. Geiser. 2016. The reactive strength index modified is a valid measure of explosiveness in collegiate female volleyball players. *J Strength Cond Res* 30:1341-7.

113. Konor, M.M., S. Morton, J.M. Eckerson, and T.L. Grindstaff. 2012. Reliability of three measures of ankle dorsiflexion range of motion. *Int J Sports Phys Ther* 7:279-87.

114. Koziris, L.P., R.C. Hickson, R.T. Chatterton, Jr., R.T. Groseth, J.M. Christie, D.G. Goldflies, and T.G. Unterman. 1999. Serum levels of total and free IGF-I and IGFBP-3 are increased and maintained in long-term training. *J Appl Physiol* 86:1436-42.

115. Kraemer, W.J., C. Dunn-Lewis, B.A. Comstock, G.A. Thomas, J.E. Clark, and B.C. Nindl. 2010. Growth hormone, exercise, and athletic performance: A continued evolution of complexity. *Curr Sports Med Rep* 9:242-52.

116. Kraemer, W.J., A.C. Fry, M.R. Rubin, T. Triplett-McBride, S.E. Gordon, L.P. Koziris, J.M. Lynch, J.S. Volek, D.E. Meuffels, R.U. Newton, and S.J. Fleck. 2001. Physiological and performance responses to tournament wrestling. *Med Sci Sports Exerc* 33:1367-78.

117. Kraemer, W.J., and N.A. Ratamess. 2005. Hormonal responses and adaptations to resistance exercise and training. *Sports Med* 35:339-61.

118. Lamberts, R.P., K.A. Lemmink, J.J. Durandt, and M.I. Lambert. 2004. Variation in heart rate during submaximal exercise: Implications for monitoring training. *J Strength Cond Res* 18:641-5.

119. Lamberts, R.P., G.J. Rietjens, H.H. Tijdink, T.D. Noakes, and M.I. Lambert. 2010. Measuring submaximal performance parameters to monitor fatigue and predict cycling performance: A case study of a world-class cyclo-cross cyclist. *Eur J Appl Physiol* 108:183-90.

120. Lamberts, R.P., J. Swart, B. Capostagno, T.D. Noakes, and M.I. Lambert. 2010. Heart rate recovery as a guide to monitor fatigue and predict changes in performance parameters. *Scand J Med Sci Sports* 20:449-57.

121. Lamberts, R.P., J. Swart, T.D. Noakes, and M.I. Lambert. 2011. A novel submaximal cycle test to monitor fatigue and predict cycling performance. *Br J Sports Med* 45:797-804.

122. Lane, A.R., and A.C. Hackney. 2015. Relationship between salivary and serum testosterone levels in response to different exercise intensities. *Hormones* 14:258-64.

123. Lane, A.R., C.B. O'Leary, and A.C. Hackney. 2015. Menstrual cycle phase effects free testosterone responses to prolonged aerobic exercise. *Acta Physiol Hung* 102:336-41.

124. Lattier, G., G.Y. Millet, A. Martin, and V. Martin. 2004. Fatigue and recovery after high-intensity exercise part I: Neuromuscular fatigue. *Int J Sports Med* 25:450-6.

125. Louder, T., M. Bressel, and E. Bressel. 2015. The kinetic specificity of plyometric training: Verbal cues revisited. *J Hum Kinet* 49:201-8.

126. Maloney, S.J., I.M. Fletcher, and J. Richards. 2015. A comparison of methods to determine bilateral asymmetries in vertical leg stiffness. *J Sports Sci*:1-7.

127. Maloney, S.J., I.M. Fletcher, and J. Richards. 2015. Reliability of unilateral vertical leg stiffness measures assessed during bilateral hopping. *J Appl Biomech* 31:285-91.

128. Mann, J.B., P.J. Ivey, W.F. Brechue, and J.L. Mayhew. 2015. Validity and reliability of hand and electronic timing for 40-yd sprint in college football players. *J Strength Cond Res* 29:1509-14.

129. Mann, T.N., C.E. Platt, R.P. Lamberts, and M.I. Lambert. 2015. Faster heart rate recovery with increased RPE: Paradoxical responses after an 87-km ultramarathon. *J Strength Cond Res* 29:3343-52.

130. Maso, F., G. Lac, E. Filaire, O. Michaux, and A. Robert. 2004. Salivary testosterone and cortisol in rugby players: Correlation with psychological overtraining items. *Br J Sports Med* 38:260-3.

131. Matuszak, M.E., A.C. Fry, L.W. Weiss, T.R. Ireland, and M.M. McKnight. 2003. Effect of rest interval length on repeated 1 repetition maximum back squats. *J Strength Cond Res* 17:634-7.

132. McCall, A., M. Nedelec, C. Carling, F. Le Gall, S. Berthoin, and G. Dupont. 2015. Reliability and sensitivity of a simple isometric posterior lower limb muscle test in professional football players. *J Sports Sci* 33:1298-304.

133. McCall, G.E., W.C. Byrnes, S.J. Fleck, A. Dickinson, and W.J. Kraemer. 1999. Acute and chronic hormonal responses to resistance training designed to promote muscle hypertrophy. *Can J Appl Physiol* 24:96-107.

134. McCunn, R., K. Aus der Funten, H.H. Fullagar, I. McKeown, and T. Meyer. 2016. Reliability and association with injury of movement screens: A critical review. *Sports Med 46:763-81.*

135. McCurdy, K., and G.A. Langford. 2005. Comparison of unilateral squat strength between the dominant and non-dominant leg in men and women. *J Sports Sci Med* 5:282-88.

136. McGill, S.M., J.T. Andersen, and A.D. Horne. 2012. Predicting performance and injury resilience from movement quality and fitness scores in a basketball team over 2 years. *J Strength Cond Res* 26:1731-9.

137. McGuigan, M.R., S. Cormack, and N.D. Gill. 2013. Strength and power profiling of athletes. *Strength Cond J* 35:7-14.

138. McGuigan, M.R., T.L. Doyle, M. Newton, D.J. Edwards, S. Nimphius, and R.U. Newton. 2006. Eccentric utilization ratio: Effect of sport and phase of training. *J Strength Cond Res* 20:992-5.

139. McGuigan, M.R., J.M. Sheppard, S.J. Cormack, and K. Taylor. 2013. Strength and power assessment protocols. In *Physiological tests for elite athletes*, edited by R.K. Tanner and C.J. Gore. Champaign, IL: Human Kinetics.

140. McKeown, I., D.W. Chapman, K. Taylor, and N. Ball. 2016. Time course of improvements in power characteristics in elite development netball players entering a full time training program. *J Strength Cond Res* 30:1308-15.

141. McKeown, I., K. Taylor-McKeown, C. Woods, and N. Ball. 2014. Athletic ability assessment: A movement assessment protocol for athletes. *Int J Sports Phys Ther* 9:862-73.

142. McLean, B.D., C. Petrucelli, and E.F. Coyle. 2012. Maximal power output and perceptual fatigue responses during a Division I female collegiate soccer season. *J Strength Cond Res* 26:3189-96.

143. McMahon, J.J., P. Comfort, and S. Pearson. 2012. Lower limb stiffness: Effect on performance and training considerations. *Strength Cond J* 34:94-101.

144. McMahon, T.J., and G.C. Cheng. 1990. The mechanics of running: How does stiffness couple with speed? *J Biomech* 23 (Supplement I):65-78.

145. Meeusen, R., M. Duclos, C. Foster, A. Fry, M. Gleeson, D. Nieman, J. Raglin, G. Rietjens, J. Steinacker, A. Urhausen, S. European College of Sport Science, and American College of Sports Medicine. 2013. Prevention, diagnosis, and treatment of the overtraining syndrome: Joint consensus statement of the European College of Sport Science and the American College of Sports Medicine. *Med Sci Sports Exerc* 45:186-205.

146. Milanez, V.F., S.P. Ramos, N.M. Okuno, D.A. Boullosa, and F.Y. Nakamura. 2014. Evidence of a non-linear dose-response relationship between training load and stress markers in elite female futsal players. *J Sports Sci Med* 13:22-29.

147. Miller, T. 2012. *NSCA's guide to tests and assessments*, edited by T. Miller. Champaign, IL: Human Kinetics.

148. Moreira, A., N.R. de Moura, A. Coutts, E.C. Costa, T. Kempton, and M.S. Aoki. 2013. Monitoring internal training load and mucosal immune responses in futsal athletes. *J Strength Cond Res* 27:1253-9.

149. Morin, J.B., and P. Samozino. 2016. Interpreting power-force-velocity profiles for individualized and specific training. *Int J Sports Physiol Perform* 11:267-72.

150. Mosler, A.B., R. Agricola, A. Weir, P. Holmich, and K.M. Crossley. 2015. Which factors differentiate athletes with hip/groin pain from those without? A systematic review with meta-analysis. *Br J Sports Med* 49:810.

151. Nagahara, R., J.B. Morin, and M. Koido. 2016. Impairment of sprint mechanical properties in an actual soccer match: A pilot study. *Int J Sports Physiol Perform.*

152. Nakamura, Y., K. Aizawa, T. Imai, I. Kono, and N. Mesaki. 2011. Hormonal responses

to resistance exercise during different menstrual cycle states. *Med Sci Sports Exerc* 43:967-73.

153. Neary, J.P., L. Malbon, and D.C. McKenzie. 2002. Relationship between serum, saliva and urinary cortisol and its implication during recovery from training. *J Sci Med Sport* 5:108-14.

154. Neville, V., M. Gleeson, and J.P. Folland. 2008. Salivary IgA as a risk factor for upper respiratory infections in elite professional athletes. *Med Sci Sports Exerc* 40:1228-36.

155. Newton, R., and E. Dugan. 2002. Application of strength diagnosis. *Strength Cond J* 24:50-59.

156. Neyroud, D., J. Temesi, G.Y. Millet, S. Verges, N.A. Maffiuletti, B. Kayser, and N. Place. 2015. Comparison of electrical nerve stimulation, electrical muscle stimulation and magnetic nerve stimulation to assess the neuromuscular function of the plantar flexor muscles. *Eur J Appl Physiol* 115:1429-39.

157. Nindl, B.C., W.J. Kraemer, P.J. Arciero, N. Samatallee, C.D. Leone, M.F. Mayo, and D.L. Hafeman. 2002. Leptin concentrations experience a delayed reduction after resistance exercise in men. *Med Sci Sports Exerc* 34:608-13.

158. Nunes, J.A., B.T. Crewther, C. Ugrinowitsch, V. Tricoli, L. Viveiros, D. de Rose, Jr., and M.S. Aoki. 2011. Salivary hormone and immune responses to three resistance exercise schemes in elite female athletes. *J Strength Cond Res* 25:2322-7.

159. O'Connor, P.J., and D.L. Corrigan. 1987. Influence of short-term cycling on salivary cortisol levels. *Med Sci Sports Exerc* 19:224-8.

160. O'Connor, P.J., W.P. Morgan, J.S. Raglin, C.M. Barksdale, and N.H. Kalin. 1989. Mood state and salivary cortisol levels following overtraining in female swimmers. *Psychoneuroendocrinol* 14:303-10.

161. Oliver, J.L., R.S. Lloyd, and A. Whitney. 2015. Monitoring of in-season neuromuscular and perceptual fatigue in youth rugby players. *Eur J Sport Sci* 15:514-22.

162. Oosthuyse, T., and A.N. Bosch. 2010. The effect of the menstrual cycle on exercise metabolism: Implications for exercise performance in eumenorrhoeic women. *Sports Med* 40:207-27.

163. Opar, D.A., T. Piatkowski, M.D. Williams, and A.J. Shield. 2013. A novel device using the Nordic hamstring exercise to assess eccentric knee flexor strength: A reliability and retrospective injury study. *J Orthop Sports Phys Ther* 43:636-40.

164. Papacosta, E., M. Gleeson, and G.P. Nassis. 2013. Salivary hormones, IgA, and performance during intense training and tapering in judo athletes. *J Strength Cond Res* 27:2569-80.

165. Parchmann, C.J., and J.M. McBride. 2011. Relationship between functional movement screen and athletic performance. *J Strength Cond Res* 25:3378-84.

166. Paul, D.J., and G.P. Nassis. 2015. Testing strength and power in soccer players: The application of conventional and traditional methods of assessment. *J Strength Cond Res* 29:1748-58.

167. Plews, D.J., P.B. Laursen, A.E. Kilding, and M. Buchhcit. 2012. Heart rate variability in elite triathletes, is variation in variability the key to effective training? A case comparison. *Eur J Appl Physiol* 112:3729-41.

168. Plews, D.J., P.B. Laursen, A.E. Kilding, and M. Buchheit. 2013. Evaluating training adaptation with heart-rate measures: A methodological comparison. *Int J Sports Physiol Perform* 8:688-91.

169. Plews, D.J., P.B. Laursen, J. Stanley, A.E. Kilding, and M. Buchheit. 2013. Training adaptation and heart rate variability in elite endurance athletes: Opening the door to effective monitoring. *Sports Med* 43:773-81.

170. Pruyn, E.C., M.L. Watsford, and A.J. Murphy. 2015. Differences in lower-body stiffness between levels of netball competition. *J Strength Cond Res* 29:1197-202.

171. Pruyn, E.C., M.L. Watsford, and A.J. Murphy. 2015. Validity and reliability of three methods of stiffness assessment. *J Sport Health Sci*.

172. Pruyn, E.C., M.L. Watsford, A.J. Murphy, M.J. Pine, R.W. Spurrs, M.L. Cameron, and R.J. Johnston. 2012. Relationship between leg stiffness and lower body injuries in professional Australian football. *J Sports Sci* 30:71-8.

173. Putlur, P., C. Foster, J.A. Miskowski, M.K. Kane, S.E. Burton, T.P. Scheett, and M.R. McGuigan. 2004. Alteration of immune function in women collegiate soccer players and college students. *J Sports Sci Med* 3:234-43.

174. Raastad, T., T. Glomsheller, T. Bjoro, and J. Hallen. 2003. Recovery of skeletal muscle contractility and hormonal responses to strength exercise after two weeks of high-volume strength training. *Scand J Med Sci Sports* 13:159-68.

175. Randell, A.D., J.B. Cronin, J.W. Keogh, N.D. Gill, and M.C. Pedersen. 2011. Effect of instantaneous performance feedback during 6 weeks of velocity-based resistance training on sport-specific performance tests. *J Strength Cond Res* 25:87-93.

176. Ratamess, N.A. 2012. *ACSM's foundations of strength training and conditioning*. Philadelphia: Lippincott Williams and Wilkins.

177. Rietjens, G.J., H. Kuipers, J.J. Adam, W.H. Saris, E. van Breda, D. van Hamont, and H.A. Keizer. 2005. Physiological, biochemical and psychological markers of strenuous training-induced fatigue. *Int J Sports Med* 26:16-26.

178. Robson-Ansley, P.J., M. Gleeson, and L. Ansley. 2009. Fatigue management in the preparation of Olympic athletes. *J Sports Sci* 27:1409-20.

179. Roe, G.A., P.J. Phibbs, K. Till, B.L. Jones, D.B. Read, J.J. Weakley, and J.D. Darrall-Jones. 2016. Changes in adductor strength after competition in academy rugby union players. *J Strength Cond Res* 30:344-50.

180. Sakamaki-Sunaga, M., S. Min, K. Kamemoto, and T. Okamoto. 2016. Effects of menstrual phase-dependent resistance training frequency on muscular hypertrophy and strength. *J Strength Cond Res* 30:1727-34.

181. Sanchez-Medina, L., and J.J. Gonzalez-Badillo. 2011. Velocity loss as an indicator of neuromuscular fatigue during resistance training. *Med Sci Sports Exerc* 43:1725-34.

182. Saw, A.E., L.C. Main, and P.B. Gastin. 2016. Monitoring the athlete training response: Subjective self-reported measures trump commonly used objective measures: A systematic review. *Br J Sports Med* 50:281-91.

183. Schelling, X., J. Calleja-Gonzalez, L. Torres-Ronda, and N. Terrados. 2015. Using testosterone and cortisol as biomarker for training individualization in elite basketball: A 4-year follow-up study. *J Strength Cond Res* 29:368-78.

184. Schmikli, S.L., M.S. Brink, W.R. de Vries, and F.J. Backx. 2011. Can we detect non-functional overreaching in young elite soccer players and middle-long distance runners using field performance tests? *Br J Sports Med* 45:631-6.

185. Schmitt, L., J. Regnard, and G.P. Millet. 2015. Monitoring fatigue status with HRV measures in elite athletes: An avenue beyond RMSSD? *Front Physiol* 6:343.

186. Sheppard, J., D. Chapman, and K.L. Taylor. 2011. An evaluation of a strength qualities assessment method for the lower body. *J Aust Strength Cond* 19:4-10.

187. Simsch, C., W. Lormes, K.G. Petersen, S. Baur, Y. Liu, A.C. Hackney, M. Lehmann, and J.M. Steinacker. 2002. Training intensity influences leptin and thyroid hormones in highly trained rowers. *Int J Sports Med* 23:422-7.

188. Smith, L.L. 2000. Cytokine hypothesis of overtraining: A physiological adaptation to excessive stress? *Med Sci Sports Exerc* 32:317-31.

189. Smith, L.L. 2004. Tissue trauma: The underlying cause of overtraining syndrome? *J Strength Cond Res* 18:185-93.

190. Steinacker, J.M., W. Lormes, S. Reissnecker, and Y. Liu. 2004. New aspects of the hormone and cytokine response to training. *Eur J Appl Physiol* 91:382-91.

191. Suchomel, T.J., C.A. Bailey, C.J. Sole, J.L. Grazer, and G.K. Beckham. 2015. Using reactive strength index-modified as an explosive performance measurement tool in Division I athletes. *J Strength Cond Res* 29:899-904.

192. Suchomel, T.J., C.J. Sole, C.A. Bailey, J.L. Grazer, and G.K. Beckham. 2015. A comparison of reactive strength index-modified between six U.S. collegiate athletic teams. *J Strength Cond Res* 29:1310-6.

193. Sung, E., A. Han, T. Hinrichs, M. Vorgerd, C. Manchado, and P. Platen. 2014. Effects of

follicular versus luteal phase-based strength training in young women. *Springerplus* 3:668.

194. Taylor, K.L., D.W. Chapman, J.B. Cronin, M.J. Newton, and N. Gill. 2012. Fatigue monitoring in high performance sport: A survey of current trends. *J Aust Strength Cond* 20:12-23.

195. Taylor, K.L., J. Cronin, N.D. Gill, D.W. Chapman, and J. Sheppard. 2010. Sources of variability in iso-inertial jump assessments. *Int J Sports Physiol Perform* 5:546-58.

196. Teo, W., M.R. McGuigan, and M.J. Newton. 2011. The effects of circadian rhythmicity of salivary cortisol and testosterone on maximal isometric force, maximal dynamic force, and power output. *J Strength Cond Res* 25:1538-45.

197. Thomas, C., P.A. Jones, and P. Comfort. 2015. Reliability of the dynamic strength index in collegiate athletes. *Int J Sports Physiol Perform* 10:542-5.

198. Thomson, R.L., C.R. Bellenger, P.R. Howe, L. Karavirta, and J.D. Buckley. 2016. Improved heart rate recovery despite reduced exercise performance following heavy training: A within-subject analysis. *J Sci Med Sport* 19:255-9.

199. Thorpe, J.L., and K.T. Ebersole. 2008. Unilateral balance performance in female collegiate soccer athletes. *J Strength Cond Res* 22:1429-33.

200. Thorpe, R.T., A.J. Strudwick, M. Buchheit, G. Atkinson, B. Drust, and W. Gregson. 2015. Monitoring fatigue during the in-season competitive phase in elite soccer players. *Int J Sports Physiol Perform* 10:958-64.

201. Tidow, G. 1990. Aspects of strength training in athletics. *New Stud Athlet* 1:93-110.

202. Tomasi, T.B., F.B. Trudeau, D. Czerwinski, and S. Erredge. 1982. Immune parameters in athletes before and after strenuous exercise. *J Clin Immunol* 2:173-8.

203. Urhausen, A., H. Gabriel, and W. Kindermann. 1995. Blood hormones as markers of training stress and overtraining. *Sports Med* 20:251-76.

204. VanBruggen, M.D., A.C. Hackney, R.G. McMurray, and K.S. Ondrak. 2011. The relationship between serum and salivary cortisol levels in response to different intensities of exercise. *Int J Sports Physiol Perform* 6:396-407.

205. Vesterinen, V., L. Hokka, E. Hynynen, J. Mikkola, K. Hakkinen, and A. Nummela. 2014. Heart rate-running speed index may be an efficient method of monitoring endurance training adaptation. *J Strength Cond Res* 28:902-8.

206. Vesterinen, V., A. Nummela, S. Ayramo, T. Laine, E. Hynynen, J. Mikkola, and K. Hakkinen. 2016. Monitoring training adaptation with a submaximal running test in field conditions. *Int J Sports Physiol Perform* 11:393-99.

207. Veugelers, K.R., G. Naughton, C. Duncan, D. Burgess, and S. Graham. 2016. Validity and reliability of a submaximal intermittent running test in elite Australian football players. *J Strength Cond Res* 30:3347-53.

208. Viru, A., and M. Viru. 2000. *Biochemical monitoring of sport training*. Champaign, IL: Human Kinetics.

209. Watsford, M.L., A.J. Murphy, K.A. McLachlan, A.L. Bryant, M.L. Cameron, K.M. Crossley, and M. Makdissi. 2010. A prospective study of the relationship between lower body stiffness and hamstring injury in professional Australian rules footballers. *Am J Sports Med* 38:2058-64.

210. Wehbe, G., T.J. Gabett, D. Dwyer, C. McLellan, and S. Coad. 2015. Monitoring neuromuscular fatigue in team-sport athletes using a cycle-ergometer test. *Int J Sports Physiol Perform* 10:292-7.

211. Wehbe, G.M., T.J. Gabbett, T.B. Hartwig, and C.P. McLellan. 2015. Reliability of a cycle ergometer peak power test in running-based team sport athletes: A technical report. *J Strength Cond Res* 29:2050-5.

212. Weir, J.P. 2005. Quantifying test-retest reliability using the intraclass correlation coefficient and the sem. *J Strength Cond Res* 19:231-40.

213. West, D.W., N.A. Burd, J.E. Tang, D.R. Moore, A.W. Staples, A.M. Holwerda, S.K. Baker, and S.M. Phillips. 2010. Elevations in ostensibly anabolic hormones with resistance exercise enhance neither training-induced muscle hypertrophy nor strength of the elbow flexors. *J Appl Physiol* 108:60-7.

214. West, D.W., and S.M. Phillips. 2012. Associations of exercise-induced hormone profiles and gains in strength and hypertrophy in a large cohort after weight training. *Eur J Appl Physiol* 112:2693-702.

215. Wilson, G.J., A.J. Murphy, and J.F. Pryor. 1994. Musculotendinous stiffness: Its relationship to eccentric, isometric, and concentric performance. *J Appl Physiol* 76:2714-9.

216. Young, K.P., G.G. Haff, R.U. Newton, T.J. Gabbett, and J.M. Sheppard. 2015. Assessment and monitoring of ballistic and maximal upper-body strength qualities in athletes. *Int J Sports Physiol Perform* 10:232-7.

217. Young, K.P., G.G. Haff, R.U. Newton, and J.M. Sheppard. 2014. Reliability of a novel testing protocol to assess upper-body strength qualities in elite athletes. *Int J Sports Physiol Perform* 9:871-5.

218. Young, W., A. Russell, P. Burge, A. Clarke, S. Cormack, and G. Stewart. 2008. The use of sprint tests for assessment of speed qualities of elite Australian rules footballers. *Int J Sports Physiol Perform.* 3:199-206.

219. Zielinski, J., and K. Kusy. 2015. Hypoxanthine: A universal metabolic indicator of training status in competitive sports. *Exerc Sport Sci Rev* 43:214-21.

220. Zoladz, J.A., A.J. Sargeant, J. Emmerich, J. Stoklosa, and A. Zychowski. 1993. Changes in acid-base status of marathon runners during an incremental field test. Relationship to mean competitive marathon velocity. *Eur J Appl Physiol Occup Physiol* 67:71-6.

Chapter 6

1. Abbiss, C.R., M.J. Quod, G. Levin, D.T. Martin, and P.B. Laursen. 2009. Accuracy of the Velotron ergometer and SRM power meter. *Int J Sports Med* 30:107-12.

2. Agostinho, M.F., A.G. Philippe, G.S. Marcolino, E.R. Pereira, T. Busso, R.B. Candau, and E. Franchini. 2015. Perceived training intensity and performance changes quantification in judo. *J Strength Cond Res* 29:1570-7.

3. Akenhead, R., and G.P. Nassis. 2016. Training load and player monitoring in high-level football: Current practice and perceptions. *Int J Sports Physiol Perform* 11:587-93.

4. An, W.W., V. Wong, and R.T. Cheung. 2015. Lower limb reaction force asymmetry in rowers with and without a history of back injury. *Sports Biomech* 14:375-83.

5. Baguet, A., I. Everaert, P. Hespel, M. Petrovic, E. Achten, and W. Derave. 2011. A new method for non-invasive estimation of human muscle fiber type composition. *PLoS One* 6:e21956.

6. Bailey, C.A., K. Sato, A. Burnett, and M.H. Stone. 2015. Force-production asymmetry in male and female athletes of differing strength levels. *Int J Sports Physiol Perform* 10:504-8.

7. Balsalobre-Fernandez, C., M. Glaister, and R.A. Lockey. 2015. The validity and reliability of an iPhone app for measuring vertical jump performance. *J Sports Sci* 33:1574-9.

8. Balsalobre-Fernandez, C., M. Kuzdub, P. Poveda-Ortiz, and J.D. Campo-Vecino. 2016. Validity and reliability of the PUSH wearable device to measure movement velocity during the back squat exercise. *J Strength Cond Res* 30:1968-74.

9. Bandodkar, A.J., W. Jia, C. Yardimci, X. Wang, J. Ramirez, and J. Wang. 2015. Tattoo-based noninvasive glucose monitoring: A proof-of-concept study. *Anal Chem* 87:394-8.

10. Bandodkar, A.J., and J. Wang. 2014. Non-invasive wearable electrochemical sensors: A review. *Trends Biotechnol* 32:363-71.

11. Banissy, M.J., and N.G. Muggleton. 2013. Transcranial direct current stimulation in sports training: Potential approaches. *Front Hum Neurosci* 7:129.

12. Banister, E.W., T.W. Calvert, M.V. Savage, and T. Bach. 1975. A system model of training for athletic performance. *Aust J Sports Med* 7:170-76.

13. Barreira, P., B. Drust, M.A. Robinson, and J. Vanrenterghem. 2015. Asymmetry after hamstring injury in English premier league: Issue resolved, or perhaps not? *Int J Sports Med* 36:455-9.

14. Barrett, S., A. Midgley, and R. Lovell. 2014. Playerload: Reliability, convergent validity, and influence of unit position during treadmill running. *Int J Sports Physiol Perform* 9:945-52.

15. Bassett, D.R., Jr. 2002. Scientific contributions of A.V. Hill: Exercise physiology pioneer. *J Appl Physiol* 93:1567-82.

16. Bastani, A., and S. Jaberzadeh. 2012. Does anodal transcranial direct current stimulation enhance excitability of the motor cortex and motor function in healthy individuals and subjects with stroke: A systematic review and meta-analysis. *Clin Neurophysiol* 123:644-57.

17. Beckham, G., T. Suchomel, and S. Mizuguchi. 2014. Force plate use in performance monitoring and sport science testing. *New Stud Athlet* 29:25-37.

18. Bellenger, C.R., J.T. Fuller, R.L. Thomson, K. Davison, E.Y. Robertson, and J.D. Buckley. 2016. Monitoring athletic training status through autonomic heart rate regulation: A systematic review and meta-analysis. *Sports Med* 46:1461-86.

19. Bergeron, M.F., R. Bahr, P. Bartsch, L. Bourdon, J.A. Calbet, K.H. Carlsen, O. Castagna, J. Gonzalez-Alonso, C. Lundby, R.J. Maughan, G. Millet, M. Mountjoy, S. Racinais, P. Rasmussen, D.G. Singh, A.W. Subudhi, A.J. Young, T. Soligard, and L. Engebretsen. 2012. International Olympic Committee consensus statement on thermoregulatory and altitude challenges for high-level athletes. *Br J Sports Med* 46:770-9.

20. Bex, T., A. Baguet, E. Achten, P. Aerts, D. De Clercq, and W. Derave. 2016. Cyclic movement frequency is associated with muscle typology in athletes. *Scand J Med Sci Sports*.

21. Bini, R.R., and P.A. Hume. 2014. Assessment of bilateral asymmetry in cycling using a commercial instrumented crank system and instrumented pedals. *Int J Sports Physiol Perform* 9:876-81.

22. Blazevich, A.J., and N.C. Sharp. 2005. Understanding muscle architectural adaptation: Macro- and micro-level research. *Cells Tissues Organs* 181:1-10.

23. Borges, N.R., and M.W. Driller. 2016. Wearable lactate threshold predicting device is valid and reliable in runners. *J Strength Cond Res* 30:2212-8.

24. Bosco, C., P.V. Komi, J. Tihanyi, G. Fekete, and P. Apor. 1983. Mechanical power test and fiber composition of human leg extensor muscles. *Eur J Appl Physiol Occup Physiol* 51:129-35.

25. Bosco, C., P. Luhtanen, and P.V. Komi. 1983. A simple method for measurement of mechanical power in jumping. *Eur J Appl Physiol Occup Physiol* 50:273-82.

26. Bradbury, J.C., and S.L. Forman. 2012. The impact of pitch counts and days of rest on performance among major-league baseball pitchers. *J Strength Cond Res* 26:1181-7.

27. Buchheit, M., Y. Cholley, M. Nagel, and N. Poulos. 2016. The effect of body mass on eccentric knee flexor strength assessed with an instrumented Nordic hamstring device (Nordbord) in football players. *Int J Sports Physiol Perform* 11:721-6.

28. Buchheit, M., A. Gray, and J.B. Morin. 2015. Assessing stride variables and vertical stiffness with GPS-embedded accelerometers: Preliminary insights for the monitoring of neuromuscular fatigue on the field. *J Sports Sci Med* 14:698-701.

29. Bullock, N., D.T. Martin, A. Ross, D. Rosemond, T. Holland, and F.E. Marino. 2008. Characteristics of the start in women's world cup skeleton. *Sports Biomech* 7:351-60.

30. Busso, T., R. Candau, and J.R. Lacour. 1994. Fatigue and fitness modelled from the effects of training on performance. *Eur J Appl Physiol Occup Physiol* 69:50-4.

31. Busso, T., and L. Thomas. 2006. Using mathematical modeling in training planning. *Int J Sports Physiol Perform* 1:400-5.

32. Casto, K.V., and D.A. Edwards. 2016. Before, during, and after: How phases of competition differentially affect testosterone, cortisol, and estradiol levels in women athletes. *Adapt Hum Behav Physiol* 2:11-25.

33. Chambers, R., T.J. Gabbett, M.H. Cole, and A. Beard. 2015. The use of wearable microsensors to quantify sport-specific movements. *Sports Med* 45:1065-81.

34. Conceicao, F., J. Fernandes, M. Lewis, J.J. Gonzalez-Badillo, and P. Jimenez-Reyes. 2015. Movement velocity as a measure of exercise intensity in three lower limb exercises. *J Sports Sci*:1-8.

35. Cormie, P., J.M. McBride, and G.O. McCaulley. 2008. Power-time, force-time, and velocity-time curve analysis during the jump squat: Impact of load. *J Appl Biomech* 24:112-20.

36. Costill, D.L., J. Daniels, W. Evans, W. Fink, G. Krahenbuhl, and B. Saltin. 1976. Skeletal muscle enzymes and fiber composition in male and female track athletes. *J Appl Physiol* 40:149-54.

37. Coutts, A.J. 2014. In the age of technology, Occam's razor still applies. *Int J Sports Physiol Perform* 9:741.

38. Coutts, A.J. 2016. Working fast and working slow: The benefits of embedding research in high performance sport. *Int J Sports Physiol Perform* 11:1-2.

39. Crewther, B.T., M.R. McGuigan, and N.D. Gill. 2011. The ratio and allometric scaling of speed, power, and strength in elite male rugby union players. *J Strength Cond Res* 25:1968-75.

40. Cross, M.R., M. Brughelli, S.R. Brown, P. Samozino, N.D. Gill, J.B. Cronin, and J.B. Morin. 2015. Mechanical properties of sprinting in elite rugby union and rugby league. *Int J Sports Physiol Perform* 10:695-702.

41. Cummins, C., R. Orr, H. O'Connor, and C. West. 2013. Global positioning systems (GPS) and microtechnology sensors in team sports: A systematic review. *Sports Med* 43:1025-42.

42. de Magalhaes, F.A., G. Vannozzi, G. Gatta, and S. Fantozzi. 2015. Wearable inertial sensors in swimming motion analysis: A systematic review. *J Sports Sci* 33:732-45.

43. Derrick, T.R. 2004. Signal processing. In *Research methods in biomechanics*, edited by D.G.E. Robertson, G.E. Caldwell, J. Hamill, G. Kamen and S.N. Whittlesey, 227-38. Champaign, IL: Human Kinetics.

44. Dijkstra, H.P., N. Pollock, R. Chakraverty, and J.M. Alonso. 2014. Managing the health of the elite athlete: A new integrated performance health management and coaching model. *Br J Sports Med* 48:523-31.

45. Dorel, S., C.A. Hautier, O. Rambaud, D. Rouffet, E. Van Praagh, J.R. Lacour, and M. Bourdin. 2005. Torque and power-velocity relationships in cycling: Relevance to track sprint performance in world-class cyclists. *Int J Sports Med* 26:739-46.

46. Dowling, A.V., J. Favre, and T.P. Andriacchi. 2012. Inertial sensor-based feedback can reduce key risk metrics for anterior cruciate ligament injury during jump landings. *Am J Sports Med* 40:1075-83.

47. Driller, M.W., C.K. Argus, and C.M. Shing. 2013. The reliability of a 30-s sprint test on the Wattbike cycle ergometer. *Int J Sports Physiol Perform* 8:379-83.

48. Dugan, E.L., T.L. Doyle, B. Humphries, C.J. Hasson, and R.U. Newton. 2004. Determining the optimal load for jump squats: A review of methods and calculations. *J Strength Cond Res* 18:668-74.

49. Duncan, M.J., J. Hankey, M. Lyons, R.S. James, and A.M. Nevill. 2013. Peak power prediction in junior basketballers: Comparing linear and allometric models. *J Strength Cond Res* 27:597-603.

50. Ekegren, C.L., B.J. Gabbe, and C.F. Finch. 2016. Sports injury surveillance systems: A review of methods and data quality. *Sports Med 46:49-65*.

51. Flatt, A.A., and M.R. Esco. 2016. Evaluating individual training adaptation with smartphone-derived heart rate variability in a collegiate female soccer team. *J Strength Cond Res 30:378-85*.

52. Flatt, A.A., and M.R. Esco. 2015. Smartphone-derived heart rate variability and training load in a female soccer team. *Int J Sports Physiol Perform* 10:994-1000.

53. Fry, A.C., B.K. Schilling, R.S. Staron, F.C. Hagerman, R.S. Hikida, and J.T. Thrush. 2003. Muscle fiber characteristics and performance correlates of male Olympic-style weightlifters. *J Strength Cond Res* 17:746-54.

54. Gabbett, T.J., and S. Ullah. 2012. Relationship between running loads and soft-tissue injury in elite team sport athletes. *J Strength Cond Res* 26:953-60.

55. Gaffney, M., M. Walsh, B. O'Flynn, and C.O. Mathuna. 2015. A highly automated, wireless inertial measurement unit based system for monitoring gym-based push-start training sessions by bob-skeleton athletes. *Sensors Transducers* 184:26-38.

56. Gao, W., S. Emaminejad, H.Y. Nyein, S. Challa, K. Chen, A. Peck, H.M. Fahad, H. Ota, H. Shiraki, D. Kiriya, D.H. Lien, G.A. Brooks, R.W. Davis, and A. Javey. 2016. Fully integrated wearable sensor arrays for multiplexed in situ perspiration analysis. *Nature* 529:509-14.

57. Giandolini, M., S. Pavailler, P. Samozino, J.B. Morin, and N. Horvais. 2015. Foot strike pattern and impact continuous measurements during a trail running race: Proof of concept in a world-class athlete. *Footwear Sci* 7:127-37.

58. Giandolini, M., T. Poupard, P. Gimenez, N. Horvais, G.Y. Millet, J.B. Morin, and P. Samozino. 2014. A simple field method to identify foot strike pattern during running. *J Biomech* 47:1588-93.

59. Gomes, B.B., N.V. Ramos, F.A. Conceicao, R.H. Sanders, M.A. Vaz, and J.P. Vilas-Boas. 2015. Paddling force profiles at different stroke rates in elite sprint kayaking. *J Appl Biomech* 31:258-63.

60. Goodall, S., G. Howatson, L. Romer, and E. Ross. 2014. Transcranial magnetic stimulation in sport science: A commentary. *Eur J Sport Sci* 14 Suppl 1:S332-40.

61. Halperin, I., S. Hughes, and D.W. Chapman. 2016. Physiological profile of a professional boxer preparing for title bout: A case study. *J Sports Sci*:1-8.

62. Halson, S.L. 2014. Monitoring training load to understand fatigue in athletes. *Sports Med* 44 Suppl 2:S139-47.

63. Hamill, J., G.E. Caldwell, and T.R. Derrick. 1997. Reconstructing digital signals using Shannon's sampling theorem. *J Appl Biomech* 13:226-38.

64. Hanstock, H.G., N.P. Walsh, J.P. Edwards, M.B. Fortes, S.L. Cosby, A. Nugent, T. Curran, P.V. Coyle, M.D. Ward, and X.H. Yong. 2016. Tear fluid SIgA as a noninvasive biomarker of mucosal immunity and common cold risk. *Med Sci Sports Exerc* 48:569-77.

65. Haugen, T., and M. Buchheit. 2016. Sprint running performance monitoring: Methodological and practical considerations. *Sports Med* 46:641-56.

66. Haugen, T., E. Tonnessen, and S. Seiler. 2015. Correction factors for photocell sprint timing with flying start. *Int J Sports Physiol Perform* 10:1055-7.

67. Hautier, C.A., M.T. Linossier, A. Belli, J.R. Lacour, and L.M. Arsac. 1996. Optimal velocity for maximal power production in non-isokinetic cycling is related to muscle fibre type composition. *Eur J Appl Physiol Occup Physiol* 74:114-8.

68. Henry, F.M. 1952. Force-time characteristics of the sprint start. *Res Q Exerc Sport* 23:301-18.

69. Henry, F.M., and I.R. Tranton. 1951. The velocity curve of sprint running with some observations on the muscle viscosity factors. *Res Q* 22:409-22.

70. Hill, A. 1927. *Muscular movement in man: The factors governing speed and recovery from fatigue.* New York: McGraw-Hill.

71. Hori, N., R.U. Newton, N. Kawamori, M.R. McGuigan, W.J. Kraemer, and K. Nosaka. 2009. Reliability of performance measurements derived from ground reaction force data during countermovement jump and the influence of sampling frequency. *J Strength Cond Res* 23:874-82.

72. Jia, W., A.J. Bandodkar, G. Valdes-Ramirez, J.R. Windmiller, Z. Yang, J. Ramirez, G. Chan, and J. Wang. 2013. Electrochemical tattoo biosensors for real-time noninvasive lactate monitoring in human perspiration. *Anal Chem* 85:6553-60.

73. Jobson, S.A., L. Passfield, G. Atkinson, G. Barton, and P. Scarf. 2009. The analysis and utilization of cycling training data. *Sports Med* 39:833-44.

74. Johnston, R.J., M.L. Watsford, S.J. Kelly, M.J. Pine, and R.W. Spurrs. 2014. Validity and interunit reliability of 10 Hz and 15 Hz GPS units for assessing athlete movement demands. *J Strength Cond Res* 28:1649-55.

75. Jordan, M.J., P. Aagaard, and W. Herzog. 2015. Lower limb asymmetry in mechanical muscle function: A comparison between ski racers with and without ACL reconstruction. *Scand J Med Sci Sports* 25:e301-9.

76. Jovanavic, M., and E. Flanagan. 2014. Researched applications of velocity based strength training. *J Aust Strength Cond* 22:58-69.

77. Kahnemann, D. 2011. *Thinking, fast and slow*: Macmillan.

78. Kim, J., G. Valdes-Ramirez, A.J. Bandodkar, W. Jia, A.G. Martinez, J. Ramirez, P. Mercier, and J. Wang. 2014. Non-invasive mouthguard biosensor for continuous salivary monitoring of metabolites. *Analyst* 139:1632-6.

79. Kinugasa, T., E. Cerin, and S. Hooper. 2004. Single-subject research designs and data analyses for assessing elite athletes' conditioning. *Sports Med* 34:1035-50.

80. Krogh, A. 1913. A bicycle ergometer and respiration apparatus for the experimental study of muscular work. *Skandinavisches Archiv Für Physiologie* 30:375-94.

81. Krogh, A., and J. Lindhard. 1913. The regulation of respiration and circulation during the initial stages of muscular work. *J Physiol* 47:112-36.

82. Le Meur, Y., J. Louis, A. Aubry, J. Gueneron, A. Pichon, K. Schaal, J.B. Corcuff, S.N. Hatem, R. Isnard, and C. Hausswirth. 2014. Maximal exercise limitation in functionally overreached triathletes: Role of cardiac adrenergic stimulation. *J Appl Physiol* 117:214-22.

83. Lindsay, T.R., J.A. Yaggie, and S.J. McGregor. 2016. A wireless accelerometer node for reliable and valid measurement of lumbar accelerations during treadmill running. *Sports Biomech*:1-12.

84. Mangine, G.T., J.R. Hoffman, A.M. Gonzalez, A.J. Wells, J.R. Townsend, A.R. Jajtner, W. McCormack, E.H. Robinson, M.S. Fragala, D.H. Fukuda, and J.R. Stout. 2014. Speed, force and power values produced from a non-motorized treadmill test are related to sprinting performance. *J Strength Cond Res* 28:1812-9.

85. Marsland, F., K. Lyons, J. Anson, G. Waddington, C. Macintosh, and D. Chapman. 2012. Identification of cross-country skiing movement patterns using micro-sensors. *Sensors* 12:5047-66.

86. Marsland, F., C. Mackintosh, J. Anson, K. Lyons, G. Waddington, and D.W. Chapman. 2015. Using micro-sensor data to quantify macro kinematics of classical cross-country skiing during on-snow training. *Sports Biomech* 14:435-47.

87. Martinez-Marti, F., J.L. Gonzalez-Montesinos, D.P. Morales, J.R. Santos, J. Castro-Pinero, M.A. Carvajal, and A.J. Palma. 2016. Validation of instrumented insoles for measuring height in vertical jump. *Int J Sports Med* 37:374-81.

88. Mason, B., J. Lenton, J. Rhodes, R. Cooper, and V. Goosey-Tolfrey. 2014. Comparing the activity profiles of wheelchair rugby using a miniaturised data logger and radio-frequency tracking system. *BioMed Res Int* 2014:348048.

89. Matzeu, G., C. Fay, A. Vaillant, S. Coyle, and D. Diamond. 2015. A wearable device for monitoring sweat rates via image analysis. *IEEE Trans Biomed Eng.*

90. Matzeu, G., L. Florea, and D. Diamond. 2015. Advances in wearable chemical sensor design for monitoring biological fluids. *Sensors and Actuators B: Chemical* 211:403-18.

91. McArdle, W.D., F.I. Katch, and V.L. Katch. 2014. *Exercise physiology: Energy, nutrition, and human performance.* 8th ed. Baltimore: Lippincott Williams & Wilkins.

92. McBride, J.M., T. Triplett-McBride, A.J. Davie, P.J. Abernethy, and R.U. Newton. 2003. Characteristics of titin in strength and power athletes. *Eur J Appl Physiol* 88:553-7.

93. McCall, A., C. Carling, M. Davison, M. Nedelec, F. Le Gall, S. Berthoin, and G. Dupont. 2015. Injury risk factors, screening tests and preventative strategies: A systematic review of the evidence that underpins the perceptions and practices of 44 football (soccer) teams from various premier leagues. *Br J Sports Med* 49:583-9.

94. McCall, A., C. Carling, M. Nedelec, M. Davison, F. Le Gall, S. Berthoin, and G. Dupont. 2014. Risk factors, testing and preventative strategies for non-contact injuries in professional football: Current perceptions and practices of 44 teams from various premier leagues. *Br J Sports Med* 48:1352-7.

95. McGuigan, M.R., S. Cormack, and N.D. Gill. 2013. Strength and power profiling of athletes. *Strength Cond J* 35:7-14.

96. McKenna, M., and P.E. Riches. 2007. A comparison of sprinting kinematics on two types of treadmill and over-ground. *Scand J Med Sci Sports* 17:649-55.

97. McLean, B.D., A.J. Coutts, V. Kelly, M.R. McGuigan, and S.J. Cormack. 2010. Neuromuscular, endocrine, and perceptual fatigue responses during different length between-match microcycles in professional rugby league players. *Int J Sports Physiol Perform* 5:367-83.

98. McMaster, D.T., N. Gill, J. Cronin, and M. McGuigan. 2014. A brief review of strength

and ballistic assessment methodologies in sport. *Sports Med* 44:603-23.

99. McMiken, D.F., and J.T. Daniels. 1976. Aerobic requirements and maximum aerobic power in treadmill and track running. *Med Sci Sports* 8:14-7.

100. Meister, S., K. Aus der Funten, and T. Meyer. 2014. Repeated monitoring of blood parameters for evaluating strain and overload in elite football players: Is it justified? *J Sports Sci* 32:1328-31.

101. Mendiguchia, J., P. Edouard, P. Samozino, M. Brughelli, M. Cross, A. Ross, N. Gill, and J.B. Morin. 2016. Field monitoring of sprinting power-force-velocity profile before, during and after hamstring injury: Two case reports. *J Sports Sci* 34:535-41.

102. Mendiguchia, J., P. Samozino, E. Martinez-Ruiz, M. Brughelli, S. Schmikli, J.B. Morin, and A. Mendez-Villanueva. 2014. Progression of mechanical properties during on-field sprint running after returning to sports from a hamstring muscle injury in soccer players. *Int J Sports Med* 35:690-5.

103. Montgomery, P.G., D.J. Green, N. Etxebarria, D.B. Pyne, P.U. Saunders, and C.L. Minahan. 2009. Validation of heart rate monitor-based predictions of oxygen uptake and energy expenditure. *J Strength Cond Res* 23:1489-95.

104. Moreira, A., J.C. Bilsborough, C.J. Sullivan, M. Ciancosi, M.S. Aoki, and A.J. Coutts. 2015. Training periodization of professional Australian football players during an entire Australian football league season. *Int J Sports Physiol Perform* 10:566-71.

105. Morel, B., and C.A. Hautier. 2016. The neuromuscular fatigue induced by repeated scrums generates instability that can be limited by appropriate recovery. *Scand J Med Sci Sports*.

106. Morin, J.B., and P. Samozino. 2016. Interpreting power-force-velocity profiles for individualized and specific training. *Int J Sports Physiol Perform* 11:267-72.

107. Morin, S., S. Ahmaidi, and P.M. Lepretre. 2016. Relevance of damped harmonic oscillation for modeling the training effects on daily physical performance capacity in team sport. *Int J Sports Physiol Perform*.

108. Muro-de-la-Herran, A., B. Garcia-Zapirain, and A. Mendez-Zorrilla. 2014. Gait analysis methods: An overview of wearable and non-wearable systems, highlighting clinical applications. *Sensors (Basel)* 14:3362-94.

109. Myers, A.C., H. Huang, and Y. Zhu. 2015. Wearable silver nanowire dry electrodes for electrophysiological sensing. *RSC Advances* 5:11627-32.

110. Narici, M., M. Franchi, and C. Maganaris. 2016. Muscle structural assembly and functional consequences. *J Exp Biol* 219:276-84.

111. Newton, R., and E. Dugan. 2002. Application of strength diagnosis. *Strength Cond J* 24:50-59.

112. Opar, D.A., T. Piatkowski, M.D. Williams, and A.J. Shield. 2013. A novel device using the Nordic hamstring exercise to assess eccentric knee flexor strength: A reliability and retrospective injury study. *J Orthop Sports Phys Ther* 43:636-40.

113. Orchard, J.W., P. Blanch, J. Paoloni, A. Kountouris, K. Sims, J.J. Orchard, and P. Brukner. 2015. Cricket fast bowling workload patterns as risk factors for tendon, muscle, bone and joint injuries. *Br J Sports Med* 49:1064-8.

114. Orchard, J.W., P. Blanch, J. Paoloni, A. Kountouris, K. Sims, J.J. Orchard, and P. Brukner. 2015. Fast bowling match workloads over 5-26 days and risk of injury in the following month. *J Sci Med Sport* 18:26-30.

115. Peritz, D.C., A. Howard, M. Ciocca, and E.H. Chung. 2015. Smartphone ECG aids real time diagnosis of palpitations in the competitive college athlete. *J Electrocardiol* 48:896-9.

116. Pette, D., and R.S. Staron. 2000. Myosin isoforms, muscle fiber types, and transitions. *Microsc Res Tech* 50:500-9.

117. Pinot, J., and F. Grappe. 2011. The record power profile to assess performance in elite cyclists. *Int J Sports Med* 32:839-44.

118. Quod, M.J., D.T. Martin, J.C. Martin, and P.B. Laursen. 2010. The power profile predicts road cycling MMP. *Int J Sports Med* 31:397-401.

119. Reed, R., P. Scarf, S.A. Jobson, and L. Passfield. 2016. Determining optimal cadence for an individual road cyclist from field data. *Eur J Sport Sci*:1-9.

120. Robertson, D.G.E., G.E. Caldwell, J. Hamill, G. Kamen, and S.N. Whittlesey. 2014. *Research methods in biomechanics*. 2nd ed. Champaign, IL: Human Kinetics.

121. Saltin, B., and P.O. Astrand. 1967. Maximal oxygen uptake in athletes. *J Appl Physiol* 23:353-8.

122. Samozino, P., G. Rabita, S. Dorel, J. Slawinski, N. Peyrot, E. Saez de Villarreal, and J.B. Morin. 2016. A simple method for measuring power, force, velocity properties, and mechanical effectiveness in sprint running. *Scand J Med Sci Sports* 26:648-58.

123. Sanchez-Medina, L., J.J. Gonzalez-Badillo, C.E. Perez, and J.G. Pallares. 2014. Velocity- and power-load relationships of the bench pull vs. Bench press exercises. *Int J Sports Med* 35:209-16.

124. Sargent, C., M. Lastella, S.L. Halson, and G.D. Roach. 2016. The validity of activity monitors for measuring sleep in elite athletes. *J Sci Med Sport*.

125. Sato, K., W.A. Sands, and M.H. Stone. 2012. The reliability of accelerometry to measure weightlifting performance. *Sports Biomech* 11:524-31.

126. Sato, K., S.L. Smith, and W.A. Sands. 2009. Validation of an accelerometer for measuring sport performance. *J Strength Cond Res* 23:341-7.

127. Saw, A.E., L.C. Main, and P.B. Gastin. 2016. Monitoring the athlete training response: Subjective self-reported measures trump commonly used objective measures: A systematic review. *Br J Sports Med* 50:281-91.

128. Saw, A.E., L.C. Main, and P.B. Gastin. 2015. Role of a self-report measure in athlete preparation. *J Strength Cond Res* 29:685-91.

129. Sayers, S.P., D.V. Harackiewicz, E.A. Harman, P.N. Frykman, and M.T. Rosenstein. 1999. Cross-validation of three jump power equations. *Med Sci Sports Exerc* 31:572-7.

130. Schmitt, L., J. Regnard, and G.P. Millet. 2015. Monitoring fatigue status with HRV measures in elite athletes: An avenue beyond RMSSD? *Front Physiol* 6:343.

131. Shanley, E., L. Bailey, M.P. Sandago, A. Pinkerton, S.B. Singleton, and C.A. Thigpen. 2015. The use of a pitch count estimator to calculate exposure in collegiate baseball pitchers. *Phys Ther Sport* 16:344-8.

132. Shull, P.B., W. Jirattigalachote, M.A. Hunt, M.R. Cutkosky, and S.L. Delp. 2014. Quantified self and human movement: A review on the clinical impact of wearable sensing and feedback for gait analysis and intervention. *Gait Posture* 40:11-9.

133. Simons, C., and E.J. Bradshaw. 2016. Reliability of accelerometry to assess impact loads of jumping and landing tasks. *Sports Biomech*:1-10.

134. Simperingham, K.D., J.B. Cronin, and A. Ross. 2016. Advances in sprint acceleration profiling for field-based team-sport athletes: Utility, reliability, validity and limitations. *Sports Med* 46:1619-45.

135. Sirotic, A.C., and A.J. Coutts. 2008. The reliability of physiological and performance measures during simulated team-sport running on a non-motorised treadmill. *J Sci Med Sport* 11:500-9.

136. Skiba, P.F., D. Clarke, A. Vanhatalo, and A.M. Jones. 2014. Validation of a novel intermittent W' model for cycling using field data. *Int J Sports Physiol Perform* 9:900-4.

137. Smith, M.S., R.J. Dyson, T. Hale, and L. Janaway. 2000. Development of a boxing dynamometer and its punch force discrimination efficacy. *J Sports Sci* 18:445-50.

138. Steinacker, J.M., W. Lormes, S. Reissnecker, and Y. Liu. 2004. New aspects of the hormone and cytokine response to training. *Eur J Appl Physiol* 91:382-91.

139. Strohrmann, C., H. Harms, C. Kappeler-Setz, and G. Troster. 2012. Monitoring kinematic changes with fatigue in running using body-worn sensors. *IEEE Trans Inf Technol Biomed* 16:983-90.

140. Tao, W., T. Liu, R. Zheng, and H. Feng. 2012. Gait analysis using wearable sensors. *Sensors (Basel)* 12:2255-83.

141. Taylor, K.L., D.W. Chapman, J.B. Cronin, M.J. Newton, and N. Gill. 2012. Fatigue monitoring in high performance sport: A survey of current trends. *J Aust Strength Cond* 20:12-23.

142. Thomas, N., I. Lähdesmäki, and B.A. Parviz. 2012. A contact lens with an integrated lactate sensor. *Sensors and Actuators B: Chemical* 162:128-34.

143. Thompson, W.R. 2016. Worldwide survey of fitness trends for 2017. *ACSMs Health Fit J* 20:8-17.

144. Tipton, C. 2014. *History of exercise physiology*. Champaign, IL: Human Kinetics.

145. Tonnessen, E., V. Rasdal, I.S. Svendsen, T.A. Haugen, E. Hem, and O. Sandbakk. 2016. Concurrent development of endurance capacity and explosiveness: The training characteristics of world-class Nordic combined athletes. *Int J Sports Physiol Perform* 11:643-51.

146. Tonnessen, E., I.S. Svendsen, B.R. Ronnestad, J. Hisdal, T.A. Haugen, and S. Seiler. 2015. The annual training periodization of 8 world champions in orienteering. *Int J Sports Physiol Perform* 10:29-38.

147. Tran, J., A.J. Rice, L.C. Main, and P.B. Gastin. 2015. Profiling the training practices and performances of elite rowers. *Int J Sports Physiol Perform* 10:572-80.

148. Trappe, S., N. Luden, K. Minchev, U. Raue, B. Jemiolo, and T.A. Trappe. 2015. Skeletal muscle signature of a champion sprint runner. *J Appl Physiol* 118:1460-6.

149. Turner, A. 2014. Total score of athleticism: A strategy for assessing an athlete's athleticism. *UK Strength Cond Assoc J* 33:13-17.

150. Ullah, S., T.J. Gabbett, and C.F. Finch. 2014. Statistical modelling for recurrent events: An application to sports injuries. *Br J Sports Med* 48:1287-93.

151. Urhausen, A., H. Gabriel, and W. Kindermann. 1995. Blood hormones as markers of training stress and overtraining. *Sports Med* 20:251-76.

152. van der Worp, H., J.W. Vrielink, and S.W. Bredeweg. 2016. Do runners who suffer injuries have higher vertical ground reaction forces than those who remain injury-free? A systematic review and meta-analysis. *Br J Sports Med*.

153. Varley, M.C., I.H. Fairweather, and R.J. Aughey. 2012. Validity and reliability of GPS for measuring instantaneous velocity during acceleration, deceleration, and constant motion. *J Sports Sci* 30:121-7.

154. Viru, A., and M. Viru. 2000. *Biochemical monitoring of sport training*. Champaign, IL: Human Kinetics.

155. Walilko, T.J., D.C. Viano, and C.A. Bir. 2005. Biomechanics of the head for Olympic boxer punches to the face. *Br J Sports Med* 39:710-9.

156. Watari, R., B. Hettinga, S. Osis, and R. Ferber. 2016. Validation of a torso-mounted accelerometer for measures of vertical oscillation and ground contact time during treadmill running. *J Appl Biomech 32:306-10*.

157. Wehbe, G., T.J. Gabett, D. Dwyer, C. McLellan, and S. Coad. 2015. Monitoring neuromuscular fatigue in team-sport athletes using a cycle-ergometer test. *Int J Sports Physiol Perform* 10:292-7.

158. Wheeler, J.W., P.B. Shull, and T.F. Besier. 2011. Real-time knee adduction moment feedback for gait retraining through visual and tactile displays. *J Biomech Eng* 133:041007.

159. Wood, G.A. 1982. Data smoothing and differentiation procedures in biomechanics. *Exerc Sport Sci Rev* 10:308-62.

160. Yao, H., A.J. Shum, M. Cowan, I. Lahdesmaki, and B.A. Parviz. 2011. A contact lens with embedded sensor for monitoring tear glucose level. *Biosens Bioelectron* 26:3290-6.

Chapter 7

1. Akenhead, R., and G.P. Nassis. 2016. Training load and player monitoring in high-level football: Current practice and perceptions. *Int J Sports Physiol Perform* 11:587-93.

2. Amonette, W., K. English, and W.J. Kraemer. 2016. *Evidence-based practice in exercise science: The six-step approach*. Champaign, IL: Human Kinetics.

3. Argus, C.K., N.D. Gill, J.W. Keogh, and W.G. Hopkins. 2011. Acute effects of verbal feedback on upper-body performance in elite athletes. *J Strength Cond Res* 25:3282-7.

4. Arnold, R., D. Fletcher, and L. Molyneux. 2012. Performance leadership and management in elite sport: Recommendations, advice and suggestions from national performance directors. *Euro Sport Manage Quart* 12:317-36.

5. Bemben, M.G., J.L. Clasey, and B.H. Massey. 1990. The effect of the rate of muscle contraction on the force-time curve parameters of male and female subjects. *Res Q Exerc Sport* 61:96-9.

6. Benz, A., N. Winkelman, J. Porter, and S. Nimphius. 2016. Coaching instructions and cues for enhancing sprint performance. *Strength Cond J* 38:1-11.

7. Bishop, D. 2008. An applied research model for the sport sciences. *Sports Med* 38:253-63.

8. Borresen, J., and M. Lambert. 2006. Validity of self-reported training duration. *Int J Sports Sci Coaching* 1:353-59.

9. Botek, M., A.J. McKune, J. Krejci, P. Stejskal, and A. Gaba. 2014. Change in performance in response to training load adjustment based on autonomic activity. *Int J Sports Med* 35:482-8.

10. Claudino, J.G., J.B. Cronin, B. Mezencio, J.P. Pinho, C. Pereira, L. Mochizuki, A.C. Amadio, and J.C. Serrao. 2016. Auto-regulating jump performance to induce functional overreaching. *J Strength Cond Res* 30:2242-9.

11. Collins, D., H.J. Carson, and A. Cruickshank. 2015. Blaming Bill Gates again! Misuse, overuse and misunderstanding of performance data in sport. *Sport, Education and Society* 20:1088-99.

12. Cormack, S.J., R.U. Newton, M.R. McGuigan, and P. Cormie. 2008. Neuromuscular and endocrine responses of elite players during an Australian rules football season. *Int J Sports Physiol Perform* 3:439-53.

13. Dijkstra, H.P., N. Pollock, R. Chakraverty, and J.M. Alonso. 2014. Managing the health of the elite athlete: A new integrated performance health management and coaching model. *Br J Sports Med* 48:523-31.

14. Dowling, A.V., J. Favre, and T.P. Andriacchi. 2011. A wearable system to assess risk for anterior cruciate ligament injury during jump landing: Measurements of temporal events, jump height, and sagittal plane kinematics. *J Biomech Eng* 133:071008.

15. Dowling, A.V., J. Favre, and T.P. Andriacchi. 2012. Inertial sensor-based feedback can reduce key risk metrics for anterior cruciate ligament injury during jump landings. *Am J Sports Med* 40:1075-83.

16. Ducharme, S.W., W.F. Wu, K. Lim, J.M. Porter, and F. Geraldo. 2016. Standing long jump performance with an external focus of attention is improved as a result of a more effective projection angle. *J Strength Cond Res* 30:276-81.

17. Duchateau, J., and S. Baudry. 2014. Maximal discharge rate of motor units determines the maximal rate of force development during ballistic contractions in human. *Front Hum Neurosci* 8:234.

18. Farrow, D. 2013. Teaching sport skills. In *Coaching excellence*, edited by F. Pyke, 171-84. Champaign, IL: Human Kinetics.

19. Fernandez-Del-Olmo, M., D. Rio-Rodriguez, E. Iglesias-Soler, and R.M. Acero. 2014. Startle auditory stimuli enhance the performance of fast dynamic contractions. *PLoS One* 9:e87805.

20. Figoni, S.F., and A.F. Morris. 1984. Effects of knowledge of results on reciprocal, isokinetic strength and fatigue. *J Orthop Sports Phys Ther* 6:190-7.

21. Foster, C., K.M. Heimann, P.L. Esten, G. Brice, and J.P. Porcari. 2001. Differences in perceptions of training by coaches and athletes. *South Afr J Sports Med* 8:3-7.

22. Goncalves, B., R. Marcelino, L. Torres-Ronda, C. Torrents, and J. Sampaio. 2016. Effects of emphasising opposition and cooperation on collective movement behaviour during football small-sided games. *J Sports Sci*:1-9.

23. Gonzalez-Badillo, J.J., F. Pareja-Blanco, D. Rodriguez-Rosell, J.L. Abad-Herencia, J.J. Del Ojo-Lopez, and L. Sanchez-Medina. 2015. Effects of velocity-based resistance training on young soccer players of different ages. *J Strength Cond Res* 29:1329-38.

24. Graves, J.E., and R.J. James. 1990. Concurrent augmented feedback and isometric force generation during familiar and unfamiliar muscle movements. *Res Q Exerc Sport* 61:75-9.

25. Gudmundsson, J., and M. Horton. 2016. Spatio-temporal analysis of team sports—a survey. http://arxiv.org/abs/1602.06994.

26. Hakkinen, K., A. Pakarinen, M. Alen, H. Kauhanen, and P.V. Komi. 1988. Neuromuscular and hormonal adaptations in athletes to strength training in two years. *J Appl Physiol* 65:2406-12.

27. Horschig, A.D., T.E. Neff, and A.J. Serrano. 2014. Utilization of autoregulatory progressive resistance exercise in transitional

rehabilitation periodization of a high school football-player following anterior cruciate ligament reconstruction: A case report. *Int J Sports Phys Ther* 9:691-8.

28. Ille, A., I. Selin, M.C. Do, and B. Thon. 2013. Attentional focus effects on sprint start performance as a function of skill level. *J Sports Sci* 31:1705-12.

29. Izquierdo, M., J.J. Gonzalez-Badillo, K. Hakkinen, J. Ibanez, W.J. Kraemer, A. Altadill, J. Eslava, and E.M. Gorostiaga. 2006. Effect of loading on unintentional lifting velocity declines during single sets of repetitions to failure during upper and lower extremity muscle actions. *Int J Sports Med* 27:718-24.

30. Jidovtseff, B., N.K. Harris, J.M. Crielaard, and J.B. Cronin. 2011. Using the load-velocity relationship for 1RM prediction. *J Strength Cond Res* 25:267-70.

31. Jovanavic, M., and E. Flanagan. 2014. Researched applications of velocity based strength training *J Aust Strength Cond* 22:58-69.

32. Julian, R., T. Meyer, H.H. Fullagar, S. Skorski, M. Pfeiffer, M. Kellmann, A. Ferrauti, and A. Hecksteden. 2016. Individual patterns in blood-borne indicators of fatigue—trait or chance. *J Strength Cond Res*.

33. Keller, M., B. Lauber, D. Gehring, C. Leukel, and W. Taube. 2014. Jump performance and augmented feedback: Immediate benefits and long-term training effects. *Hum Mov Sci* 36:177-89.

34. Kellis, E., and V. Baltzopoulos. 1996. Resistive eccentric exercise: Effects of visual feedback on maximum moment of knee extensors and flexors. *J Orthop Sports Phys Ther* 23:120-4.

35. Kilduff, L.P., C.V. Finn, J.S. Baker, C.J. Cook, and D.J. West. 2013. Preconditioning strategies to enhance physical performance on the day of competition. *Int J Sports Physiol Perform* 8:677-81.

36. Kinugasa, T., E. Cerin, and S. Hooper. 2004. Single-subject research designs and data analyses for assessing elite athletes' conditioning. *Sports Med* 34:1035-50.

37. Kiviniemi, A.M., A.J. Hautala, H. Kinnunen, J. Nissila, P. Virtanen, J. Karjalainen, and M.P. Tulppo. 2010. Daily exercise prescription on the basis of HR variability among men and women. *Med Sci Sports Exerc* 42:1355-63.

38. Kiviniemi, A.M., A.J. Hautala, H. Kinnunen, and M.P. Tulppo. 2007. Endurance training guided individually by daily heart rate variability measurements. *Eur J Appl Physiol* 101:743-51.

39. Knight, K.L. 1979. Knee rehabilitation by the daily adjustable progressive resistive exercise technique. *Am J Sports Med* 7:336-7.

40. Kooiman, T.J., M.L. Dontje, S.R. Sprenger, W.P. Krijnen, C.P. van der Schans, and M. de Groot. 2015. Reliability and validity of ten consumer activity trackers. *BMC Sports Sci Med Rehabil* 7:24.

41. Kraemer, W.J., and S.J. Fleck. 2008. *Optimizing strength training. Designing nonlinear periodization workouts*. Champaign, IL: Human Kinetics.

42. Kristiansen, E., S.E. Tomten, D.V. Hanstad, and G.C. Roberts. 2012. Coaching communication issues with elite female athletes: Two Norwegian case studies. *Scand J Med Sci Sports* 22:e156-67.

43. Lloyd, R.S., J.B. Cronin, A.D. Faigenbaum, G.G. Haff, R. Howard, W.J. Kraemer, L.J. Micheli, G.D. Myer, and J.L. Oliver. 2016. The National Strength and Conditioning Association position statement on long-term athletic development. *J Strength Cond Res* 30:1491-509.

44. Louder, T., M. Bressel, and E. Bressel. 2015. The kinetic specificity of plyometric training: Verbal cues revisited. *J Hum Kinet* 49:201-8.

45. Maffiuletti, N.A., P. Aagaard, A.J. Blazevich, J. Folland, N. Tillin, and J. Duchateau. 2016. Rate of force development: Physiological and methodological considerations. *Eur J Appl Physiol 116:1091-116*.

46. Makaruk, H., and J.M. Porter. 2014. Focus of attention for strength and conditioning coaches. *Strength Cond J* 36:16-22.

47. Mann, J.B., J.P. Thyfault, P.A. Ivey, and S.P. Sayers. 2010. The effect of autoregulatory progressive resistance exercise vs. Linear periodization on strength improvement in college athletes. *J Strength Cond Res* 24:1718-23.

48. Meyer, E. 2014. *The culture map: Breaking through the invisible boundaries of global business*. New York: Public Affairs.

49. Miranda, D.L., W.H. Hsu, D.C. Gravelle, K. Petersen, R. Ryzman, J. Niemi, and N. Lesniewski-Laas. 2016. Sensory enhancing insoles improve athletic performance during a hexagonal agility task. *J Biomech 49:1058-63*.

50. Molinsky, A. 2013. *Global dexterity: How to adapt your behavior across cultures without losing yourself in the process*. Boston, MA: Harvard Business Review Press.

51. Nickerson, R.S. 1998. Confirmation bias: A ubiquitous phenomenon in many guises. *Rev Gen Psych* 2:175-220.

52. Nimmerichter, A., R.G. Eston, N. Bachl, and C. Williams. 2011. Longitudinal monitoring of power output and heart rate profiles in elite cyclists. *J Sports Sci* 29:831-40.

53. Padulo, J., P. Mignogna, S. Mignardi, F. Tonni, and S. D'Ottavio. 2012. Effect of different pushing speeds on bench press. *Int J Sports Med* 33:376-80.

54. Pareja-Blanco, F., D. Rodriguez-Rosell, L. Sanchez-Medina, E.M. Gorostiaga, and J.J. Gonzalez-Badillo. 2014. Effect of movement velocity during resistance training on neuromuscular performance. *Int J Sports Med* 35:916-24.

55. Pareja-Blanco, F., D. Rodriguez-Rosell, L. Sanchez-Medina, J. Sanchis-Moysi, C. Dorado, R. Mora-Custodio, J.M. Yanez-Garcia, D. Morales-Alamo, I. Perez-Suarez, J.A. Calbet, and J.J. Gonzalez-Badillo. 2016. Effects of velocity loss during resistance training on athletic performance, strength gains and muscle adaptations. *Scand J Med Sci Sports*.

56. Pinot, J., and F. Grappe. 2015. A six-year monitoring case study of a top-10 cycling grand tour finisher. *J Sports Sci* 33:907-14.

57. Porter, J.M., P.M. Anton, and W.F. Wu. 2012. Increasing the distance of an external focus of attention enhances standing long jump performance. *J Strength Cond Res* 26:2389-93.

58. Porter, J.M., R.P. Nolan, E.J. Ostrowski, and G. Wulf. 2010. Directing attention externally enhances agility performance: A qualitative and quantitative analysis of the efficacy of using verbal instructions to focus attention. *Front Psychol* 1:216.

59. Porter, J.M., E.J. Ostrowski, R.P. Nolan, and W.F. Wu. 2010. Standing long-jump performance is enhanced when using an external focus of attention. *J Strength Cond Res* 24:1746-50.

60. Porter, J.M., and B. Sims. 2013. Altering focus of attention influences elite sprinting performance. *Int J Coach Sci* 8:22-27.

61. Porter, J.M., W.F. Wu, R.M. Crossley, S.W. Knopp, and O.C. Campbell. 2015. Adopting an external focus of attention improves sprinting performance in low-skilled sprinters. *J Strength Cond Res* 29:947-53.

62. Porter, J.M., W.F. Wu, and J.A. Partridge. 2010. Focus of attention and verbal instructions: Strategies of elite track and field coaches and athletes. *Sport Sci Review* 19:199-211.

63. Randell, A.D., J.B. Cronin, J.W. Keogh, N.D. Gill, and M.C. Pedersen. 2011. Effect of instantaneous performance feedback during 6 weeks of velocity-based resistance training on sport-specific performance tests. *J Strength Cond Res* 25:87-93.

64. Randell, A.D., J.B. Cronin, J.W. Keogh, N.D. Gill, and M.C. Pedersen. 2011. Reliability of performance velocity for jump squats under feedback and nonfeedback conditions. *J Strength Cond Res* 25:3514-8.

65. Rodriguez-Marroyo, J.A., J. Medina, J. Garcia-Lopez, J.V. Garcia-Tormo, and C. Foster. 2014. Correspondence between training load executed by volleyball players and the one observed by coaches. *J Strength Cond Res* 28:1588-94.

66. Rosenberger, M.E., M.P. Buman, W.L. Haskell, M.V. McConnell, and L.L. Carstensen. 2016. 24 hours of sleep, sedentary behavior, and physical activity with nine wearable devices. *Med Sci Sports Exerc* 48:547-65.

67. Sahaly, R., H. Vandewalle, T. Driss, and H. Monod. 2001. Maximal voluntary force and rate of force development in humans—importance of instruction. *Eur J Appl Physiol* 85:345-50.

68. Salas, E., R. Grossman, A.M. Hughes, and C.W. Coultas. 2015. Measuring team cohesion: Observations from the science. *Hum Factors* 57:365-74.

69. Sanchez-Medina, L., and J.J. Gonzalez-Badillo. 2011. Velocity loss as an indicator of neuromuscular fatigue during resistance training. *Med Sci Sports Exerc* 43:1725-34.

70. Saw, A.E., L.C. Main, and P.B. Gastin. 2015. Monitoring athletes through self-report: Factors influencing implementation. *J Sports Sci Med* 14:137-46.

71. Saw, A.E., L.C. Main, and P.B. Gastin. 2015. Role of a self-report measure in athlete preparation. *J Strength Cond Res* 29:685-91.

72. Sotiriadou, P., and V. De Bosscher. 2013. *Managing high performance sport*. Milton Park, UK: Routledge.

73. Stoszkowski, J., and D. Collins. 2016. Sources, topics and use of knowledge by coaches. *J Sports Sci* 34:794-802.

74. Taylor, K.L., D.W. Chapman, J.B. Cronin, M.J. Newton, and N. Gill. 2012. Fatigue monitoring in high performance sport: A survey of current trends. *J Aust Strength Cond* 20:12-23.

75. Thomas, J.R., J.K. Nelson, and S.J. Silverman. 2015. *Research methods in physical activity*. 7th ed. Champaign, IL.: Human Kinetics.

76. Thompson, W.R. 2016. Worldwide survey of fitness trends for 2017. *ACSMs Health Fit J* 20:8-17.

77. Torres-Ronda, L., B. Goncalves, R. Marcelino, C. Torrents, E. Vicente, and J. Sampaio. 2015. Heart rate, time-motion, and body impacts when changing the number of teammates and opponents in soccer small-sided games. *J Strength Cond Res* 29:2723-30.

78. Urhausen, A., H. Gabriel, and W. Kindermann. 1995. Blood hormones as markers of training stress and overtraining. *Sports Med* 20:251-76.

79. Vesterinen, V., A. Nummela, I. Heikura, T. Laine, E. Hynynen, J. Botella, and K. Hakkinen. 2016. Individual endurance training prescription with heart rate variability. *Med Sci Sports Exerc* 48:1347-54.

80. Walchli, M., J. Ruffieux, Y. Bourquin, M. Keller, and W. Taube. 2016. Maximizing performance: Augmented feedback, focus of attention, and/or reward? *Med Sci Sports Exerc* 48:714-19.

81. Wheeler, J.W., P.B. Shull, and T.F. Besier. 2011. Real-time knee adduction moment feedback for gait retraining through visual and tactile displays. *J Biomech Eng* 133:041007.

82. Williams, S., and A. Manley. 2014. Elite coaching and the technocratic engineer: Thanking the boys at Microsoft! *Sport, Education and Society*.

83. Zourdos, M.C., E. Jo, A.V. Khamoui, S.R. Lee, B.S. Park, M.J. Ormsbee, L.B. Panton, R.J. Contreras, and J.S. Kim. 2016. Modified daily undulating periodization model produces greater performance than a traditional configuration in powerlifters. *J Strength Cond Res* 30:784-91.

84. Zourdos, M.C., A. Klemp, C. Dolan, J.M. Quiles, K.A. Schau, E. Jo, E. Helms, B. Esgro, S. Duncan, S. Garcia Merino, and R. Blanco. 2016. Novel resistance training-specific rating of perceived exertion scale measuring repetitions in reserve. *J Strength Cond Res* 30:267-75.

Chapter 8

1. Adams, R., J. Adams, H. Qin, T. Bilbrey, and J.M. Schussler. 2015. Virtual coaching for the high-intensity training of a powerlifter following coronary artery bypass grafting. *Proc (Bayl Univ Med Cent)* 28:75-7.

2. Agostinho, M.F., A.G. Philippe, G.S. Marcolino, E.R. Pereira, T. Busso, R.B. Candau, and E. Franchini. 2015. Perceived training intensity and performance changes quantification in judo. *J Strength Cond Res* 29:1570-7.

3. Appleby, B., R.U. Newton, and P. Cormie. 2012. Changes in strength over a 2-year period in professional rugby union players. *J Strength Cond Res* 26:2538-46.

4. Black, J.T., P.S. Romano, B. Sadeghi, A.D. Auerbach, T.G. Ganiats, S. Greenfield, S.H. Kaplan, M.K. Ong, and B.-H.R. Group. 2014. A remote monitoring and telephone nurse coaching intervention to reduce readmissions among patients with heart failure: Study protocol for the better effectiveness after transition—heart failure (BEAT-HF) randomized controlled trial. *Trials* 15:124.

5. Brandon, R. 2016. Managing pre-season and in-season training. In *Sports injury prevention and rehabilitation: Integration medicine and science for performance solutions*, edited by D. Joyce and D. Lewindon, 377. London: Routledge.

6. Brearley, M., I. Norton, D. Kingsbury, and S. Maas. 2014. Responses of elite road motorcyclists to racing in tropical conditions: A case study. *Int J Sports Physiol Perform* 9:887-90.

7. Bullock, N., D.T. Martin, A. Ross, D. Rosemond, T. Holland, and F.E. Marino. 2008. Characteristics of the start in women's world cup skeleton. *Sports Biomech* 7:351-60.

8. Edmonds, R.C., W.H. Sinclair, and A.S. Leicht. 2013. Effect of a training week on heart rate variability in elite youth rugby league players. *Int J Sports Med* 34:1087-92.

9. Enoka, R.M., and J. Duchateau. 2016. Translating fatigue to human performance. *Med Sci Sports Exerc*.

10. Farley, O.R., C.R. Abbiss, and J.M. Sheppard. 2016. Performance analysis of surfing: A review. *J Strength Cond Res*.

11. Foster, C., J.A. Florhaug, J. Franklin, L. Gottschall, L.A. Hrovatin, S. Parker, P. Doleshal, and C. Dodge. 2001. A new approach to monitoring exercise training. *J Strength Cond Res* 15:109-15.

12. Gabbett, T.J. 2016. The training-injury prevention paradox: Should athletes be training smarter and harder? *Br J Sports Med*.

13. Gagge, A.P., J.A. Stolwijk, and J.D. Hardy. 1967. Comfort and thermal sensations and associated physiological responses at various ambient temperatures. *Environ Res* 1:1-20.

14. Gathercole, R.J., T. Stellingwerff, and B.C. Sporer. 2015. Effect of acute fatigue and training adaptation on countermovement jump performance in elite snowboard cross athletes. *J Strength Cond Res* 29:37-46.

15. Halperin, I., S. Hughes, and D.W. Chapman. 2016. Physiological profile of a professional boxer preparing for title bout: A case study. *J Sports Sci*:1-8.

16. Hopkins, W.G. 1991. Quantification of training in competitive sports. Methods and applications. *Sports Med* 12:161-83.

17. Impellizzeri, F.M., E. Rampinini, N. Maffiuletti, and S.M. Marcora. 2007. A vertical jump force test for assessing bilateral strength asymmetry in athletes. *Med Sci Sports Exerc* 39:2044-50.

18. Jimison, H.B., S. Hagler, G. Kurillo, R. Bajcsy, and M. Pavel. 2015. Remote health coaching for interactive exercise with older adults in a home environment. *Conf Proc IEEE Eng Med Biol Soc* 2015:5485-8.

19. Kinugasa, T. 2013. The application of single-case research designs to study elite athletes' conditioning: An update. *J Appl Sport Psychol* 25:157-66.

20. Langman-Evans, C., G.L. Close, and J.P. Morton. 2011. Making weight in combat sports. *Strength Cond J* 33:25-39.

21. Laux, P., B. Krumm, M. Diers, and H. Flor. 2015. Recovery-stress balance and injury risk in professional football players: A prospective study. *J Sports Sci* 33:2140-8.

22. Lundgren, L.E., T.T. Tran, S. Nimphius, E. Raymond, J.L. Secomb, O.R. Farley, R.U. Newton, J.R. Steele, and J.M. Sheppard. 2015. Development and evaluation of a simple, multifactorial model based on landing performance to indicate injury risk in surfing athletes. *Int J Sports Physiol Perform* 10:1029-35.

23. McGuigan, M.R., S. Cormack, and N.D. Gill. 2013. Strength and power profiling of athletes. *Strength Cond J* 35:7-14.

24. Morin, J.B., and P. Samozino. 2016. Interpreting power-force-velocity profiles for individualized and specific training. *Int J Sports Physiol Perform* 11:267-72.

25. Newton, R.U., and E. Dugan. 2002. Application of strength diagnosis. *Strength Cond J* 24:50-59.

26. Pinot, J., and F. Grappe. 2015. A six-year monitoring case study of a top-10 cycling grand tour finisher. *J Sports Sci* 33:907-14.

27. Plews, D.J., P.B. Laursen, J. Stanley, A.E. Kilding, and M. Buchheit. 2013. Training adaptation and heart rate variability in elite endurance athletes: Opening the door to effective monitoring. *Sports Med* 43:773-81.

28. Potkanowicz, E.S. 2015. A real-time case study in driver science: Physiological strain and related variables. *Int J Sports Physiol Perform* 10:1058-60.

29. Potkanowicz, E.S., and R.W. Mendel. 2013. The case for driver science in motorsport: A review and recommendations. *Sports Med* 43:565-74.

30. Ratamess, N.A., J.R. Hoffman, W.J. Kraemer, R.E. Ross, C.P. Tranchina, S.L. Rashti, N.A. Kelly, J.L. Vingren, J. Kang, and A.D. Faigenbaum. 2013. Effects of a competitive wrestling season on body composition, endocrine markers, and anaerobic exercise performance in NCAA collegiate wrestlers. *Eur J Appl Physiol* 113:1157-68.

31. Raysmith, B.P., and M.K. Drew. 2016. Performance success or failure is influenced by weeks lost to injury and illness in elite Australian track and field athletes: A 5-year prospective study. *J Sci Med Sport* 19:778-83.

32. Saw, A.E., L.C. Main, and P.B. Gastin. 2016. Monitoring the athlete training response: Subjective self-reported measures trump commonly used objective measures: A systematic review. *Br J Sports Med* 50:281-91.

33. Sleivert, G.G. 2007. Using microtechnology to monitor thermal strain and enhance performance in the field. *Int J Sports Physiol Perform* 2:98-102.

34. Sotiriadou, P., and V. De Bosscher. 2013. *Managing high performance sport*. Milton Park, UK: Routledge.

35. Storey, A.G., N.P. Birch, V. Fan, and H.K. Smith. 2016. Stress responses to short-term intensified and reduced training in competitive weightlifters. *Scand J Med Sci Sports* 26:29-40.

36. Sundgot-Borgen, J., N.L. Meyer, T.G. Lohman, T.R. Ackland, R.J. Maughan, A.D. Stewart, and W. Muller. 2013. How to minimise the health risks to athletes who compete in weight-sensitive sports review and position statement on behalf of the ad hoc research working group on body composition, health and performance, under the auspices of the IOC medical commission. *Br J Sports Med* 47:1012-22.

37. Svendsen, I.S., I.M. Taylor, E. Tonnessen, R. Bahr, and M. Gleeson. 2016. Training-related and competition-related risk factors for respiratory tract and gastrointestinal infections in elite cross-country skiers. *Br J Sports Med* 50:809-15.

38. Tjelta, L.I. 2016. The training of international level distance runners. *Int J Sports Sci Coaching* 11:122-34.

39. Tonnessen, E., I.S. Svendsen, B.R. Ronnestad, J. Hisdal, T.A. Haugen, and S. Seiler. 2015. The annual training periodization of 8 world champions in orienteering. *Int J Sports Physiol Perform* 10:29-38.

40. Tonnessen, E., O. Sylta, T.A. Haugen, E. Hem, I.S. Svendsen, and S. Seiler. 2014. The road to gold: Training and peaking characteristics in the year prior to a gold medal endurance performance. *PLoS One* 9:e101796.

41. Tran, J., A.J. Rice, L.C. Main, and P.B. Gastin. 2014. Development and implementation of a novel measure for quantifying training loads in rowing: The T2minute method. *J Strength Cond Res* 28:1172-80.

42. Tran, J., A.J. Rice, L.C. Main, and P.B. Gastin. 2015. Convergent validity of a novel method for quantifying rowing training loads. *J Sports Sci* 33:268-76.

43. Tran, J., A.J. Rice, L.C. Main, and P.B. Gastin. 2015. Profiling the training practices and performances of elite rowers. *Int J Sports Physiol Perform* 10:572-80.

44. Wiewelhove, T., C. Raeder, T. Meyer, M. Kellmann, M. Pfeiffer, and A. Ferrauti. 2016. Effect of repeated active recovery during a high-intensity interval training shock microcycle on markers of fatigue. *Int J Sports Physiol Perform*.

Chapter 9

1. Andersen, L., P. Orme, R. Di Michele, G.L. Close, J. Milsom, R. Morgans, B. Drust, and J.P. Morgan. 2016. Quantification of seasonal long physical load in soccer players with different starting status from the English Premier League: Implications for maintaining squad physical fitness. *Int J Sports Physiol Perf*.

2. Argus, C.K., N.D. Gill, J.W. Keogh, W.G. Hopkins, and C.M. Beaven. 2009. Changes in strength, power, and steroid hormones during a professional rugby union competition. *J Strength Cond Res* 23:1583-92.

3. Argus, C.K., N.D. Gill, J.W. Keogh, M.R. McGuigan, and W.G. Hopkins. 2012. Effects of two contrast training programs on jump performance in rugby union players during a competition phase. *Int J Sports Physiol Perform* 7:68-75.

4. Baker, D. 2001. The effects of an in-season of concurrent training on the maintenance of maximal strength and power in professional and college-aged rugby league football players. *J Strength Cond Res* 15:172-7.

5. Bengtsson, H., J. Ekstrand, and M. Hagglund. 2013. Muscle injury rates in professional football increase with fixture congestion: An 11-year follow-up of the UEFA Champions League injury study. *Br J Sports Med* 47:743-7.

6. Blanch, P., and T.J. Gabbett. 2016. Has the athlete trained enough to return to play safely? The acute:chronic workload ratio permits clinicians to quantify a player's risk of subsequent injury. *Br J Sports Med* 50:471-75.

7. Buchheit, M., W. Morgan, J. Wallace, M. Bode, and N. Poulos. 2015. Physiological, psychometric, and performance effects of the Christmas break in Australian football. *Int J Sports Physiol Perform* 10:120-3.

8. Buchheit, M., S. Racinais, J.C. Bilsborough, P.C. Bourdon, S.C. Voss, J. Hocking, J. Cordy, A. Mendez-Villanueva, and A.J. Coutts. 2013. Monitoring fitness, fatigue and running performance during a pre-season training camp in elite football players. *J Sci Med Sport* 16:550-5.

9. Carling, C., F. Le Gall, and G. Dupont. 2012. Are physical performance and injury risk in a professional soccer team in match-play affected over a prolonged period of fixture congestion? *Int J Sports Med* 33:36-42.

10. Carling, C., A. McCall, F. Le Gall, and G. Dupont. 2015. What is the extent of exposure to periods of match congestion in professional soccer players? *J Sports Sci* 20:2116-24.

11. Cohen, S., T. Kamarck, and R. Mermelstein. 1983. A global measure of perceived stress. *J Health Soc Behav* 24:385-96.

12. Cross, M.J., S. Williams, G. Trewartha, S.P. Kemp, and K.A. Stokes. 2016. The influence of in-season training loads on injury risk in professional rugby union. *Int J Sports Physiol Perform* 11:350-55.

13. Dellal, A., C. Lago-Penas, E. Rey, K. Chamari, and E. Orhant. 2015. The effects of a congested fixture period on physical performance, technical activity and injury rate during matches in a professional soccer team. *Br J Sports Med* 49:390-4.

14. Dembe, A.E., J.B. Erickson, R.G. Delbos, and S.M. Banks. 2005. The impact of overtime and long work hours on occupational injuries and illnesses: New evidence from the United States. *Occup Environ Med* 62:588-97.

15. Drew, M.K., and C.F. Finch. 2016. The relationship between training load and injury, illness and soreness: A systematic and literature review. *Sports Med* 28:1-23.

16. Dupont, G., K. Akakpo, and S. Berthoin. 2004. The effect of in-season, high-intensity interval training in soccer players. *J Strength Cond Res* 18:584-9.

17. Fowler, P., R. Duffield, K. Howle, A. Waterson, and J. Vaile. 2015. Effects of northbound long-haul international air travel on sleep quantity and subjective jet lag and wellness in professional Australian soccer players. *Int J Sports Physiol Perform* 10:648-54.

18. Fowler, P., R. Duffield, A. Waterson, and J. Vaile. 2015. Effects of regular away travel on training loads, recovery, and injury rates in professional Australian soccer players. *Int J Sports Physiol Perform* 10:546-52.

19. Fowler, P.M., R. Duffield, D. Lu, J.A. Hickmans, and T.J. Scott. 2016. Effects of long-haul transmeridian travel on subjective jet-lag and self-reported sleep and upper respiratory symptoms in professional rugby league players. *Int J Sports Physiol Perform* 24:1-24.

20. Fuller, C.W., A.E. Taylor, and M. Raftery. 2015. Does long-distance air travel associated with the sevens world series increase players' risk of injury? *Br J Sports Med* 49:458-64.

21. Gabbett, T.J. 2016. The training-injury prevention paradox: Should athletes be training smarter and harder? *Br J Sports Med*.

22. Gageler, W.H., S. Wearing, and D.A. James. 2015. Automatic jump detection method for athlete monitoring and performance in volleyball. *Int J Perform Anal Sport* 15:284-96.

23. Gastin, P.B., D. Meyer, and D. Robinson. 2013. Perceptions of wellness to monitor adaptive responses to training and competition in elite Australian football. *J Strength Cond Res* 27:2518-26.

24. Gonzalez, A.M., J.R. Hoffman, J.P. Rogowski, W. Burgos, E. Manalo, K. Weise, M.S. Fragala, and J.R. Stout. 2013. Performance changes in NBA basketball players vary in

starters vs. nonstarters over a competitive season. *J Strength Cond Res* 27:611-5.

25. Hagglund, M., M. Walden, H. Magnusson, K. Kristenson, H. Bengtsson, and J. Ekstrand. 2013. Injuries affect team performance negatively in professional football: An 11-year follow-up of the UEFA Champions League injury study. *Br J Sports Med* 47:738-42.

26. Hecksteden, A., S. Skorski, S. Schwindling, D. Hammes, M. Pfeiffer, M. Kellmann, A. Ferrauti, and T. Meyer. 2016. Blood-borne markers of fatigue in competitive athletes—results from simulated training camps. *PLoS One* 11:e0148810.

27. Hodun, M., R. Clarke, M. De Ste Croix, and J.D. Hughes. 2016. Global positioning system analysis of running performance in female field sports: A review of the literature. *Strength Cond J* 38:49-56.

28. Hrysomallis, C. 2010. Upper-body strength and power changes during a football season. *J Strength Cond Res* 24:557-9.

29. Hrysomallis, C., and D. Buttifant. 2012. Influence of training years on upper-body strength and power changes during the competitive season for professional Australian rules football players. *J Sci Med Sport* 15:374-8.

30. Hulin, B.T., T.J. Gabbett, P. Blanch, P. Chapman, D. Bailey, and J.W. Orchard. 2014. Spikes in acute workload are associated with increased injury risk in elite cricket fast bowlers. *Br J Sports Med* 48:708-12.

31. Hulin, B.T., T.J. Gabbett, D.W. Lawson, P. Caputi, and J.A. Sampson. 2016. The acute:chronic workload ratio predicts injury: High chronic workload may decrease injury risk in elite rugby league players. *Br J Sports Med* 50:231-36.

32. Johnston, M.J., C.J. Cook, D. Drake, L. Costley, J.P. Johnston, and L.P. Kilduff. 2016. The neuromuscular, biochemical and endocrine responses to a single session verses double session training day in elite athletes. *J Strength Cond Res*.

33. Jones, T.W., A. Smith, L.S. Macnaughton, and D.N. French. 2016. Strength and conditioning and concurrent training practices in elite rugby union. *J Strength Cond Res* 30:3354-66.

34. Kelly, V.G., and A.J. Coutts. 2007. Planning and monitoring training loads during the competition phase in team sports. *Strength Cond J* 29:32-37.

35. Laurent, C.M., A.M. Fullenkamp, A.L. Morgan, and D.A. Fischer. 2014. Power, fatigue, and recovery changes in national collegiate athletic association Division I hockey players across a competitive season. *J Strength Cond Res* 28:3338-45.

36. McGuigan, M.R., S. Cormack, and N.D. Gill. 2013. Strength and power profiling of athletes. *Strength Cond J* 35:7-14.

37. McMaster, D.T., N. Gill, J. Cronin, and M. McGuigan. 2013. The development, retention and decay rates of strength and power in elite rugby union, rugby league and American football: A systematic review. *Sports Med* 43:367-84.

38. McMaster, D.T., N.D. Gill, J.B. Cronin, and M.R. McGuigan. 2016. Force-velocity-power assessment in semiprofessional rugby union players. *J Strength Cond Res* 30:1118-26.

39. Murray, N.B., T.J. Gabbett, and K. Chamari. 2014. Effect of different between-match recovery times on the activity profiles and injury rates of national rugby league players. *J Strength Cond Res* 28:3476-83.

40. Nimphius, S., M.R. McGuigan, and R.U. Newton. 2012. Changes in muscle architecture and performance during a competitive season in female softball players. *J Strength Cond Res* 26:2655-66.

41. Nindl, B.C., C.D. Leone, W.J. Tharion, R.F. Johnson, J.W. Castellani, J.F. Patton, and S.J. Montain. 2002. Physical performance responses during 72 h of military operational stress. *Med Sci Sports Exerc* 34:1814-22.

42. Nindl, B.C., T.J. Williams, P.A. Deuster, N.L. Butler, and B.H. Jones. 2013. Strategies for optimizing military physical readiness and preventing musculoskeletal injuries in the 21st century. *US Army Med Dep J*:5-23.

43. Pitchford, N.W., S.J. Robertson, C. Sargent, J. Cordy, D.J. Bishop, and J.D. Bartlett. 2016. A change in training environment alters sleep quality but not quantity in elite Australian rules football players. *Int J Sports Physiol Perform*.

44. Racinais, S., M. Buchheit, J. Bilsborough, P.C. Bourdon, J. Cordy, and A.J. Coutts. 2014. Physiological and performance responses to a training camp in the heat in professional Australian football players. *Int J Sports Physiol Perform* 9:598-603.

45. Rogalski, B., B. Dawson, J. Heasman, and T.J. Gabbett. 2013. Training and game loads and injury risk in elite Australian footballers. *J Sci Med Sport* 16:499-503.

46. Samuels, C.H. 2012. Jet lag and travel fatigue: A comprehensive management plan for sport medicine physicians and high-performance support teams. *Clin J Sport Med* 22:268-73.

47. Saw, A.E., L.C. Main, and P.B. Gastin. 2016. Monitoring the athlete training response: Subjective self-reported measures trump commonly used objective measures: A systematic review. *Br J Sports Med* 50:281-91.

48. Scofield, D.E., and J.R. Kardouni. 2015. The tactical athlete: A product of 21st century strength and conditioning. *Strength Cond J* 37:2-7.

49. Taylor, L., B.C. Chrismas, B. Dascombe, K. Chamari, and P.M. Fowler. 2016. The importance of monitoring sleep within adolescent athletes: Athletic, academic, and health considerations. *Front Physiol* 7:101.

50. Thorpe, R.T., A.J. Strudwick, M. Buchheit, G. Atkinson, B. Drust, and W. Gregson. 2015. Monitoring fatigue during the in-season competitive phase in elite soccer players. *Int J Sports Physiol Perform* 10:958-64.

51. Veugelers, K.R., G. Naughton, C. Duncan, D. Burgess, and S. Graham. 2016. Validity and reliability of a submaximal intermittent running test in elite Australian football players. *J Strength Cond* Res 30:3347-53.

52. Welsh, T.T., J.A. Alemany, S.J. Montain, P.N. Frykman, A.P. Tuckow, A.J. Young, and B.C. Nindl. 2008. Effects of intensified military field training on jumping performance. *Int J Sports Med* 29:45-52.

53. Williams, S., G. Trewartha, S.P. Kemp, J.H. Brooks, C.W. Fuller, A.E. Taylor, M.J. Cross, and K.A. Stokes. 2016. Time loss injuries compromise team success in elite rugby union: A 7-year prospective study. *Br J Sports Med 50:651-6.*

54. Windt, J., T.J. Gabbett, D. Ferris, and K.M. Khan. 2016. Training load—injury paradox: Is greater preseason participation associated with lower in-season injury risk in elite rugby league players? *Br J Sports Med.*

INDEX

ABOUT THE AUTHOR

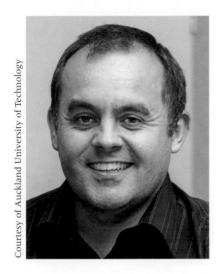

Courtesy of Auckland University of Technology

Mike McGuigan, PhD, CSCS, is a professor of strength and conditioning at Auckland University of Technology (AUT) in New Zealand and a member of the strength and conditioning research group in AUT's Sports Performance Research Institute New Zealand. He is one of the world's leading scientific researchers on athlete monitoring and is highly regarded internationally for his work on resistance training and strength and power development.

Before working at AUT, McGuigan was at Edith Cowan University and the University of Wisconsin–La Crosse and worked as a sport scientist for High Performance Sport New Zealand. He also has vast experience as an athlete monitoring consultant for elite athletes and coaches, working with high-profile New Zealand sport teams such as the All Blacks and the Silver Ferns.

McGuigan is a strength and conditioning specialist certified by the National Strength and Conditioning Association (NSCA). He received the NSCA's Outstanding Young Investigator of the Year Award in 2007 and the William J. Kraemer Most Outstanding Sport Scientist Award in 2016. He serves as an associate editor of the *Journal of Australian Strength and Conditioning*, the *Journal of Strength and Conditioning Research*, and the *International Journal of Sports Physiology and Performance*.

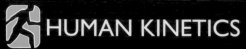
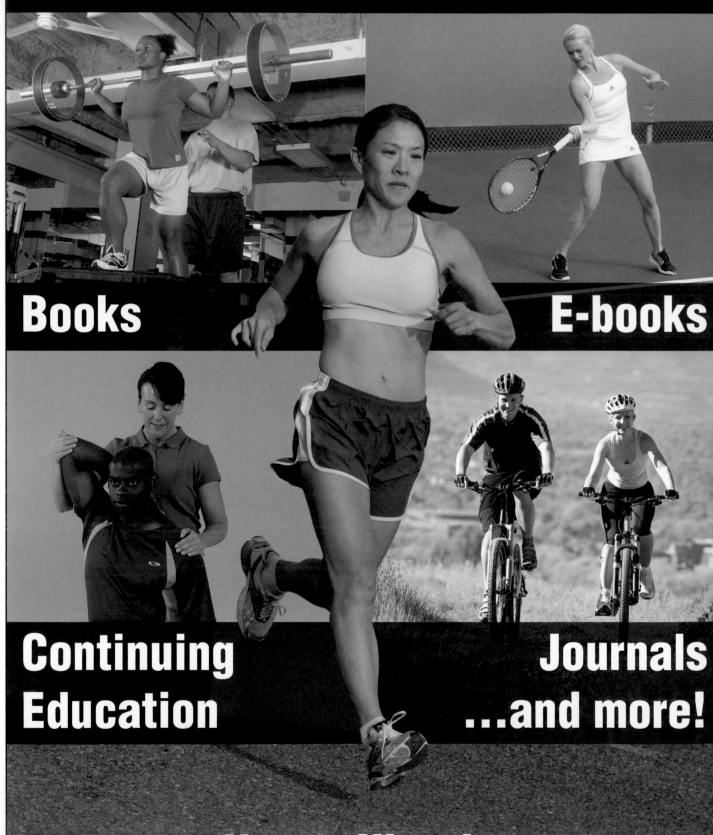